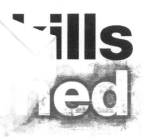

WITHDRAWN

Clinical Skills Explained

Muhammed Akunjee and Nazmul Akunjee
GP Principals, London, UK

Zeshaan Maan,
Surgical Trainee, London, UK

and Mina Ally
Foundation Doctor, Dartford, UK

Scion

© Scion Publishing Ltd, 2012

ISBN 978 1 904842 78 1

First published in 2012

A CIP catalogue record for this book is available from the British Library.

Scion Publishing Limited
The Old Hayloft, Vantage Business Park, Bloxham Road, Banbury, Oxfordshire
OX16 9UX
www.scionpublishing.com

Important Note from the Publisher
The information contained within this book was obtained by Scion Publishing Limited from sources believed by us to be reliable. However, while every effort has been made to ensure its accuracy, no responsibility for loss or injury whatsoever occasioned to any person acting or refraining from action as a result of information contained herein can be accepted by the authors or publishers.

Although every effort has been made to ensure that all owners of copyright material have been acknowledged in this publication, we would be pleased to acknowledge in subsequent reprints or editions any omissions brought to our attention.

Readers should remember that medicine is a constantly evolving science and while the authors and publishers have ensured that all dosages, applications and practices are based on current indications, there may be specific practices which differ between communities. You should always follow the guidelines laid down by the manufacturers of specific products and the relevant authorities in the country in which you are practising.

Artwork by Nazmul Akunjee, London, UK
Cover design by amdesign, Banbury, UK
Typeset by Manila Typesetting Company, Philippines
Printed by Ashford Colour Press Ltd. UK

Contents

Section 3 – Procedures

Foreword

It is often said within medical education that 'assessment drives learning'. This means that regardless of what a student has been taught throughout the year, they will focus on those topics that actually come up in the exam at the end of the year. With the widespread uptake of OSCEs in medical schools to assess clinical skills, students have now adapted accordingly. All across the world students walk into cubicles on exam day and mindlessly repeat '*I would like to wash my hands*' before being told it is unnecessary. They will religiously chant '*There is no clubbing or cyanosis*', while ignoring the patient's amputated digit. The focused, snapshot style of the OSCE has made many students perform in an artificial and robotic way. This style is reinforced by the many exam-oriented '*Pass MBBS!*' books available on the market, books that tell students the 'secrets' of what to say to get through the exam. Medical educators across the world are increasingly recognizing this problem, and are trying to find ways to avoid such checklist-induced performances.

Given this background, this book, *Clinical Skills Explained* comes as a timely and welcome breath of fresh air. The philosophy behind this book is that there is more to learning clinical skills that simply ticking off boxes on a checklist. At the same time students must learn within a context and style that enables them to do well in their exams. It bridges the gap between the detailed textbooks on physical examination and the books on how to 'do' OSCEs. Students can learn clinical examination in a natural and practical way, whilst at the same time developing their awareness of what they need to be able to do to pass their clinical exams.

The authors are talented at summarizing what one needs to know in clear, simple language. The colourful diagrams and summary boxes make quick review and revision much easier. Medical students in their early years will benefit greatly from the integrated approach that these doctors have used in this handbook. With a bit of luck, this integrated approach will eventually find its way into the OSCEs themselves. At that point both our teaching and assessment will realign to what they are originally supposed to do: produce good doctors.

Dr Deen M Mirza
Assistant Professor Family Medicine, UAE University
GP Appraiser (Sutton and Merton PCT)
International Editor for the *London Journal of Primary Care*

Preface

Medical school education has undergone a number of evolutionary changes in the past few decades. Gone are the days of didactic, lecture-based pre-clinical teaching held in constrained lecture theatres, detached from day to day clinical practice. Replacing this is a new integrated curriculum allowing for hands-on practical and clinical skills experience right from the outset. The examination process has also changed to reflect this, with Objective Structured Clinical Examination (OSCE) stations substituting the now defunct subjective vivas that more often than not were based on chance rather than individual skill and knowledge.

Unfortunately, the OSCE system has not necessarily been the perfect replacement for vivas. Increasingly, medical educators are realizing that a generation of student doctors are now focusing more on how to pass exams rather than how to be good clinicians. Their efforts and knowledge are concentrated more on shortcuts that may be crammed just prior to the examinations rather than actually knowing what they are doing, why they are doing it and its implications. Many students are beginning to fear opening up the large textbooks that contain much detail on aetiology, physiology and pathology, preferring the short, sharp *crash course-esque* books on how to pass exams.

Clinical Skills Explained endeavours to try and bridge between these two approaches. As the name suggests, it aims to explain the complexities of the common medical skills, examinations and procedures that doctors will be employing on a regular basis and attempts to clarify the rationale behind each task. It has been designed and formatted in an easily understandable way, peppered with useful information such as top tips, colourful pictures, the latest medical guidelines and then common case scenarios to revise and test your understanding. Each chapter is presented with background knowledge and relevant pathophysiology before moving on to a comprehensive systematic approach on how to tackle the skill at hand.

We have written the book to cover the essential topics and common skills that you would be expected to face in the first three clinical years at medical school. Hence, we have intentionally left out skills such as female catheterization, setting up a syringe driver, breast examination, injection techniques etc. such that the book neither becomes too cumbersome, nor irrelevant to the course material tested in the earlier clinical years.

We hope that *Clinical Skills Explained* will be a valuable text that will accompany you on your clinical journey throughout the years of medical school. We believe that it will help you excel in your exams and also go on to be not only a competent, but a distinguished medical practitioner.

Muhammed Akunjee and Nazmul Akunjee
London, December 2011

About the authors

Dr Muhammed Akunjee (MBBS, MRCGP, PGCME, PGCDM) is currently a GP Principal in North London (since 2007) and Clinical Director for the local PCT. He qualified from Guy's, Kings and St. Thomas's Medical School in 2002 and completed his MRCGP gaining a distinction in 2006. During this time he was also awarded first prize for the Roche / RCGP Registrar award. As an undergraduate he was awarded the War Memorial Prize and distinction in Psychology / Sociology. He was also awarded a number of bursaries and research awards including the Leukaemia Research Fund Bursary, the Rayne Institute Research Prize, the British Medical & Dental Student's Fund Bursary, and the King's College Lightfoot Award. Dr Akunjee is actively involved in medical student teaching and is currently a clinical skills tutor as well as an OSCE examiner at a London university. He has been involved in the publication of a number of papers and medical revision books including the award-winning *Easy Guide to OSCE's* series.

Dr Nazmul Akunjee (MBBS, MRCGP) has recently completed his GP vocational training and is currently a GP Principal. He qualified from GKT medical school in 2005 and has published a number of articles related to examination skills in OSCEs in peer-reviewed journals. He completed the London Deanery's *Introduction to Teaching in Primary Care* course in June 2011, and is currently teaching medical students at a London university. He is also a course facilitator for the *CSAPrep course* that helps GP Registrars pass their MRCGP Clinical Skills Assessment examinations. He is also a co-author of the award-winning *Easy Guide to OSCE's* series of medical revision books.

Dr Mina Ally (MBBS, BSc) is currently a Year 1 Core Medical Trainee at Whipps Cross University Hospital. She completed an intercalated BSc in Nutrition with Basic Medical Sciences with first class honours at King's College London in 2007. She qualified with distinction in clinical sciences and clinical practice from King's College London Medical School in 2009; she had the highest academic ranking on qualification and, was awarded the King's College London School of Medicine Gold Medal and the Todd Prize in Clinical Medicine, as well as the Haberdasher Company Prize. At medical school she became part of the 'peer led teaching scheme', in which she formally taught medical students in the years below in preparation for their clinical examinations. She currently teaches medical students through ward-based activities and structured topic teaching for the OSCE. She has examined mock OSCEs for final year medical students and was an examiner for the MBBS Year 2 Finals OSCE at King's College London in 2011.

Mr Zeshaan Maan (MBBS, MRCS, MSc) is currently a Year 2 Core Surgical Trainee working at St Andrews Centre for Plastic Surgery and Burns. He was recognised as a National Merit Scholar and AP Scholar with Distinction while studying at Bellarmine College Preparatory in San Jose, California. He qualified from King's College London School of Medicine in 2008 and has completed a Diploma in Philosophy of Medicine, a surgical MSc at Imperial College London and obtained Membership of the Royal College of Surgeons. At medical school he was involved in organising a number of teaching sessions for students in the years below. During clinical training, he organised teaching programmes for medical students and junior doctors and taught on courses at the RSM and Imperial College. He has also examined the MBBS Year 2 Finals OSCE at King's College London.

Acknowledgments

Reviewers

Dr Asif Ali is a GP Principal at Langley Health Centre and is the Medical Director for Berkshire East Community Health Services, providing a leading role in shaping community health services. He graduated from Guy's King's and St Thomas's (GKT) Medical School, London with a distinction in clinical sciences and was awarded the Cancer Research UK prize (2001) and the Rayne Institute Prize (2001) for research on the effects of war and sanctions on health care systems. He has attained the Diploma of Child Health (2005), Diploma of Royal College of Obstetrics and Gynaecology (2005) and Membership of the Royal College of General Practitioners with distinction (2006). Dr Ali has a great passion for training and education at both undergraduate and postgraduate level. He is an Oxford Deanery accredited GP trainer (Postgraduate Certificate of Medical Education, Oxford Brookes 2009) and has been teaching FY2 doctors and medical students from Oxford University and Guy's, King's and St Thomas's Medical Schools since 2009.

Dr Hafiz Syed is a Consultant in Geriatric and Stroke medicine at the Newham University Hospital. He is also supervisor for the Intermediate Care and Community Stroke Team based in Newham PCT as well as playing a part at the Hyperacute Stroke Unit at the Royal London Hospital. His research interests include post stroke oxygen kinetics (University of East London). He is an avid medical student teacher and trainer and is involved with the Year 2 Medicine in Society Module for the Bart's and London Medical Schools.

We would also like to extend our thanks to the following people who helped contribute to specific chapters in the writing of this book: Mr Majid Chowdhry, ST3 in Trauma & Orthopaedic Surgery, South Thames Rotation; Dr Mohammed Enayat, Foundation Year 1 doctor at St Thomas' Hospital; and Zack Ally, Year 4 medical student at Brighton and Sussex Medical School.

We would also like to acknowledge the work and effort made by Dr Matee Ullah, Senior House Officer at the Neurosciences Intensive Care Unit department, John Radcliffe Hospital, Oxford, for his contributions to some of the introductory history chapters.

Abbreviations

A&E	Accident and Emergency department
ACE	angiotensin converting enzyme
AIDS	acquired immunodeficiency syndrome
AMD	age-related macular degeneration
AUDIT-C	Alcohol Use Disorders Identification Test
COPD	chronic obstructive pulmonary disease
COX-1	cyclo-oxygenase-1
CT	computed tomography
CTPA	computed tomography pulmonary angiogram
DKA	diabetic ketoacidosis
DVLA	Driver & Vehicle Licensing Agency
DVT	deep vein thrombosis
ECG	electrocardiogram
FAST	Fast Alcohol Screening Test
GORD	gastro-oesophageal reflux disease
HGV	heavy goods vehicle
HIV	human immunodeficiency virus
HNPCC	hereditary non-polyposis colorectal carcinoma
HRT	hormone replacement therapy
IBS	irritable bowel syndrome
ICD-10	10th revision of the International Classification of Disease
LSD	lysergic acid diethylamide
MDMA	3,4-methylenedioxymethamphetamine
MRC	Medical Research Council
MS	multiple sclerosis
NSAIDs	non-steroidal anti-inflammatory drugs
OGD	oesophago-gastro-duodenoscopy
OTC	over the counter
PE	pulmonary embolism
SLE	systemic lupus erythematosus
SSRI	selective serotonin re-uptake inhibitor
SVT	supra-ventricular tachycardia
TB	tuberculosis
TURP	trans-urethral resection of the prostate
UTI	urinary tract infection

Chapter 1.1
Chest pain

What to do . . .

- Introduce yourself to the patient – establish rapport
- Ask the patient's name, age and occupation
- Ask the patient relevant questions about their chest pain, using SOCRATES to guide your questioning
- Ask about any associated symptoms, e.g. shortness of breath, coughing, haemoptysis, nausea, vomiting, fever
- Establish any risk factors for ACS or PE
- Ask about any past medical history, e.g. DM, HTN, AF, HF
- Ask about any drug history and for any drug allergies
- Ask about any social history – enquire if the patient smokes or drinks alcohol
- Ask about any family history, specifically for ischaemic heart disease or PE
- Perform a brief systems review and sum up your findings
- Establish a list of investigations required to refine your diagnosis, e.g. CXR and ECG
- Thank the patient and conclude the consultation

Chest pain is one of the most common presenting complaints that a doctor will be expected to manage. It is particularly common and of most concern in middle-aged and elderly patients. It is important to exclude sinister, but uncommon, causes of chest pain, such as myocardial infarction, aortic dissection and pneumothorax, whilst eliciting the patient history.

Patients often use the term chest pain to describe any pain, pressure, numbness, squeezing, or choking sensation felt in the chest, neck or upper abdomen. It may last from a few seconds to several days or weeks, and it may occur frequently or sporadically. When trying to localize the source of the chest pain it is important to take into consideration the local structures contained within the thoracic cage, including the heart, lungs, aorta, oesophagus, ribs, muscle and skin. It should not be forgotten that pain may originate from other structures outside the thorax and radiate into the chest.

Keep in mind that chest pain is merely a symptom and not a diagnosis.

1.1.1 Taking the history

Introduce yourself to the patient by stating your name and your job title. At this stage it is important to explain to the patient that you need to ask a number of questions to ascertain the nature of the chest pain.

Ask the patient for their name, age and occupation before proceeding to take a detailed history. The patient's gender and age are very important in both risk stratification and consideration of appropriate differential diagnoses:
- elderly males who present with chest pain are more likely to be suffering from an ischaemic event

TOP TIP!

In the OSCEs you are likely to encounter a patient suffering with angina (Fig 1.1 a-c), pulmonary embolism or musculoskeletal-like pain (Fig 1.1). Devote some time eliciting the character of the pain so that you are able to develop an accurate working diagnosis.

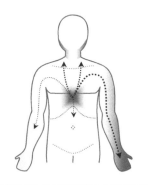

Fig 1.1a Angina pain

Central crushing chest pain that radiates to the left arm, neck and jaw. Pain can also radiate to right arm. It is often described as a 'tightening of the chest'.

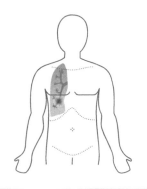

Fig 1.1b Pulmonary embolism

Sudden onset of pleuritic chest pain along with shortness of breath. In severe cases patients may have excessive coughing with haemoptysis. Recent travel, surgery, oral contraceptive pill use or cancers are risk factors

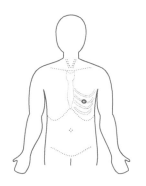

Fig 1.1c Musculoskeletal pain

Localized chest pain that is worse on inspiration. Pain varies with intensity. Localized tenderness on examination which reproduces the pain.

- young females on the oral contraceptive pill are more likely to suffer from a pulmonary embolism
- males also have a higher incidence of heart disease than females before the menopause

Occupational history actually plays a fairly limited role in the cardiac history. However, it is still important to elicit whether the patient is in current employment or retired. If employed, is the job office-based or does it involve manual work?

- physical jobs are more likely to cause musculoskeletal pain
- stressful jobs may cause anxiety-related symptoms, angina-like pain or heartburn

It is essential to establish rapport with the patient by asking open questions regarding their symptoms. This will allow the conversation to flow freely and may help the patient relax and feel at ease. Further on in your history taking, you may need to ask closed and pertinent questions to refine your working diagnosis related to their chest pain.

To maintain rapport with the patient, avoid the use of medical jargon which may confuse the patient and lead to misunderstanding. You must also listen attentively to the patient, watching out for any verbal or non-verbal cues which may reveal a hidden agenda.

1.1.2 Ideas, concerns and expectations

After appropriately introducing yourself and establishing rapport, it is useful to elicit the patient's own views of their symptoms. By asking the patient directly about their ideas and concerns, their problems are personalized and this provides a more holistic understanding of the context in which the patient presents. Also enquire about the patient's own expectations of what they hope to gain from the consultation. Use what the patient has told you as a guide to tailor your history taking, and to allay any misplaced anxiety and fears. Common anxieties expressed by patients experiencing chest pain include fear of death, strokes and disability.

Use open questions to ask the patient how the symptoms have impacted on their life. In particular, ask about specific activities and hobbies such as walking, sports activities, which they may no longer be able to perform.

1.1.3 History of the presenting complaint

Now that you have put the patient at ease and hopefully gained their trust and established rapport, you can begin to take a more detailed history about their presenting complaint. Use open questions to allow the patient to express their symptoms in their own words, such as:

- 'What seems to be the problem?'
- 'What brought you here to see a doctor today?'

You can then begin to ask more focused questions about the chest pain. You can use the mnemonic SOCRATES as a tool to guide you in taking a thorough and complete chest pain history.

Site

Ask the patient where the pain is and request them to point to it if necessary. Knowing the site of the pain may give you some indication as to the cause of the pain. For example, a patient complaining of a retrosternal chest pain is likely to be suffering with ischaemia, whereas a patient complaining of a localized, reproducible, superficial pain is probably suffering from a musculoskeletal problem (see *Fig 1.1c*).

Onset

It is important to elicit when the chest pain started and whether it is chronic or acute. Some knowledge about the time of onset of the chest pain may help to distinguish between potential causes. For example, a sudden onset of sharp localized chest pain in a tall thin male is likely to be due to a pneumothorax. Chronic stable angina, on the other hand, is usually described as a slow and often insidious course of chest pain which is worse on exertion and relieved by rest (see *Fig 1.1a*).

Character

The character of the pain is perhaps the most important element to elicit in the chest pain history. Allow the patient to express themselves freely, describing their symptoms in their own words. Do not lead the patient by putting words into their mouth. However, if the patient is unable to express the exact nature of their pain, consider offering a number of descriptions to them to choose from.

Patients may describe their chest pain in a number of ways, such as crushing, tearing, burning, squeezing. They may also describe it as sharp, dull, or as a weight-like sensation or pressure over their chest:
- 'feels like a ton of bricks sitting on my chest'
- 'I feel like I am being stabbed with a knife'

Though the description given by the patient may point to an obvious cause, it is essential to re-confirm the sensation with the patient to avoid misinterpretation or ambiguity.
- A crushing retrosternal chest pain is commonly described in patients suffering with an ischaemic event.
- A sudden persisting sharp tearing pain is likely to be caused by an aortic dissection. (see *Fig 1.2a*).
- A burning sensation often points towards a gastro-intestinal cause such as reflux disease (GORD) (see *Fig 1.2b*).

Radiation

Determining whether or not the pain radiates is helpful in narrowing down the list of possible causes:
- pain classically radiating to the left arm or jaw is ischaemic in nature until proven otherwise
- pain radiating up from the epigastric area to the throat is likely to be due to reflux disease
- a sharp pain radiating to the back, often between the shoulder blades, is probably due to a dissecting aortic aneurysm and needs to be managed immediately

Associated symptoms

Chest pain frequently presents in conjunction with other symptoms and eliciting these may help confirm or negate your working diagnosis. Common associated symptoms include difficulty in breathing, palpitations, dizziness, nausea and vomiting, coughing and haemoptysis, sweating and feeling feverish.
- A patient who is feeling cold, nauseous and sweaty alongside their pain should make you think of a possible myocardial infarction.

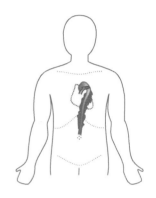

Fig 1.2a Aortic dissection

Sudden onset of severe, tearing chest pain radiating to the back. May be associated with hypertension, connective tissue disorders and vasculitis. Patients with Marfan's syndrome are at an increased risk of developing it.

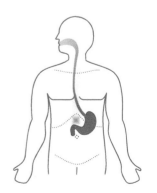

Fig 1.2b Reflux disease

Burning pain that is felt in the epigastrium radiating up to the throat. Can be associated with certain foods such as chilli, caffeine and fatty or spicy foods. Patient may complain of excessive saliva in their mouth (water brash) and bitter, sour taste (acid brash).

- A patient suffering with fever and productive cough with their pain is likely to be developing a chest infection.
- A patient suffering from tightness of the chest, palpitations and shortness of breath may be suffering from anxiety or a panic attack.

Timing

Establish when the pain occurs and how long it lasts for, whether it occurs at a particular time of day and if it occurs at rest or on physical exertion.
- A retrosternal crushing chest pain that occurs during exercise should make you consider angina as a possible cause.
- On the other hand, a similar pain occurring at rest should be regarded as acute coronary syndrome (ACS) and requires immediate medical attention.

Exacerbating and relieving factors

A thorough chest pain history is not complete without establishing what factors exacerbate or relieve the pain:
- chest pain worsened on deep inspiration is defined as being pleuritic in nature and is indicative of pulmonary embolism, pneumothorax or pneumonia
- musculoskeletal pain may be confused with pleuritic chest pain as the patient often describes it in a similar way; however, in musculoskeletal pain, you often will find a local area of tenderness exacerbated by movement, but relieved by rest
- sharp pain associated with movement, such as leaning forwards, and intensified when taking a deep breath in, usually points towards pericarditis
- pain made worse after eating a heavy meal, exercise, stress, emotion or in cold weather is likely to be due to angina; such pain should stop on ceasing activity or by taking a puff of GTN spray
- pain exacerbated by hunger or lying down and relieved after taking alkaline substances such as antacids is probably due to reflux disease

Severity

Eliciting the severity of the pain is often overlooked by medical students and qualified doctors alike. However, it is important to ask the patient how severe their pain is. A quantitative way of doing this is to ask the patient to rank the severity on a scale of one to ten; ten being the worst pain they have ever experienced, and one signifying the least. Asking the severity of their pain may also help develop the rapport between yourself and the patient as well as helping you to empathize with their experience.

Risk factors

Depending on your possible working diagnosis, it is important to elicit associated risk factors the patient may have which would help reinforce your clinical hypothesis. For chest pain these include ACS and pulmonary embolism (PE).

Acute coronary syndrome
If you suspect an ischaemic aetiology to the chest pain, it is helpful to stratify the patient's risk of developing a cardiovascular event by eliciting a number of different factors and co-morbidities. Major cardiovascular risk factors include high blood pressure, diabetes, high cholesterol, obesity, smoking and lack of

exercise. Other risk factors include previous ischaemic heart disease and a strong family history of cardiac disease. Such variables will help to ascertain a Framingham risk score for the patient, defining the likelihood of developing a cardiac event in the next ten years.

Pulmonary embolism

If you believe that the patient's chest pain is pleuritic in nature and may be due to a pulmonary embolism, you should elicit the relevant risk factors which can be used to support your diagnosis. Major risk factors for the development of a PE include deep vein thrombosis (DVT), immobility, prolonged bed rest, recent major surgical or orthopaedic procedure, cancers, pregnancy, oestrogen supplement (contraceptive pill, HRT), smoking, obesity, atrial fibrillation, and hypercoagulability disorders (thrombophilia).

1.1.4 **Past medical history**

Once you are finished taking a thorough history of the presenting complaint, you should move on to ask about the patient's past medical history, including their medical illnesses and any prior hospital admissions. Enquire about any previous cardiac investigations such as exercise treadmill, angiogram and myocardial perfusions scans, and operations such as coronary artery bypass graft (CABG). Specifically enquire about diabetes, hypertension, coronary artery disease, atrial fibrillation, heart failure, valvular disease and cardiomyopathy. Due to the improvement in the hygiene of the general population, as well as increased and widespread use of antibiotics, rheumatic fever is now uncommon in the developed world, but it is still important to consider in the elderly or immigrant populations.

1.1.5 **Drug history**

Taking a complete drug history may reveal some pointers or clues towards a likely diagnosis. Ask the patient what medication they are currently on or have taken in the past. Try to include over-the-counter medications (OTC) and herbal remedies. Enquire specifically as to whether the patient has used a GTN spray and if it helped resolve their chest pain because this may point towards cardiac ischaemia. In women, do not forget to ask about usage of the oral contraceptive pill, or HRT in menopausal women, since they have both been shown to increase the risk of developing a PE. It is vital to ask about drug allergies or intolerances to avoid any potential problems such as anaphylaxis or adverse drug reaction.

A patient presenting with chest pain who is already taking a number of cardiac medications, such as beta blockers, aspirin, ACE inhibitors or nitrates, may have a worsening ischaemic aetiology and may well require titration of their medication. Burning chest pain in a patient who has recently been started on one of the non-steroidal anti-inflammatory drugs (NSAIDs), such as ibuprofen or diclofenac, may be indicative of reflux disease.

1.1.6 **Social history**

A detailed social history is crucial in ascertaining predisposing factors in cardiac disease. Ask the patient if they have ever smoked and, if so, how many cigarettes or roll-ups a day and for how long. Smoking is the most important cause of atherosclerosis development in young people and also affects cardiovascular risk due to its effect on blood pressure and tendency for blood to clot.

DIFFERENTIAL DIAGNOSIS

Cardiovascular
- Acute Coronary Syndrome (ACS)
- Acute myocardial infarction
- Aortic dissection
- Pericarditis

Pulmonary
- Spontaneous pneumothorax
- Pneumonia
- Pulmonary embolism
- Pulmonary hypertension

Other
- Reflux oesophagitis (GORD)
- Musculoskeletal pain (MSK)
- Herpes zoster
- Panic disorder

Medical Guidelines
Recommended Lifestyle Advice

Diet: Encourage patients to eat a Mediterranean-style low fat diet

Smoking: Advise smokers to quit and offer assistance from a smoking cessation service

Alcohol: Advise patients to keep weekly alcohol consumption within safe limits (<21 units per wk for men, <14 units per wk for women).

Avoid binge drinking

Weight: Advise patients to maintain a healthy weight and offer weight loss advice if relevant

NICE guidelines: MI: secondary prevention (2007)

Enquire whether the patient drinks alcohol and, if so, what type and how many units a week. Heavy consumption of alcohol has been found to have a direct toxic effect on the heart by raising blood pressure, raising cholesterol levels and causing cardiomyopathy.

Discreetly ask about illicit use of drugs such as cocaine and marijuana, the effects of which can masquerade as ischaemic chest pain.

You should take the opportunity to enquire about the patient's dietary and exercising habits. Ask about intake of fatty food, red meat, sugar and salt. Enquire about the patient's level of activity to establish whether they undertake a basic level of exercise; the British Heart Foundation recommends a minimum of 30 minutes of brisk exercise at least five times a week.

Ask the patient about any recent travel, including long haul flights or uninterrupted long distance bus journeys, which are risk factors for the development of PEs.

1.1.7 Family history

Common cardiac disorders such as coronary artery disease have a strong genetic element. It is essential, therefore, to enquire as to whether the patient has any first-degree relatives who suffered from an early death or premature coronary heart disease, i.e. below the age of 50 years. Similarly, PE also has a familial element and you should enquire specifically about any veno-thromboembolic disease occurring in a first-degree relative before the age of 50 years.

1.1.8 Systems review

Complete your chest pain history with a brief systems review. This may give an insight into the patient's general health and also allow you to revisit and re-evaluate your differential diagnosis. Ask the patient if they have experienced any change in their bowel habits, noticed any swelling in their ankles, or any aches or pains in their muscles or joints. Have they felt dizzy, lost consciousness or noted any weakness in their limbs?

1.1.9 Summing up

Give yourself time at the end of the consultation to summarize your findings back to the patient. Specifically ask the patient if there is anything in the history that they would like to add or amend. This helps to minimize the chance of any misinterpretation or misunderstandings. This exercise also engenders trust in the patient as it demonstrates that you have been attentive to what they have been saying.

Having completed taking your chest pain history you should now be in a position to deliver a list of relevant and potential differential diagnoses that the patient may be suffering from. This list would usually be refined further based on the results of additional investigations you undertake (see *Chapter 2.3*). Reassure your patient by agreeing a shared plan about what the next steps will be. This may include informing the patient what you believe is the cause of their chest pain, explaining what investigations you will be undertaking and the possible treatment options. In addition, you may wish to offer the patient any relevant information leaflets if appropriate. Thank the patient for their time and conclude the interview amicably.

1.1.10 **Common clinical scenarios**

The following are a list of common chest pain cases which you may encounter.
For each one, consider:

- what the possible differential diagnosis could be
- what key features you would look for
- what questions you would ask to refine or confirm your diagnosis

You could use role play with a friend, using the histories in the cases below as
a framework.

CASE 1	A 48 year old bus driver presents with 'pressure' over his chest when walking long distances, worsening over the last few months. He also notes that the chest pain occurs when he is angry or when out in the cold. The pain is relieved on rest and when taking his GTN spray. He is obese, smokes 20 cigarettes a day, drinks 30 units of alcohol a week and suffers with hypercholesterolaemia. He has a family history of diabetes and his mother has hypertension.
CASE 2	A 59 year old builder with a history of sudden onset retrosternal chest pain radiating to his jaw and his left arm at rest. The pain is not relieved by GTN spray and lasts for 20 minutes. He is also complaining of feeling nauseous, cold and breaking into a sweat. He is known to suffer from diabetes, hypertension and hypercholesterolaemia. He is currently taking aspirin, bisoprolol, nicorandil, ramipril, ISMN, simvastatin and metformin. His brother died aged 49 from a heart attack.
CASE 3	A 39 year old gentleman who suffers from Marfan syndrome presents with sudden onset of severe tearing central chest pain which radiates to the back and is persistent in nature. His past medical history includes hypertension. He is a known smoker but has been teetotal for his whole life.
CASE 4	A 25 year old pregnant lady recently returned from a long haul flight from Thailand complaining of right calf pain and swelling. She has recently developed sharp onset chest pain, worse on deep inspiration and associated with slight haemoptysis and shortness of breath. She does not complain of any pain on movement or mention any recent falls or trauma.
CASE 5	A 28 year old lady complaining of acute onset of retrosternal chest pain that radiates to her left shoulder. She has recently suffered with a viral infection. The pain is made worse on deep inspiration and lying down, whilst it is relieved on sitting forward and taking ibuprofen. She is not taking the pill. There is no relevant family history.
CASE 6	A 34 year old gentleman who works in an Indian restaurant. He complains of a burning sensation in the lower chest that radiates to his throat. The pain is worse on lying down and after meals but improves on leaning forward. He also notes a bitter taste in his mouth with extra salivation in the mornings. He drinks 6 cups of coffee every day and is a heavy drinker. He smokes 2 packs of cigarettes a day. He also states that he has been taking ibuprofen for a recent cold.

CASE 7

A 32 year old delivery man complaining of an acute onset of aching pain localized on the right chest wall. It is made worse on inspiration, movement and lifting, and is tender to touch. There is no radiation nor any associated symptoms such as shortness of breath, palpitations or haemoptysis. There is no relevant past medical, family or drug history. He is a social drinker.

Chapter 1.2
History of palpitations

What to do . . .

- Introduce yourself to the patient – establish rapport
- Ask the patient's name, age and occupation
- Ask the patient relevant questions about their palpitations such as their nature and aggravating and relieving factors
- Ask about any associated symptoms, e.g. chest pain, shortness of breath, syncope, anxiety
- Ask about any past medical history including previous investigations or operations
- Ask about any drug history and for any drug allergies
- Ask about any social history – establish if the patient smokes or drinks alcohol
- Take a brief dietary history to include caffeine, chocolate and red wine
- Ask about any family history and specifically for premature death
- Perform a brief systems review and sum up your findings
- Thank the patient and conclude the consultation

A palpitation is a subjective abnormal awareness of the heart beating. It can often be described as a missed beat, extra beat or felt as a heavy thud. It may occur in bradycardia, tachycardia or even at rest with a normal heart rate. Its presence does not automatically suggest serious underlying cardiac pathology because most occur sporadically and resolve spontaneously. Uncomplicated palpitations can be experienced after a bout of exercise, excessive caffeine, in anxiety states, or in conditions such as anaemia. However, if a patient complains of recurrent or persisting symptoms, or there is an association with haemodynamic instability, this would warrant further investigation.

Palpitations may be caused by three different mechanisms (see *Table 1.1*):
- arrhythmias – in cardiac electrical dysfunction there is a disruption of the normal conduction pathways that conduct impulses from the sinoatrial node to the rest of the heart; in conditions such as atrial fibrillation and supraventricular tachycardia, this may lead to abnormal heart beats and arrhythmias that give rise to palpitations

TOP TIP!

Although palpitations comprise up to 40% of cardiology referrals, in most cases no significant organic pathology is found.

Table 1.1 **Causes of palpitations**	
Arrhythmias	Atrial fibrillation, supraventricular tachycardia, ventricular tachycardia, ventricular fibrillation, heart block
Hyperdynamic circulation	Valvular incompetence, thyrotoxicosis, hypercapnia, pyrexia, anaemia, pregnancy
Sympathetic overdrive	Panic disorders, hypoglycaemia, hypoxia, levocetirizine antihistamines, anaemia, heart failure

- increased stroke volume – valvular incompetence and thyrotoxicosis can result in increased stroke volume, causing premature beats
- raised sympathetic drive – increased sympathetic drive due to panic attacks and hypoxia, for example, can induce a rapid heart rate causing palpitations

1.2.1 Taking the history

Introduce yourself by mentioning your name, job title and the reason you are asking the patient the questions. Ask the patient some background questions such as their name, age and occupation before asking about their palpitations. This information can be handy later on when you formulate your list of differentials. The patient's age and gender can play a role in the consideration of an appropriate differential diagnosis. For example, the elderly are more likely to be aware of their heartbeat, but they are also more likely to have cardiac disease. Younger patients are more likely to have psychosomatic causes for their palpitations. Patients with palpitations associated with episodes of syncope should be advised to inform the DVLA and told not to drive.

1.2.2 Ideas, concerns and expectations

After appropriately introducing yourself and establishing rapport, this is usually a good time to ask the patient what they think may be the cause of their abnormal heartbeat. Cardiac symptoms normally generate quite intense anxiety in patients. Common concerns include fear of having a heart attack, cardiac arrest and incapacity. Spend some time enquiring about how the symptoms have affected the patient's life and elicit whether their symptoms have prevented them from performing any particular activity. Establish the patient's expectations: the patient's symptoms may lead them to expect further investigations to rule out their concerns and fears. These expectations may range from having a few blood tests to undergoing an exercise ECG.

1.2.3 History of the presenting complaint

Before diving in and taking a thorough history of the patient's presenting symptoms, clarify what they mean when they use the word 'palpitations'. Patients may often misuse this word to mean an episode of chest pain, tightness or shortness of breath. You may wish to ask them, *'What do you mean by palpitations? Can you describe what you felt?'*

Nature

It is useful to check with the patient whether their palpitations were regular or irregular and the duration. Ask them if they felt any missed beats, extra beats or the sensation of a singular heavy thud. Note whether the palpitations were persistent or simply fleeting in nature. If the patient is having difficulty expressing the nature of the palpitations it may be useful to ask them to tap out the rhythm of the beat on a hard surface.

A sudden onset, rapid, short-lived palpitation may suggest a supraventricular tachycardia. Patients may describe elaborate techniques they use to terminate their episodes. Such techniques are often not too dissimilar to the Valsalva manoeuvre such as holding their breath, or perhaps rubbing their neck (carotid massage).

DIFFERENTIAL DIAGNOSIS

Cardiac causes of palpitations
Regular
Rapid
- SVT
- VT
- Atrial flutter
- Sinus tachycardia

Slow
- Bradycardia
- Heart block

Irregular
Persistent
- Atrial fibrillation
- Heart block (Wenckebach, complete)

Intermittent
- Ectopic beats
- Paroxysm AF

A singular heavy thud or a feeling of an extra beat occurring randomly with no associated symptoms is highly suggestive of an innocent ventricular ectopic beat. The sensation is not because of the extrasystole itself but is due to the prolonged pause and more intense subsequent irregular beat which results.

Exacerbating and relieving factors

Ask the patient what they were doing just before the palpitations began because this may reveal an obvious precipitant factor. Enquire particularly about recent consumption of alcohol or caffeine. Caffeine content may vary depending on the drink consumed: coffee is renowned to contain more caffeine than tea, and drinks such as cola or energy drinks contain large amounts of caffeine.

Some types of abnormal heart rhythms may be induced by exercise or particular positions. In the case of postural tachycardias, a simple change in posture such as bending down or leaning forward may precipitate a rapid abnormal heartbeat. In such cases, simply sitting back down or resting may terminate the event.

Some palpitations may be more noticeable when the patient is lying down to sleep. This is believed to be caused by the heart slowing down at night, creating a lower resting heartbeat, and thus making an ectopic beat more pronounced.

Associated symptoms

Establish whether the palpitations occur on their own or if they are associated with any other symptoms. Common symptoms that may occur include chest pain, shortness of breath, dizziness, blackout or a feeling of nausea or anxiety. If any of these symptoms do exist it is important to take a more detailed history about them and their relationship to the palpitations; such as do they occur before, during or after the palpitations? Chest pain and syncope may indicate serious pathology and should be considered as red flag symptoms – this is particularly important as it may be the first clear indication of cardiac dysfunction. If the patient has had blackout syncope then this means that there is insufficient cerebral perfusion due to poor cardiac output; possible causes of this may be a tachyarrhythmia or a complete heart block.

Palpitations may also occur in psychological states such as anxiety or panic disorders. Patients who suffer from panic attacks may complain of short-lived chest tightness, a feeling of the heart thumping in their chest, impending doom, or a dry mouth. They may also suffer with hyperventilation and perioral paraesthesia. At times, however, it may be difficult to tease out whether the patient suffered from anxiety initially and that brought on the palpitations, or whether the palpitations led to the panic attack.

TOP TIP!

It is often thought that caffeine is the main cause of palpitations in those consuming energy drinks. However, such drinks also contain taurine that plays an important role in heart muscle contraction and nervous system stimulation, causing palpitations.

QUESTIONS TO ASK . . .

- With your finger, tap out on the table the nature of the palpitation
- Is there anything that brings on an attack?
- Does your heart beat regularly or irregularly?
- When you feel the palpitations is there anything that you can do to stop them?
- How long does the episode last for?
- Do you notice any other symptoms with the palpitations?

BOX 1.1 **Causes of atrial fibrillation**

- Hypertension
- Infection (pneumonia, pericarditis)
- Ischaemic heart disease
- Mitral valve disease
- Thyrotoxicosis
- Alcohol
- Cardiomyopathy
- Ventricular hypertrophy

Other causes of palpitations such as thyrotoxicosis may present with florid symptoms that should be explored. Weight loss, sweating, poor heat tolerance and eye symptoms should point you to investigate for possible hyperthyroidism. Thyrotoxicosis in its own right can cause atrial fibrillation that may present with palpitations.

1.2.4 Past medical history

Take a detailed past medical history including any previous medical illness and hospital admissions. Enquire about previous episodes of palpitations and treatments. Patients may have had several A&E attendances for treatment of a possible reversible SVT. Previous treatments could include chemical or electrical cardioversion, as well as insertion of a pacemaker and cardiac ablation. Ask if the patient has any other medical conditions such as pre-existing heart disease, hypertension, diabetes, stroke, thyroid disease and anaemia. Do not forget to explore for any previous psychiatric illness including anxiety disorders.

Drug history

Ask the patient what medication they are taking, including any over-the-counter (OTC) preparations; this is particularly important as a number of cold and cough remedies contain sympathomimetic agents (i.e. ephedrine) which have been shown to precipitate palpitations. There are a number of agents that can predispose to palpitations including tricyclic antidepressants, theophylline, phenothiazines, antihistamine and verapramil. Do not forget to ask about drug allergies or intolerances.

Social history

Enquire whether the patient is a smoker and if so, establish the number of pack years. Cigarette smoking is a major contributor to palpitations due to the stimulant effect of nicotine on the heart. Also ask the patient if they drink alcohol and if so, how many units per week. Alcohol has also been implicated in the development of palpitations via cardiomyopathy and AF. It can cause palpitations directly by depleting the body's magnesium stores which play a vital role in regulating the heartbeat. Discreetly ask about illicit drug use as use of substances such as cocaine, ecstasy (MDMA) and cannabis can induce palpitations.

If you have not already done so, ensure that you take a thorough dietary history which should include asking about tea, coffee, chocolate (dark) and red wine consumption. Also enquire about the patient's social circumstances, looking for any evidence of adverse life events that may impact upon the patient's state of mind.

Family history

It is important to enquire when taking a palpitation history whether the patient has any first-degree relatives who suffer or have suffered from similar symptoms. Enquire specifically if there is any family history of sudden premature death which may be due to hypertrophic obstructive cardiomyopathy (HOCM) or prolonged QT syndrome. Ask about any valvular disorders (aortic stenosis) or ischaemic heart disease.

Medical Guidelines
Diagnosing and investigating AF

In patients presenting with any of the following:

- breathlessness/dyspnoea
- palpitations
- syncope/dizziness
- chest discomfort
- stroke/TIA

Annual pulse palpation – should be performed to assess for the presence of an irregular pulse that may indicate underlying AF. An electrocardiogram (ECG) should be performed in all patients, whether symptomatic or not, in whom AF is suspected because an irregular pulse has been detected.

24-hour ambulatory ECG monitoring – should be used in those with suspected asymptomatic episodes or symptomatic episodes less than 24 hours apart.

Event recorder ECG – should be used in those with symptomatic episodes more than 24 hours apart.

Echo – should be performed in patients with AF in the following circumstances: a young patient in need of a baseline echo for long-term management, for any patient in whom cardioversion is considered, or when there is suspicion of underlying structural heart disease (e.g. heart failure, heart murmur).

NICE Guidelines: Atrial fibrillation (2006)

1.2.5 **Systems review**

Complete your palpitation history with a brief systems review. Ask about any neurological symptoms such as fits, faints, weakness in the arms or legs, and any problems with their vision or hearing. Also enquire about relevant cardiac symptoms such as chest pain, shortness of breath and pedal oedema.

1.2.6 **Summing up**

Summarize your findings back to the patient and ask if they would like to add anything that you may have missed. It may be useful to summarize once you have completed the history of the presenting complaint because this may give you some time to reflect upon the information gathered so far.

Reassure your patient by coming to an agreement with them about what the next steps will be, checking to make sure they understand what is going on. Ask them if they have any questions they would like you to answer. In addition, offer the patient information leaflets and discuss when you (or another health professional) will see them next. End the interview by thanking the patient.

1.2.7 **Common clinical scenarios**

The following are a list of common palpitation cases which you may encounter. For each one, consider:
• what the possible differential diagnosis could be
• what key features you would look for
• what questions you would ask to refine or confirm your diagnosis

You could use role play with a friend, using the histories in the cases below as a framework.

CASE 1

A 48 year old shop manager presents in the A&E department complaining of shortness of breath, swelling of the ankles and palpitations. In addition he states that his heart thumps rapidly. Also, he has been getting tired and short of breath after walking 100 metres and sometimes wakes up at night gasping for breath. He does not have any significant past medical history nor any hospital admissions. He is not on any medications and has no known allergies. He smokes 15 cigarettes and drinks 3 pints of beer daily.

CASE 2

A 25 year old athlete complains to his GP that whilst running 2 days ago he felt his heart race for some time. When he ceased running the heart continued to beat rapidly for a few minutes before returning to normal. He has never had this before and is normally fit and well. He does not have any significant past medical history nor any hospital admissions. He is not on any medications and has no drug allergies. He does not smoke or drink.

CASE 3   A 23 year old medical student revising for finals presents to A&E with what she describes as palpitations. It was a one-off episode where she had not slept well the previous night. She does not have any past psychiatric history. She also complains of chest tightness, breathlessness and a sense of impending doom. The episode lasted a few minutes. She is otherwise fit and well.

CASE 4   A 38 year old lady presents who is 33 weeks pregnant. She brings her pregnancy book with her which reveals no complications in the current pregnancy. She complains of random episodes of a fast heartbeat that last for a few minutes before spontaneously resolving. They are worse on exertion and lying down. She denies chest or calf pain.

CASE 5   A 38 year old woman complains of acute loss of weight. She also complains of soft and frequent stools, oily skin and blurring of vision along with palpitations. She has noticed that she is comfortable in her summer clothing in the winter months.

CASE 6   A 75 year old man complains of a 5 day history of a productive cough with fever and sweats. He brings up a thick brownish-green phlegm whenever he coughs. He taps out the rhythm on the table and states that it was irregular in nature. He has no other medical problems of note and lives a healthy lifestyle. On examination he has right-sided basal crepitations.

Chapter 1.3
Shortness of breath

What to do . . .

- Introduce yourself to the patient – establish rapport
- Ask the patient's name, age and occupation
- Ask the patient relevant questions relating to their shortness of breath, such as onset, nature, aggravating and relieving factors, exercise and sleep
- Ask about any associated symptoms, e.g. coughing, fever, haemoptysis, weight loss, night sweats
- Ask about any recent travel history
- Ask about any past medical history including previous investigations or operations
- Ask about any drug history and for any drug allergies
- Ask about any social history – enquire if the patient smokes or drinks alcohol
- Ask about any family history, specifically for atopic conditions
- Perform a brief systems review and sum up your findings
- Thank the patient and conclude the consultation

Shortness of breath, otherwise known as breathlessness or dyspnoea, can at times be quite a frightening symptom for the patient. Throughout our daily lives we may experience short episodes of breathlessness, particularly when undertaking high levels of activity such as exercising or playing sport, but these bouts tend to be short lived and do not interfere with a patient's ability to manage their daily affairs. However, when the shortness of breath is prolonged and persistent, it is likely to have an underlying medical aetiology.

Although it is easy to assume that all episodes of shortness of breath have a respiratory origin, this is often an incorrect assumption. Dyspnoea may be caused by dysfunction of virtually any system in the body including the heart (heart failure, arrhythmia, myocardial infarction), lung (asthma, COPD, pulmonary embolism), metabolic (diabetic ketoacidosis, drug overdose), or endocrine (thyrotoxicosis) systems. In addition, psychogenic disorders such as panic attack or anxiety may also precipitate difficulty in breathing.

1.3.1 Taking the history

Begin by introducing yourself to the patient by stating your full name, grade and the purpose of the consultation. Attempt to establish rapport by asking open questions such as how the patient is feeling today. Ask some background questions such as their name, age and occupation before asking about their shortness of breath. It is important to establish the patient's occupational history, including current and previous jobs, because there are a variety of different occupations that may be implicated in dyspnoea (*Box 1.2*). Patients

BOX 1.2 **Occupational lung disease**

Pneumoconiosis
- Asbestosis (exposure to asbestos)
- Berylliosis (exposure to beryllium – found in fluorescent light bulbs)
- Chalicosis (exposure to stone; seen in stone cutters)
- Coalworker's pneumoconiosis (coal miners)
- Siderosis (exposure to iron, e.g. in welders or foundry workers)
- Silicosis (exposure to silicon, e.g. in stone masons when sand blasting)

Hypersensitivity pneumonitis
- Bird fancier's lung (from pigeons, parrots, budgies)
- Farmer's lung (from hay, mould)

Occupational asthma

who work in or around farms or in close contact with birds or hay can develop bird fancier's lung or farmer's lung. Others who have worked in coal mines or as stone masons run the risk of developing pneumoconiosis. Builders, roofers or dock workers who used to be in employment in the mid-twentieth century may have been exposed to asbestos that can cause lung cancer (mesothelioma). Breathing in and being exposed to certain dusts (flour), gases, vapours (spray paints) or fumes (soldering fumes) may cause asthma that is mainly symptomatic at work (occupational asthma).

1.3.2 Ideas, concerns and expectations

After appropriately introducing yourself and establishing rapport, it is useful to elicit the patient's own health beliefs about their breathlessness. Try to establish what the patient thinks is going on and what concerns they may have; these concerns are commonly the possibility of lung cancer, work-related dyspnoea or myocardial infarction. Spend some time enquiring about how the problem has affected the patient's life and establish whether it is interfering with their normal daily activities, hobbies or pastimes (sports, walking).

1.3.3 History of the presenting complaint

Next move on to take a more detailed history about the patient's breathlessness. Initially start by asking open questions before moving on to more focused closed questions.

Onset

Establish when the patient first noticed their breathlessness and the speed at which it came on. Acute onset of unexplained shortness of breath should always point you towards more serious aetiology; for example, a young child who has attended a party and who now complains of acute onset and worsening shortness of breath with stridor should make you consider an acute airway obstruction by a foreign body such as a peanut. Similarly, a patient attending with acute dyspnoea with stridor, urticarial rash and pruritus after being stung by a bee should alert you to an anaphylactic shock. Other causes of acute shortness of breath include pneumothorax which can occur spontaneously in a tall thin adult male.

Insidious onset of slowly worsening shortness of breath, particularly in an elderly smoker, should have COPD excluded as a possible cause. A similar presentation in a patient with ischaemic heart disease and gradually deteriorating breathlessness on lying flat should alert you to heart failure.

Nature

Determine the nature of the breathlessness by asking whether it is present all the time or comes and goes. Breathlessness that is ever present is more likely to be caused by respiratory conditions such as COPD or cardiac dysfunction such as heart failure or anaemia. Intermittent breathlessness may be due to arrhythmias, occupational lung disease or as a psychogenic symptom of an acute stress reaction or to a panic attack.

Exercise

Establishing a relationship between the patient's dyspnoea and their ability to exercise is a good indicator of the severity. First, try to establish the patient's level of exercise tolerance prior to the development of their symptom. Compare this with their current level of exercise tolerance – ask the patient how far they can walk before getting breathless.

Enquire about the effects the breathlessness has had on the patient, such as how it is affecting their ability to climb up and down stairs or, worse still, does it affect simple activities such as talking or getting dressed? The latter would indicate a severe debilitating dyspnoea. Use the MRC dyspnoea scale (*Box 1.3*) to objectively score their symptoms. Heart failure can also present with

---

BOX 1.3 **Medical Research Council dyspnoea scale**

1   Not troubled by breathlessness except on strenuous exercise
2   Short of breath when hurrying or walking up a slight hill
3   Walks slower than contemporaries on the level because of breathlessness, or has to stop for breath when walking at own pace
4   Stops for breath after about 100 m or after a few minutes on level ground
5   Too breathless to leave the house or breathless when dressing or undressing

---

BOX 1.4 **New York Heart Association functional classification**

NYHA Class	Symptoms
I	No symptoms and no limitation in ordinary physical activity, e.g. shortness of breath when walking, climbing stairs, etc.
II	Mild symptoms (mild shortness of breath and/or angina) and slight limitation during ordinary activity
III	Marked limitation in activity due to symptoms, even during less-than-ordinary activity, e.g. walking short distances (20–100 m); comfortable only at rest
IV	Severe limitations – experiences symptoms even while at rest (mostly bedbound patients)

DIFFERENTIAL DIAGNOSIS

Causes of pleuritic chest pain

- Pneumothorax
- Pneumonia
- Pleurisy
- Pulmonary embolism
- Musculoskeletal chest pain

TOP TIP!

Non-steroidal anti-inflammatory drugs (NSAIDs) have been implicated as the trigger of an asthma attack in 10% of cases of asthmatics. Other drugs that can precipitate an asthma attack include aspirin and β-blockers

breathlessness on exertion. If the patient is known to have heart failure then consider using the NYHA scale to grade severity (*Box 1.4*).

Relieving and exacerbating factors

Determine whether there are any factors that make the patient's breathlessness better or worse. Patients who find using inhalers or nebulizers relieves their symptoms probably have asthma or COPD as likely causes. Patients who improve whilst on holiday or off work and worsen on return are likely to have an occupational precipitant. Dyspnoea with wheeze that is exacerbated by dust, smoke, cold, pollen, pets or exercise may be suggestive of atopy or asthma.

Sleep

Find out how the breathlessness affects the patient's sleep. Patients who frequently wake during the night short of breath and gasping for air may be describing paroxysmal nocturnal dyspnoea which is seen in pulmonary oedema. This occurs when the lung's alveoli are filled with fluid as the patient sleeps, reducing the oxygen and carbon dioxide exchange which ultimately wakes the patient from their sleep. A similar pathology occurs in orthopnoea where the patient is breathless from simply lying flat.

An effective way to quickly assess the severity of dyspnoea is to ask the patient whether they are able to lie flat and if not, how may pillows they use. Occasionally patients with severe worsening heart failure may be forced to use more pillows to prop themselves up; they may even have to sleep upright to feel comfortable.

Associated symptoms

Breathlessness often presents in conjunction with other symptoms such as cough, fever, chest pain, wheeze, palpitations, dizziness or ankle swelling. Eliciting these will help narrow down your list of possible differentials. Patients complaining of a brief history of shortness of breath with fever, sweats and productive cough may suggest an infective origin (pneumonia), whereas a history of worsening shortness of breath with night sweats, weight loss and haemoptysis may suggest tuberculosis. Coughing up frank blood in a chronic smoker should be investigated promptly with an urgent chest X-ray for lung cancer. Acute onset of sharp pleuritic chest pain that is made worse with deep inspiration and coughing, along with post-surgical haemoptysis, should have a pulmonary embolism (see *Box 1.5* for risk factors) excluded. An irregular heart beat with palpitations in an acutely short of breath person may have a cardiac origin such as an arrhythmia.

BOX 1.5 **Risk factors for pulmonary embolism**

Immobilization (after surgery or long distance air travel)
Pregnancy
Obesity
Cancer
Oral contraceptive pill, HRT
Thrombophilia
    genetic: factor V Leiden, protein C or S deficiency
    acquired: antiphospholipid syndrome, nephrotic syndrome

1.3.4 **Past medical history**

Take a detailed past medical history including any previous illnesses and hospital admissions. Enquire about previous investigations, such as chest X-rays or CT scans (CTPA), and any recent procedures such as chest drains (may predispose to pneumothorax). Specifically establish whether the patient has had any trauma or operations within the last few weeks; complex operations such as hip replacement dramatically increase the chances of developing a pulmonary embolism, primarily due to their lack of mobilization.

Specifically enquire about pneumonia, tuberculosis, hypertension, high cholesterol, rheumatic fever, asthma, ischaemic heart disease (associated with heart failure and pulmonary oedema), PE, DVT, diabetes and cancer. In a younger patient it may be useful to ask about atopic conditions such as hayfever or eczema which may predispose them to asthma later in life.

If the patient suffers from asthma or COPD, it is important to take a more focused history regarding the number of exacerbations, use of nebulizers, oral steroids or home oxygen (COPD) and any spells in intensive care (ITU).

Travel history

Enquiring about recent travel may reveal potential causes for the patient's breathlessness. Long journeys may cause DVTs and subsequent PEs (sometimes known as 'economy class syndrome'). Foreign travel, particular to hotels with air conditioning facilities, may put the patient at risk of legionnaires' disease. Patients who have recently travelled from countries with a high prevalence of tuberculosis should be screened with a chest X-ray or Mantoux test.

Drug history

Ask the patient what medication they are currently on or have taken in the recent past (such as use of inhalers or nebulizers, oral steroids, leukotriene receptor antagonist, theophylline). Do not forget to also ask about any OTC medications or herbal remedies that the patient has tried. Specifically enquire about drugs that may adversely affect breathing such as β-blockers (asthma), amiodarone (pulmonary fibrosis), nitrofurantoin (pulmonary fibrosis) and methotrexate (pneumonitis). A common side effect of ACE inhibitors is a dry cough. In female patients it is important to establish whether they are on the pill or HRT (risk of PEs).

Social history

Enquire whether the patient is a current smoker, ex-smoker or has never smoked tobacco. If the patient does smoke, note whether they smoke cigarettes, cigars or roll-ups. In the case of cigarettes, try and calculate the number of 'pack years'. A pack year is defined as smoking 20 cigarettes a day for one year. Hence, a patient smoking 40 a day for 5 years would have 10 pack years. All forms of smoking have been implicated in worsening respiratory disease, in particular the development of COPD and lung cancer.

Briefly ask about alcohol use, noting the type and units consumed if relevant. Discreetly ask about illicit drug use. Cannabis has been shown to cause coughing, wheezing and chest tightness, whereas heroin may cause respiratory depression.

TOP TIP!

Cigar smokers have a slightly reduced prevalence of lung cancer compared to cigarette smokers because they tend not to inhale as much. Some studies have suggested that roll-ups cause greater damage than cigarettes due to their lack of a filter.

TOP TIP!

If the patient is suffering from moderate to severe shortness of breath it may be pertinent to enquire about their social circumstances. Find out whether the patient lives alone or has any carers. Enquire whether they have any stairs in the house and whether they have difficulty climbing them.

TOP TIP!

In a patient who suffers from atopic symptoms such as coughing, wheezing, sneezing and rhinitis, you should enquire whether they keep any pets and if their symptoms are exacerbated by direct contact with them. Pets such as cats, dogs and budgies have all been implicated.

DIFFERENTIAL DIAGNOSIS

Shortness of breath
Acute
- Inhaled foreign body
- Anaphylaxis
- Asthma attack
- Pulmonary embolism
- Pneumothorax
- Pulmonary oedema
- Chest injuries
- Pneumonia (days)

Chronic
- COPD
- Asthma
- Heart failure
- Lung cancer
- Anaemia
- Pneumoconiosis

Family history

It is important to enquire whether the patient has any first-degree relatives who suffer or have suffered from similar symptoms. A family history of atopy may predispose the patient to developing asthma in later life. Family members with tuberculosis who live in close proximity to the patient may put them at risk of developing the condition.

1.3.5 Systems review

Complete your breathlessness history with a brief systems review. You may wish to enquire more generally about common symptoms such as chest pain, palpitations or neurological symptoms, or any muscle or joint pain in order to check the patient's health and wellbeing.

1.3.6 Summing up

Summarize your findings back to the patient and ask if they would like to add anything that you may have missed. Reassure your patient by coming to an agreement with them about what the next step will be; remember to check to make sure they understand what is going on. Ask them if they have any questions they would like you to answer. In addition, offer the patient information leaflets and discuss when you (or another health professional) will see them next. End the interview by thanking the patient. In an examination situation, you should deliver an appropriate summary to the examiner.

1.3.7 Common clinical scenarios

The following are a list of common breathlessness cases which you may encounter. For each one, consider:
- what the possible differential diagnosis could be
- what key features you would look for
- what questions you would ask to refine or confirm your diagnosis

You could use role play with a friend, using the histories in the cases below as a framework.

CASE 1

A 25 year old Somali student has recently sought asylum in the UK. He complains of a 3 month history of tiredness, fatigue and worsening shortness of breath. On further enquiry you note that he has haemoptysis, fever and weight loss. He is a non-smoker and has not recently travelled.

CASE 2

A 55 year old former publican presents with hoarseness of voice, coughing up frank blood and 2 stone weight loss over the last few months. He is an ex-smoker who quit 5 years ago. On further enquiry he started smoking when he was 15 and has smoked 2 packets a day for the past 35 years.

CASE 3   A 65 year old retired gardener complains of worsening shortness of breath on exertion. He is unable to lie flat and has been sleeping on three pillows for the last 3 months. Previously he enjoyed strolls in the park but now he complains that he struggles to even walk 50 metres. He also notices that his shoes are tighter and more difficult to put on.

CASE 4   A 27 year old lady patient gave birth 3 weeks ago. She now complains of chest pain worse on deep inspiration. She also notes shortness of breath and a mild ache over her left lower leg. Recently there have been specks of blood in her phlegm.

CASE 5   A keen football player aged 16 years presents with exertional cough and wheeze during strenuous activity. He is generally well and currently asymptomatic. However, his mother mentions that when he was younger he suffered from eczema.

CASE 6   A 45 year old woman travelled to the Philippines for a business trip. She stayed in a hotel for much of her trip. On returning home she developed chills, muscle aches and a headache. She did not respond to OTC medication or a course of penicillin.

CASE 7   A 62 year old retired miner has been complaining of a chronic cough as well as mild shortness of breath. More recently he has noticed a productive cough that is black is colour. He is a non-smoker and has lived a healthy lifestyle.

Chapter 1.4
Cough

What to do . . .

- Introduce yourself to the patient – establish rapport
- Ask the patient's name, age and occupation
- Ask the patient relevant questions relating to their cough, such as onset, timing, character, and aggravating and relieving factors
- Ask about any associated symptoms, e.g. fever, haemoptysis, weight loss, night sweats
- Ask about any recent travel
- Ask about any past medical history including previous investigations or operations
- Ask about any drug history and for any drug allergies such as to ACE inhibitors or NSAIDs
- Ask about any social history – establish if the patient smokes or drinks alcohol
- Ask about any family history and specifically for atopic conditions including asthma
- Perform a brief systems review and sum up your findings
- Thank the patient and conclude the consultation

Coughing is a reflex action that helps clear the respiratory tract of any excess mucus, phlegm, or irritants. It represents a first line of defence against foreign bodies entering the airways. The lining of the lower respiratory tract contains sensitive nerve endings that, when triggered, send information to the medulla oblongata which modulates a co-ordinated cough response. A person is made to take a short sharp breath before the abdominal and chest muscles contract, causing a pressure increase in the thoracic cavity, forcibly exhaling air. As the air is released the lower airway is cleansed of secretions, dust and dirt.

Coughing is also a non-specific symptom and may be caused by a wide range of different conditions, for example, infections, allergies, medication, reflux and respiratory diseases can all give rise to cough.

Taking a cough history includes eliciting a wide range of associated symptoms that will help you arrive at a potential diagnosis.

1.4.1 Taking the history

Introduce yourself by mentioning your name and job description. Ask the patient some background questions such as their name, age, and whether they are in employment before moving on to enquire about their cough. The patient's age and gender can play a role in the consideration of an appropriate differential diagnosis, for example, coughs from simple viral infections, asthma and common colds often occur in children; in older patients, a cough may result from bronchitis, smoking, chronic lung disease, and pneumonia.

1.4.2 **Ideas, concerns and expectations**

After appropriately introducing yourself and establishing rapport, it is usually a good moment to ask the patient what they think is causing their cough. Also go on to establish whether the patient has any particular concerns about their cough: patient anxieties often include fear of infection and tumours. Spend some time enquiring about how the symptom has affected the patient's life and elicit whether their cough has prevented or hindered them from performing a particular activity, such as sleeping, for example.

1.4.3 **History of presenting complaint**

Take a detailed history about the patient's cough. Begin by establishing when it started, whether it comes and goes, and its character. Finally, elicit any associated symptoms as well as factors that may exacerbate or relieve it.

Onset

It is important to know when the cough first started and how often it occurs. Coughs can be classified as acute, sub-acute or chronic depending on duration. Chronic coughs tend to last more than 2 months, whereas acute onset coughs last less than 3 weeks.

- Acute coughs may be caused by viral upper respiratory tract infection, pneumonia, pulmonary oedema or pulmonary embolism. A sudden onset should alert you to the possibility of foreign body inhalation or an anaphylactic reaction.
- Chronic coughs are often seen in chronic respiratory diseases such as asthma, COPD and fibrosis.

> **TOP TIP!**
>
> Respiratory tract infections, asthma, and gastro-oesophageal reflux disease are the most common causes of chronic cough in children. Foreign body aspiration should be considered in young children

Timing

Does the cough come and go or is it there all the time? Persistent coughing may be due to a common cold, pneumonia, smoker's cough, or chronic lung and airways disease. Episodic coughs, on the other hand, may represent viral croup, asthma, heart failure or allergies. Certain coughs may present at particular times of the day. In asthma, coughs tend to have a diurnal variation, being worse in the morning and late at night. Coughs that occur seasonally may be seen in seasonal allergic rhinitis or in hayfever sufferers. Patients who report that their cough is worse when at work and improved when on holiday may have occupational asthma, which is common amongst miners, poultry farmers and people working with cement.

Character

Try to elicit the nature of the cough. Does the patient describe it as a dry cough or is it chesty? Dry coughs are usually non-productive and are due to upper airway inflammation. They may be described as a 'tickle' or a feeling of an irritation at the back of the throat. A chesty cough is usually productive in nature and is associated with phlegm and excessive mucus production.

Exacerbating and relieving factors

It is then useful to try to establish whether the cough is made worse or improved by any particular activity or situation. Patients who cough when angry or in an emotional state may be suffering from asthma; they may also notice the cough after exercising and such patients may notice a marked reduction of their cough after using a salbutamol inhaler.

Patients who only notice a cough after eating may suffer from oesophageal reflux disease whereby acid may reflux up the oesophagus and into the lower respiratory tract, inducing a cough response. A cough that is only present when the patient lies down may be indicative of a post-nasal drip.

Associated symptoms

Spend some time eliciting any symptoms that are present along with the cough. Symptoms such as fever, night sweats, haemoptysis, phlegm, wheeze and weight loss may be described by the patient. A productive cough along with fever normally indicates an infective cause affecting the upper or lower respiratory tracts.

- Upper respiratory tract infections (URTIs) are usually viral in nature and are typically self-limiting, usually resolving within 7–10 days; patients often report a runny nose, muscle aches and pains, and a generalized feeling of tiredness.
- Lower respiratory tract infections (LRTIs) may present with similar symptoms to URTIs; however, the symptoms are often more prolonged and intense. Patients may also complain of shortness of breath, pleuritic chest pain and a productive cough. LRTIs are classified into bronchitis or pneumonias. Possible pathogens that are implicated include viral, bacterial or fungal organisms. Whilst it may be difficult to distinguish between them clinically, the colour of the sputum may give an early indication:

  - viral infections often start with clear phlegm that later turns yellow or green

  - bacterial infections also present with green phlegm, but if a rusty brown coloured sputum is noted then a bacterial pneumococcal pneumonia should be excluded

  - thick black phlegm, whilst uncommon, may be indicative of an underlying fungal infection such as aspergillosis.

> **DIFFERENTIAL DIAGNOSIS**
>
> **Causes of coughing up blood**
> - Pneumonia
> - Pulmonary embolism
> - Tuberculosis
> - Bronchiectasis
> - Bronchitis
> - Lung cancer
> - Goodpasture's syndrome
> - Wegener's granulomatosis

Haemoptysis, or coughing up blood, may be an alarming symptom for the patient. You should evaluate the quantity of blood produced as well as its duration. A patient reporting a fever, sweats and cough for > 1 week with specks of blood in their phlegm may have a severe chest infection warranting a chest X-ray. A prolonged history with fever, night sweats and weight loss in an Asian or African patient should be investigated for tuberculosis. Copious haemoptysis with weight loss and hoarseness of voice in a heavy smoker should alert you to the possibility of lung cancer. If the tumour is adjacent to the bronchus, the patient may report symptoms of upper airway obstruction, including shortness of breath, wheeze and stridor. They may also suffer from complications such as pneumonia, bronchiectasis, lung abscess or lobar collapse.

1.4.4 Past medical history

Take a detailed past medical history including any previous illnesses and hospital admissions. Enquire about previous chest infections and treatments. Ask if the patient has any other medical conditions such as chronic airways and lung disease, asthma, diabetes, stroke, TB, or blood disorders.

Drug history

Ask the patient about any medication they are currently taking. Ask specifically about ACE inhibitors, NSAIDs, β-blockers and aspirin. ACE inhibitors are known to cause a persistent dry cough in 15% of cases. NSAIDs, β-blockers and aspirin may induce or worsen a person's asthma.

Don't forget to ask about drug allergies or intolerances. This is important in a cough history, because a cough could be brought on by many allergens in a hypersensitive person. These include dust, cold temperature, pollen, smoke and animal dander.

Social history

Enquire whether the patient has ever smoked and, if so, how many cigarettes a day and for how long. Smoking is directly implicated in the development of lung cancer, bronchitis and COPD.

Ask about alcohol use, noting the type of alcohol and how many units a week. Discreetly ask about illicit drug use.

Travel history

Briefly enquire whether the patient has travelled abroad recently. A stay within a hostel or hotel with air conditioning facilities may suggest legionnaires' disease. Long haul plane journeys may give rise to a pulmonary embolism. Finally, patients returning from areas that have high prevalence of TB can be at risk of developing the illness.

Family history

It is important when taking a cough history to ask whether the patient has any first-degree relatives who suffer, or have suffered, from similar symptoms. In particular, ask about asthma and chronic lung disease.

1.4.5 Systems review

Complete your cough history with a brief systems review. Ask about common symptoms such as chest pain, palpitations or change in bowel habits, or any muscle or joint pain in order to check the patient's health and wellbeing.

1.4.6 Summing up

Summarize your findings back to the patient and ask if they would like to add anything that you may have missed. Reassure your patient by coming to an agreement with them about what the next steps will be; check at each stage to make sure they understand what is going on. Ask them if they have any questions they would like you to answer. In addition, offer the patient information leaflets and discuss when you (or another health professional) will see them next. End the interview by thanking the patient. In an exam situation, you should deliver an appropriate summary to the examiner.

1.4.7 Common clinical scenarios

The following are a list of common cough cases which you may encounter. For each one, consider:

- what the level of risk could be
- what key features you would look for
- what questions you would ask to refine or confirm your diagnosis

You could use role play with a friend, using the histories in the cases below as a framework.

CASE 1

A 14 year old student complains of a cough and a wheeze over the last 3 months, particularly when playing sport. The breathlessness started during winter, and was particularly bad when playing football in the cold wind. The breathing has slowly worsened and he now finds it hard to do even short periods of exercise. The patient's sleep is now being affected by his symptoms. He suffered from hayfever and eczema as a child.

CASE 2

A 20 year old law student, who is normally fit and well, last night developed sharp pain under her left breast. The pain has no radiation and gradually worsened in intensity overnight with no relief from paracetamol. The pain is worse on movement and on deep breathing. She has coughed up two clots of fresh blood this morning but has not had any other cough, sputum or fever. She has become increasingly anxious and breathless over this period. She has recently started on a combined oral contraceptive pill and smokes 10 cigarettes a day. Her brother died 2 years ago from a clot in the lung. She returned from a 23 hour coach journey 2 days ago.

CASE 3

A 63 year old lifelong smoker and retired plumber was admitted from the outpatients clinic because of a 3 month history of weight loss and coughing up blood. Initially the sputum was brownish in colour with clots mixed in with clear sputum but now there is fresh blood and it occurs four to five times a day. He has developed a dry irritating cough with breathlessness on exertion. His exercise tolerance is about 700 m on the flat and he gets breathless after climbing 14 stairs at home. He has no history of fever, chest pain, wheeze, difficulty in breathing when lying down, or palpitations. He has lost about 12 kg in weight in the last 3 months and has felt increasingly lethargic over this time. In the last few weeks his voice has become hoarse. He has smoked 20 cigarettes a day for the last 35 years, and drinks 5–10 pints of beer each week.

CASE 4

A 61 year old retired car factory worker has been getting progressively less well over the last 2–3 years. He is a lifelong smoker, smoking 30 cigarettes a day. Every winter for the last 8–9 years he has had severe cough with thick green sputum; this has now worsened and now seems to happen all the year round. He can only walk about 100 m on the flat before stopping due to breathlessness and wheeze. He has never noticed any blood in his sputum and has not been feverish in the past few months. He does not have any chest pains, swelling of ankles or periods of breathlessness at night. His GP recently started him on some inhalers but he rarely uses them as they seem to do little good. He does not take any other medications, and is otherwise well, with systemic symptoms. He is worried that he is never going to get better.

CASE 5

A 65 year old woman presents with a 2 week history of fever, worsening shortness of breath with a productive cough. The phlegm was initially white but has turned rusty coloured. She mentions she has recently experienced pain in her chest whenever she coughs or takes a deep breath in. She is a non-smoker with no recent history of travel.

Chapter 1.5
Abdominal pain

What to do . . .

- Introduce yourself to the patient – establish rapport
- Ask the patient's name, age and occupation
- Ask the patient relevant questions about their abdominal pain, such as its site, onset, character, radiation, aggravating and relieving factors, its timing and the effect of food
- Ask about any associated symptoms, e.g. change in bowel habits, weight loss, jaundice, nausea, vomiting, fever
- Ask about any past medical history including previous investigations or operations
- Ask about any drug history and for any drug allergies
- Ask about any social history – enquire if the patient smokes or drinks alcohol
- Ask about any recent travel history
- Ask about any family history, specifically for polyposis (HNPCC)
- Perform a brief systems review and sum up your findings
- Thank the patient and conclude the consultation

Abdominal pain is pain that is felt anywhere between the chest and groin areas. It represents between 5% and 10% of all A&E admissions. There are many organs in the abdomen from which pain may arise and so it is important to consider the location of the pain in relation to the underlying structures. However, take into account that abdominal pain may also arise from outside the abdominal cavity and radiate inwards, such as from the chest (e.g. lower lobe pneumonia) or the pelvis (e.g. pelvic inflammatory disease).

The intensity of the pain does not always reflect the seriousness of the condition. Severe abdominal pain can arise from mild conditions, such as gas or the cramping spasms of viral gastroenteritis. Conversely, relatively mild pain may present in life-threatening conditions, such as cancer of the colon or early appendicitis.

Whilst abdominal pain usually presents with focal localized discomfort, if it becomes widespread and affects the whole abdomen this should be taken very seriously. A rupture of an inflamed organ, such as the appendix or an eroding peptic ulcer, may lead to general pain associated with stiffness of the abdomen and fever – this is known as peritonitis (inflammation and infection of the lining of the abdominal cavity) and is a medical emergency.

1.5.1 Taking the history

As with any history, it is essential to begin by introducing yourself, including offering your name and your job title. Ask the patient their name, age and

TOP TIP!

Offer the patient pain relief before taking a full history. Not only will this make them more comfortable, but they are likely to give you a better history when not in excruciating pain.

occupation before specifically addressing the abdominal pain. Begin by asking open questions regarding their symptoms before moving on to more direct questions relating to the nature of their pain. This will hopefully relax the patient, allow them to relate their story fully and encourage them to answer your questions more openly.

A patient's age and gender play a significant role in the consideration of an appropriate differential diagnosis, for example:

- inflammatory bowel disease has a bimodal age distribution, presenting in teenage years and peaking again in middle-age
- in women, gynaecological causes for the pain must always be considered and any woman of reproductive age presenting with abdominal pain must have a pregnancy test to rule out a possible ectopic
- although appendicitis (see *Fig 1.3*) usually presents in the extremes of age, it should always be considered in all age groups.

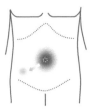

Fig 1.3 Acute appendicitis

Dull periumbilical pain that later localizes to the right iliac fossa. The pain may also be felt if the left iliac fossa is palpated (Rovsing's sign).

1.5.2 **Ideas, concerns and expectations**

After appropriately introducing yourself and establishing rapport, it is important to enquire as to what the patient believes may be the cause of their pain. This allows the patient to put their pain into context, possibly provides you with information you would not otherwise have elicited, and warns you about any misconceptions and worries they may hold.

Spend some time enquiring about how the symptoms has affected the patient's life and elicit whether their symptoms are interfering with their normal daily activities.

1.5.3 **History of presenting complaint**

As with any pain history, it is important to elicit as much information as possible about the various aspects of the patient's abdominal pain. This will help narrow down the causes of the pain and allow you to exclude less probable differentials.

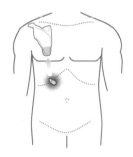

Fig 1.4 Acute cholecystitis

Colicky pain later becoming constant in the right hypochondrium or epigastrium that radiates to the right scapula and shoulder.

Site

Ask the patient where the pain is located or request that they point towards it if necessary. The site of the pain is instrumental in guiding the focus of your history, though common and serious possibilities, such as acute appendicitis, should not be discounted as they may present atypically.

Pain from pancreatitis is typically found in the epigastrium, whilst the pain of acute appendicitis classically begins around the umbilicus before localizing in the right iliac fossa (McBurney's point) after a few hours. Pain in the lower left quadrant can be due to colonic (especially sigmoid) pathology, whilst kidney pain presents in the right and left flanks. Liver disease or gallstones (see *Fig 1.4*) typically cause pain in the right upper quadrant.

Onset

It is important to elicit when the pain started and whether it has ever occurred in the past. Knowledge about the time of onset of the pain is useful in distinguishing between potential causes. For example, acute onset suggests a sudden event such as colonic ischaemia or obstruction of the bile duct by a gallstone. Sudden onset central abdominal or epigastric pain should alert you to the possibility of

QUESTIONS TO ASK . . .

- Where is the pain located? When did it start? How long did it last for?
- Does the pain move anywhere? Is it related to meals?
- Does it come and go or is it there all the time? Does the pain feel sharp or is it a dull ache? Is it burning or cramp-like?
- What symptoms are associated with the pain? How severe is the pain if you had to score the pain out of 10?

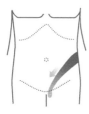

Fig 1.5 Renal colic

Intense colicky pain radiating from loin to groin and into the scrotum in males. The patient may writhe in pain from the severity.

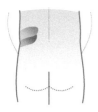

Fig 1.6 Loin pain

Loin pain is often indicative of renal disease (kidney stone or pyelonephritis). It is best located in the back just below the rib cage.

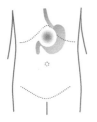

Fig 1.7 Peptic ulcer

Epigastric pain can radiate to the back and is usually related to meals. It may be associated with water brash (heartburn) and nausea.

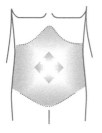

Fig 1.8 Generalized peritonitis

Sudden onset of severe pain radiating to the whole abdomen. Pain worsens with small movements but is relieved by lying still, e.g. perforated peptic ulcer.

a ruptured abdominal aortic aneurysm, especially if the patient has a history of hypertension and peripheral vascular disease.

A more insidious onset with progressive worsening of symptoms, with ascites, gynaecomastia and spider naevi may indicate chronic decompensated liver disease. Irritable bowel syndrome (IBS) can occur over months or years and may last for decades.

Character

It is very important to elicit the character of the pain so ensure that you allow the patient to freely express themselves and describe the symptoms in their own words. If the patient is unable to express the exact nature of their pain, consider offering a number of descriptions for them to choose from. Ask the patient whether the pain they are experiencing is cramping, dull or sharp, or whether it is constant or colicky in nature.

The pain associated with inflammation of the parietal peritoneum is steady and aching, and worsened by changes in movement. The pain associated with obstruction of a hollow viscus, such as the ureter, bowel or bile duct, is intermittent or 'colicky' in nature due to the waves of peristalsis around the obstruction as seen in kidney stones (see *Fig 1.5* and *Fig 1.6*) or bowel obstruction.

Radiation

It is useful to ask whether the pain moves or spreads anywhere else. The pain of renal colic typically radiates from the loin to the groin and into the scrotum in males. Pain from an ulcer (*Fig 1.7*) will often radiate through to the back, whilst pain associated with the rupture of an abdominal aortic aneurysm may radiate to the back, flank, or genitals. Pain due to gallstones may radiate to the lower tip of the right shoulder blade.

Associated symptoms

Abdominal pain can often present in conjunction with other symptoms. You should ask in particular about nausea and vomiting, loss of appetite and any change in bowel habit. If the patient is vomiting, specifically enquire about the presence of blood or a 'coffee ground' appearance (haematemesis). Note any reported blood in the stool (haematochezia) or black stools (melaena), as such symptoms suggest a possible GI bleed. Melaena is pathognomonic of a slow upper GI bleed, as haemoglobin within the blood is broken down and oxidized through the bowel to produce black tarry stools. Fresh frank blood *per rectum* is most likely due to a lower GI bleed as the blood has not had the chance to be broken down by the gut and colon, but it could also be caused by a high output upper GI bleed. If this is the case, the patient is likely to be in peri-shock if not already in shock.

Enquire about change in bowel habits such as constipation or diarrhoea, particularly in the older age groups as this may be a feature of colon cancer.

Ask the patient if they have noticed any changes to their stools such as the presence of mucus or difficulty in flushing them away. Mucus in the stool may be due to IBS, inflammatory bowel disease or bacterial infection (*Campylobacter*). Steatorrhoea is the presence of excess fat within the stool and produces pale, light, foul-smelling faeces that are difficult to flush away. This may be seen in small bowel disease preventing the absorption of fat, such as in coeliac disease and tropical sprue, or pancreatitis and gallbladder obstruction.

Abdominal pain associated with distension, vomiting and absolute constipation (absence of flatus as well as faeces) is the typical picture of intestinal obstruction. Right upper quadrant abdominal pain associated with bilious vomiting should raise your suspicion of an intestinal obstruction distal to the ampulla of Vater or cholecystitis. Lower left quadrant abdominal pain, in association with a palpable mass and blood or mucus passed *per rectum*, may indicate diverticular or inflammatory bowel disease.

Timing

Pain that comes and goes is described as colicky and is usually caused by the contraction of smooth muscle against an obstruction. Such pain is common in biliary disorders like stones in the gallbladder. This pain arises as the gallbladder intermittently contracts in the attempt to expel the stone which is often lodged in the neck of the gallbladder.

Exacerbating and relieving factors

It is important to ask about the factors that make the pain better or worse. The pain of acute pancreatitis is often relieved by leaning forward (like for pericarditis), whilst the pain from gastric oesophageal reflux disease is made worse by lying flat. The colicky pain experienced with early acute appendicitis and gastroenteritis are somewhat relieved by writhing and massage, whereas in peritonitis lying perfectly still helps to mitigate the pain (see *Fig 1.8*).

Pain associated with the ingestion of food may point towards a diagnosis of peptic ulcer disease, IBS or gallbladder disease. The pain from a gastric ulcer is usually worse shortly after eating food, whereas the pain from duodenal ulcers usually arises at night and is relieved by meals. Pain from IBS may come on at the time of eating meals and may be relieved upon defecation. Gallstone pain may be triggered after eating a large fatty meal.

Severity

Gauging the severity of the pain is vital in the immediate management (pain relief) and in determining its possible cause. A useful tool for subjectively scaling the intensity of the pain is to ask the patient to rate the pain on a scale of one to ten, one being minimal pain and ten being the worst pain ever felt. However, be aware that the severity of pain does not always equate to the underlying aetiology.

1.5.4 Past medical history

Take a detailed past medical history including any previous illnesses and hospital admissions. Enquire about any investigations that have already been undertaken, such as endoscopies or barium studies. Also ask about any previous operations that they have had. Adhesion formation after abdominal or pelvic surgery is one of the commonest causes of bowel obstruction, alongside herniae.

Specifically ask about cancer, inflammatory bowel disease, including Crohn's and ulcerative colitis, peptic ulcer disease, gallstones or any past acute abdominal events.

Medical Guidelines
Red flags for bowel cancer

Any patient who presents with the following symptoms requires urgent (2 week) specialist input:

- Patients aged 40 years old or more reporting rectal bleeding with a change of bowel habit towards looser stools and/ or increased stool frequency persisting for 6 weeks or more

- Patients aged 60 years old or more with rectal bleeding persisting for 6 weeks or more without a change in bowel habit and without anal symptoms

- Patients aged 60 years old or more with a change in bowel habit to looser stools and/or more frequent stools persisting for 6 weeks or more without rectal bleeding

- Any patient presenting with a right lower abdominal mass consistent with involvement of the large bowel

- Any patient with a palpable rectal mass

NICE Guidelines: Cancer referral pathway (2005)

DIFFERENTIAL DIAGNOSIS

Abdominal pain
Acute
- Appendicitis
- Gastroenteritis
- Bowel obstruction
- Cholangitis
- Renal stone
- Pancreatitis

Chronic
- Inflammatory bowel disease
- Irritable bowel syndrome
- Constipation
- Diverticulitis
- Pancreatitis
- Pelvic inflammatory disease

TOP TIP!

It is important not to prematurely mention cancer as a possible cause for the patient's pain as it, quite naturally, generates a lot of anxiety in the patient and may cause you to lose precious time allaying the patient's fears.

Drug history

Ask the patient what medication they are currently on or have taken in the past. Do not forget to also ask about any OTC medications or herbal remedies that the patient has tried. If the patient has taken any analgesia, ascertain its effectiveness and ask how long they have been using it. NSAIDs are particularly important here as they are commonly used and are a causative factor in peptic ulcer disease. Drugs such as statins, taken for cholesterol, have been shown occasionally to cause hepatitis, as has the oral contraceptive pill.

Remember to ask about drug allergies or intolerances. Lactose intolerance, which is common in Asian and black populations, commonly causes abdominal pain, bloating and altered bowel habit in a young child.

Social history

Enquire whether the patient has ever smoked and, if so, how many cigarettes a day and for how long. Discreetly ask about illicit drug use. Ask about alcohol use, noting the type of alcohol and how many units a week. Alcohol history is important because hepatitis, liver cirrhosis, gastric ulcers as well as oesophageal cancers can be caused by excessive alcohol consumption.

It is important in the abdominal pain history to enquire how the pain is affecting the patient's life, in particular their work or studies. Ask how many sick days / days off they have had to take. This not only gives you an indication of the severity of the pain but also helps you to tailor your treatment towards the patient.

Psychological causes of abdominal pain must also be considered as they can be exacerbated by stressful life events. Functional bowel disorders such as IBS can often be made worse by stress such as a demanding job or exams.

Travel history

Always ask about recent travel because infections such as viral hepatitis and gastroenteritis may be contracted abroad. It is also important to establish whether any close contacts have been suffering with similar symptoms, as this may suggest a possible infectious source (i.e. gastroenteritis).

Family history

It is important to ask whether the patient has any first-degree relatives who suffer or have suffered from similar symptoms. A family history of inflammatory bowel disease or bowel cancers can help point you in the right direction. Hereditary non-polyposis colorectal carcinoma (HNPCC or Lynch type II syndrome) can present with a variety of different cancers such as colorectal, endometrial and ovarian and, although not common, it is important that you consider it.

1.5.5 Systems review

Complete your abdominal pain history with a brief systems review. Ask the patient about relevant symptoms such as problems with swallowing (dysphagia), fever, jaundice or changes in bowel habit. You may also wish to enquire more generally about common symptoms such as chest pain, palpitations or neurological symptoms, or any muscle or joint pain in order to check the patient's health and wellbeing.

1.5.6 **Summing up**

Summarize your findings back to the patient and ask if they would like to add anything that you may have missed. Reassure your patient by coming to an agreement with them about what the next step will be, checking to make sure they understand what is going on. Ask them if they have any questions they would like you to answer. In addition, offer the patient information leaflets and discuss when you (or another health professional) will see them next. End the interview by thanking the patient. In an exam situation, conclude by giving an appropriate summary to the examiner.

> **TOP TIP!**
>
> In an exam, bear in mind that you may be judged on both your verbal and non-verbal communication skills by the patient as well as the examiner.

1.5.7 **Common clinical scenarios**

The following are a list of common abdominal pain cases which you may encounter. For each one, consider:
- what the level of risk could be
- what key features you would look for
- what questions you would ask to refine or confirm your diagnosis

You could use role play with a friend, using the histories in the cases below as a framework.

CASE 1
An 18 year old student complains of severe pain around the umbilicus which came on 8 hours ago and has since been moving towards to the right iliac fossa. He has a low grade fever and is feeling nauseous and has vomited once. The vomit was not bile-stained. He has never had a similar pain before and is otherwise fit and well. He is not taking any regular medications and has no relevant family history.

CASE 2
A 66 year old retired lady complains of epigastric pain and vomiting for the past 2 days. She says the pain goes through to her back and has been getting worse. The pain is worse after she eats and she has felt slightly feverish. She has suffered from gallstones in the past. She drinks 50 units of alcohol per week and smokes 10 cigarettes a day. Her urine is negative for signs of infection. She had a recent gastric endoscopy that was normal.

CASE 3
A 62 year old former athlete presents with a 5 day history of burning epigastric pain radiating through to the back. He has been having difficulty eating lately and says the pain gets worse when he eats, though it is alleviated when he drinks milk. He suffers from osteoarthritis for which he takes regular diclofenac. He smokes 20 cigarettes a day and drinks 21 units of alcohol per week.

CASE 4
A 58 year old postman presents with a 1 week history of epigastric pain radiating through to the back. He describes the pain as burning and he has been vomiting lately. On a few occasions he has noticed what he describes as 'brown bits'. The pain is worse at night and is relieved by eating. He suffers from heartburn on occasion for which he takes antacids. He is a non-smoker and drinks 12 units of alcohol per week.

CASE 5

A 21 year old builder complains of a 2 month history of intermittent abdominal pain and malaise. He has felt fatigued for the past 5 months and occasionally suffers from bouts of diarrhoea. He also complains of ulcers in the mouth and has noticed mild weight loss over the past 3 months. He has no past medical history of note. His uncle suffers from ulcerative colitis. He smokes 10 cigarettes a day and does not drink alcohol.

CASE 6

A 26 year old intravenous drug user presents to A&E with pain in the right upper quadrant which has worsened over the last month. He complains of feeling generally unwell and has lost much of his appetite. Some of his friends have mentioned that he looks 'yellow'. He has no past medical history of note. He has no recent history of travel. He drinks 25 units of alcohol per week and smokes 20 cigarettes a day.

CASE 7

A 41 year old housewife complains of a 2 hour history of left flank pain radiating down to the groin. The pain comes and goes and causes her to writhe around. She says this pain is as bad as the pain she experienced during childbirth. She drinks a glass of wine a day and does not smoke. Urine dipstick is 4+ blood.

CASE 8

A 26 year old investment banker comes into A&E with right-sided lower abdominal pain. She complains of nausea and vomiting. She says that she recently noticed some prune juice-like vaginal bleeding. She has no past medical history of note. Her last period was 7 weeks ago. She uses an IUD for contraception. She does not smoke or drink. Her urine pregnancy test is positive.

Chapter 1.6
Nausea and vomiting

What to do...
- Introduce yourself to the patient – establish rapport
- Ask the patient's name, age and occupation
- Ask the patient relevant questions about their nausea and vomiting, such as the onset, frequency and duration; note the volume and colour and whether it is projectile or not
- Ask about any associated symptoms, e.g. abdominal pain, headaches, diarrhoea, fever and weight loss
- Ask about travel history
- Ask about any past medical history e.g. DM, cancers, pregnancy
- Ask about any drug history (such as chemotherapy, opioids, antibiotics) and for any drug allergies
- Ask about any social history – enquire if the patient smokes or drinks alcohol
- Ask about any family history
- Perform a brief systems review and sum up your findings
- Thank the patient and conclude the consultation

Nausea and vomiting are unpleasant symptoms experienced by many patients. Nausea is the abnormal sensation of feeling sick whereas vomiting is the actual forceful ejection of stomach contents. Although distressing, these symptoms may act in the acute phase as a natural bio-defence mechanism to prevent toxic substances from entering the body. However, in the case of chronic nausea and vomiting, this almost always has an abnormal underlying aetiology.

The actual process of vomiting is controlled by the vomiting centre located in the medulla of the brain. It receives input from different parts of the body such as the vestibular fibres from the inner ear and visceral fibres from the GI tract and inputs from the base of the fourth ventricle. It also receives input from higher cortical centres that process stimuli from tastes, smells and pain receptors. This information is processed by the vomiting centre and can lead to a feeling of nausea and vomiting in the patient.

There are a large number of different conditions that can lead to nausea and vomiting such as infection, GI tract disorders, psychiatric illness, medications, as well as neurological conditions. In the acute setting it is important to assess the patient rapidly and to fluid resuscitate them to prevent dehydration and possible death. Once stable, use a systematic and comprehensive approach to try to differentiate between the wide variety of possible causes.

TOP TIP!

Vomiting should always be distinguished from regurgitation which occurs without the feeling of nausea.

1.6.1 **Taking the history**

Begin by introducing yourself to the patient by stating your full name and job title. Ask the patient for their name, age and occupation before proceeding to take a detailed history. The patient's gender and age are very important in consideration of appropriate differential diagnoses. Remember that pregnancy is the most common endocrine cause of nausea and must be considered in any woman of childbearing age.

Occupational history plays a fairly limited role in the nausea and vomiting history. However, it is still important to elicit whether the patient is in current employment or retired. Individuals who work with pesticides or organophosphates may be exposed to their toxic effects, and people with particularly stressful jobs and impending examinations may suffer from anxiety-related nausea and vomiting.

1.6.2 **Ideas, concerns and expectations**

After appropriately introducing yourself and establishing rapport, it may be useful to elicit the patient's own views of what is going on. Eliciting the patient's ideas and concerns about their symptoms will help to personalize the patient's problems and give you a holistic understanding of the context in which they present. Also enquire about the patient's own expectations of what they wish to gain from the consultation and use this information as a guide to tailor your history and allay any misplaced anxiety or fears. Ask the patient how their symptoms have impacted on their life, particularly with regard to whether they are still able to attend work or eat as normal – when symptoms start to affect activities of daily living they can become very distressing to the patient. Most patients who suffer from nausea and vomiting worry about food poisoning or an underlying malignancy. They may also be concerned as to whether their symptoms are contagious or, if they are in employment, when they can return to work.

1.6.3 **History of presenting complaint**

Once the patient is settled begin asking more focused questions around the nausea and vomiting. Consider splitting the history into discrete areas: the vomiting episode, preceding symptoms and associated symptoms. It is usually best to start asking about symptoms related to the GI tract to rule out the most common causes before moving on to exclude other systems.

The vomiting

Duration, onset and frequency

Try to establish when the patient's vomiting began, how long it has been going on for and how may times they have vomited in a day. The longer the patient's symptoms have been going on for and the more frequent the bouts of vomiting, the more likely the patient is to be dehydrated and unwell. Acute onset of vomiting is usually due to infections such as appendicitis, gastroenteritis, meningitis, encephalitis, or bowel obstruction. Chronic causes may be due to gastroparesis, brain tumour or pregnancy. In women of childbearing age presenting with early morning vomiting and a delayed period you should always perform a pregnancy test (Hyperemesis gravidarum). Psychiatric causes should always be considered and may present as acute or chronic vomiting due to anxiety and bulimia.

TOP TIP!

Always consider pregnancy as a cause of nausea and vomiting in a woman of childbearing age.

Medical Guidelines
Days of exclusion from school from gastroenteritis

- Children should not attend any school or other childcare facility while they have diarrhoea or vomiting caused by gastroenteritis
- Children should not go back to their school or other childcare facility until at least 48 hours after the last episode of diarrhoea or vomiting
- Children should not swim in swimming pools for 2 weeks after the last episode of diarrhoea

NICE guideline: Diarrhoea and vomiting in children (2009)

Content

Ask the patient about the content and consistency of their vomit. Note its colour and whether there was any blood present. Bilious vomiting usually presents as yellow or green fluid and may represent possible small bowel obstruction. Blood in the vomit suggests an upper GI cause in a site proximal to the duodenal-jejunal junction. Bright red fresh blood indicates that the bleed is acute because the blood did not have time to become altered by gastric acid (in which case 'coffee ground' vomit would occur). Fresh blood may indicate a Mallory–Weiss tear or bleeding oesophageal varices, whereas 'coffee ground' vomit tends to occur with bleeding peptic ulcers.

Establish whether the vomit contained food particles and if they are digested or remain undigested. Undigested particles suggest that the food has yet to enter the stomach and be broken down by its acid content. This may be due to motility disorders such as achalasia, or structural or luminal disorders such as oesophageal stricture or a pharyngeal pouch.

Quantity

Try and get the patient to roughly estimate the volume of vomit they produce. Although this may be difficult it is often useful to request that the patient tries to express the quantity in cup measures. Remember that the volume of vomit does not correlate directly with the severity of cause. However, large vomiting volume usually suggests an organic rather than a psychogenic cause.

Force

It is useful to know whether the vomiting was forceful or whether it was expelled effortlessly. Effortless vomit can be easily confused with regurgitation. A helpful way of discerning the two would be to ask whether the patient felt nauseous prior to vomiting, a feature that is often absent in regurgitation. Effortless vomiting can be a sign of oesophageal pathology. However, it may also arise in psychogenic causes. Cases where the vomiting was quite forceful, but without a discernable cause, may be psychogenic in nature and these are more often seen in young women. If someone is presenting with projectile vomiting, always consider pyloric stenosis or gastric outlet obstruction due to a malignancy or ulcer-induced stricture as a possible cause.

Events preceding symptoms

Try and get the patient to recall whether there were any preceding factors that may have contributed to their vomiting. In particular, ask if they had eaten out or had recently returned from travel. If the patient had a recent takeaway or a fast food meal you should try to establish whether others had eaten the same food and if so, whether they share the same symptoms. This may indicate food poisoning as a possible cause. There are a number of different organisms that may give rise to food poisoning with the most common being Campylobacter. Individual organisms have different incubation periods and symptoms. Knowing how long after the consumption of food the patient's symptoms started may give you a useful clue as to what the offending organism is (*Table 1.2*). The type of food consumed will also point to a possible cause; reheated rice can cause gastroenteritis induced by *Bacillus cereus*, shellfish can cause norovirus-related vomiting, whereas consuming egg-based meals can lead to salmonella. Do not forget to ask about fever and diarrhoea when considering gastroenteritis.

> **TOP TIP!**
>
> Always ask the patient to explain what they mean by projectile vomiting. Although patients may claim that their vomit was projectile in nature, a detailed history may expose this to being incorrect. Projectile vomit must travel quite a distance from the patient and may take the appearance of a 'water fountain'. Although the actual distance the vomit has to travel to be termed projectile is not clearly defined, the furthest recorded distance is 27 feet.

Medical Guidelines
Advice to avoid travellers' diarrhoea

Dietary: advise the patient to avoid eating any uncooked meats and unpeeled fruit and vegetables. Patients should not use local tap water and instead should consume bottled mineral water. Ice should always be avoided as the source is unknown. In the event that bottled water is unavailable patients should be advised to boil their water for at least 10 minutes or use water purification tablets.

Swimming pools: water from swimming pools may not be chlorinated and may thus pose a risk of infection.

Vaccines: make sure that the patient is up to date with any travel vaccines including hepatitis A, DTP, typhoid, yellow fever.

Farthing MJ (1994) Traveller's diarrhoea. Medicine International, 22: 266–71.

Table 1.2 Incubation periods and symptoms of bacterial causes of gastroenteritis

Time to presentation	Organism and typical features
1–6 hours	*Staph. aureus* (severe symptoms, acute onset, undercooked meat) *Bacillus cereus* (rice consumption, vomiting before diarrhoea)
12–48 hours	*Salmonella* (undercooked chicken or eggs) *E. coli* (travellers' diarrhoea, watery stools, abdominal pains)
48–72 hours	*Shigella* (contaminated vegetables, bloody diarrhoea, abdominal cramps) *Campylobacter* (undercooked chicken, flu-like prodromal symptoms, complications – Guillain-Barré syndrome)
> 7 days	*Giardiasis* (infected water by sewage, prolonged non-bloody diarrhoea)

Patients who have recently been abroad may have picked up an infection from contaminated foods and water from other countries. Try to establish which country they visited and the mode of transport. Typically a patient who has just come back from a cruise ship holiday where there was an outbreak of vomiting may have picked up a norovirus infection.

Associated symptoms

Try to establish whether there are any associated symptoms that present with the vomiting. Symptoms such as abdominal pain, headaches, weight loss, dizziness and anxiety, if noted, may help narrow down the list of potential causes to a particular system.

Start by asking if they felt pain, especially abdominal pain or chest pain. Do not forget that severe pain in its own right can be a cause of vomiting. Chest pain causing nausea and vomiting may be due to myocardial infarction. Pain emerging from the epigastric region could indicate oesophagitis, peptic ulcer disease, cholecystitis or pancreatitis.

Any cause of acute abdominal pain can result in vomiting. Always ask about symptoms of appendicitis, cholecystitis, biliary colic and renal colic.

Weight loss is another important symptom that may be associated with vomiting. Although some degree of weight loss is expected with chronic vomiting, a marked loss of weight should always raise suspicions of a malignancy, particularly that of a stomach cancer. Always attempt to quantify the degree of weight loss in kilograms as patients are notoriously bad at estimating their own weight.

Ask whether the weight loss was intentional or unintentional. Intentional weight loss may point towards a psychogenic cause such as anorexia nervosa and bulimia. These issues require a degree of sensitivity when probing further. You may want to ask if they ever induce vomiting themselves and if so, why. Ask about causes of stress that could lead to emotional causes of vomiting such as difficulties at work or with family life.

Check with the patient for the presence of symptoms of neurological dysfunction such as headaches, blurry vision, dizziness or vertigo. A typical migraine may begin with a throbbing headache and progress to feeling nauseous with vomiting during the episode. There may be aura (the fortification spectrum) described with visual disturbance or even progressive neurological deficits similar to those seen in a stroke.

QUESTIONS TO ASK . . .

- When did the vomiting start? How long have you been vomiting for? How often do you vomit per day?
- Do you feel nauseous before vomiting? How many cupfuls of vomit do you estimate that you bring up?
- What colour is the vomit? Have you ever seen green coloured vomit?
- Is the food digested or undigested?
- Have you ever vomited blood? If so, is it bright red or does it look like coffee grounds?

TOP TIP!

In vomiting associated with colicky abdominal pain, always consider bowel obstruction, particularly if you also notice abdominal distension and absolute constipation (no faeces or flatus being passed).

Any cause of raised intracranial pressure can lead to vomiting. A patient with a space-occupying lesion will typically have morning headache associated with vomiting, which improves throughout the course of the day. A patient suffering with meningitis or encephalitis may present with vomiting associated with fever, photophobia, headache and possibly a rash. Do not forget that a posterior circulation stroke (vertebra–basilar) can cause vomiting associated with vertigo, diplopia and cerebellar signs.

1.6.4 Past medical history

Next move on to ask about the patient's medical history including previous medical illness and hospital attendances. Specifically ask about any previous gastroenterology investigations such as OGDs (oesophago-gastro-duodenoscopy) or chemotherapy for cancers. Remember to check whether the patient suffers from diabetes because diabetic ketoacidosis (DKA) can present with vomiting and abdominal pain particularly in type 1 diabetes. Diabetics may also suffer from gastroparesis whereby there is delayed gastric emptying.

Drug history

A large number of drugs taken at their prescribed dose may cause nausea and vomiting as a potential side effect. Taking a detailed drug history including OTC medications and herbal remedies may point you towards the offending agent. If you suspect a drug may be implicated, you should try to establish whether there is a temporal correlation between starting the medication and onset of symptoms. In addition, any recent changes in dosage or addition of other medications may potentiate the vomiting. Discontinuation of the drug should cause rapid resolution of symptoms.

Enquire specifically whether the patient had been using any opiate medication such as codeine or morphine for pain, both of which can cause nausea and vomiting. Recent antibiotic use can also induce vomiting. Drugs such as erythromycin and metronidazole are most commonly implicated. If the patient has recently been diagnosed with cancer you should ask whether they have had any courses of radio- or chemotherapy.

Social history

Enquire whether the patient smokes and if so determine the number of pack years. Establish whether they drink alcohol – if they do, note the type of alcohol and how many units a week they drink. If the patient drinks above the recommended limits then they may be at risk of alcoholic liver disease. Heavy consumption of alcohol can cause peptic ulcers, liver disease (leading to oesophageal varices) and pancreatitis, all of which can result in vomiting or haematemesis.

Discreetly ask about illicit drug use such as cocaine and marijuana, some of which may cause nausea. Ask about fatty food intake, red meat, sugar and salt. Enquire about the patient's level of activity and establish whether they undertake a basic level of exercise. You can take this opportunity to ask whether the patient has any stresses at work or home, which may lead to anxiety-related nausea and vomiting.

DIFFERENTIAL DIAGNOSIS

Gastrointestinal system
Gastroenteritis – viral/bacterial
Acute abdomen
  Appendicitis
  Cholecystitis
  Pancreatitis
  Peptic ulcer disease
Obstruction
  Adhesions
  Strangulated hernia
  Tumour
  Pyloric stenosis
Endocrine system
Pregnancy
Diabetic ketoacidosis
Addison's disease
Uraemia (renal failure)
Central nervous system
Raised ICP
  Brain tumour or any SOL
  Meningitis/encephalitis
Migraine
Vestibular
  Labyrinthitis
  Ménière's disease
Psychiatric/psychological
Anorexia nervosa
Bulimia nervosa
Anxiety
Medications
Opiate analgesics
Chemotherapy agents

TOP TIP!

Inner ear disorders such as viral labyrinthitis, vestibular neuronitis and Ménière's disease can lead to vomiting associated with auditory symptoms such as hearing loss and vertigo.

TOP TIP!

A patient who presents with hyperpigmentation, particularly affecting skin folds along with non-specific symptoms such as headache, nausea, tiredness and abdominal pain, should be investigated for Addison's disease.

Family history

Family history does not usually play a large role in nausea and vomiting but you may wish to ask about history of brain tumours and check if anyone has had similar symptoms in the past. A family history of migraines may point towards a diagnosis of cyclic vomiting syndrome which is a diagnosis of exclusion. It usually presents with quite forceful episodes of vomiting interspersed with periods of normality. Symptoms usually begin in childhood but tail off in later life.

1.6.5 Systems review

Complete your nausea and vomiting history with a brief systems review. This may give an insight into the patient's general health and will also allow you to revisit and re-evaluate your differential diagnosis. You can also use this as a method of running through the systems from head to toe to ensure you have not missed a potential cause. Ask the patient if they have experienced any headaches, visual disturbances, chest or abdominal pain, shortness of breath, change in their bowel habits or weight loss. Have they felt dizzy, lost consciousness or noted any swelling, stiffness or weakness in their limbs? Are they passing urine comfortably with no burning sensation?

1.6.6 Summing up

Give yourself time at the end of the patient consultation to summarize back your findings. Specifically ask the patient if there is anything in the history they would like to add or amend as this may help to minimize the chance of any misinterpretations or misunderstandings.

Having completed taking your nausea and vomiting history you should now be in a position to deliver a list of relevant and potential differential diagnoses that the patient may be suffering from. This list would be further refined depending on the results of further investigations you may undertake.

Reassure your patient by agreeing a shared plan about what the next steps will be. This may include informing the patient what you believe is the cause of their nausea and vomiting, explaining what investigations you will be undertaking and the possible treatment options. In addition, you may wish to offer the patient any relevant information leaflets if appropriate. Thank the patient for their time and conclude the interview amicably.

1.6.7 Common clinical scenarios

The following are a list of common nausea and vomiting cases which you may encounter. For each one, consider:
• what the possible differential diagnosis of each could be
• what key features you would look for
• what questions you would ask to refine or confirm your diagnosis

You could use role play with a friend, using the histories in the cases below as a framework.

CASE 1

A 62 year old lady presents with headaches which usually occur first thing in the morning and improve as the day progresses. They can be severe enough to wake the patient up and are also associated with feelings of nausea and occasional blurred vision. Her family have noted that she has become more erratic and irritable recently and are worried about early onset dementia.

CASE 2

A 14 year old boy is admitted with colicky abdominal pain, severe nausea and vomiting and acute dehydration. He has been generally well up until the last month where he has been complaining of increased urinary frequency, thirst and unintentional weight loss.

CASE 3

A 35 year old woman has been suffering with chronic back pain following a car accident 3 years ago. She has been taking paracetamol and ibuprofen regularly for the past 5 months and they are no longer controlling the pain. Two weeks ago her GP started her on codeine phosphate to take as required. She now has a 10 day history of nausea and episodes of vomiting with no other associated symptoms. Her last menstrual period was 7 days ago.

CASE 4

A 19 year old boy has had a 2 day history of bloody diarrhoea and vomiting. Throughout the last 2 days he has also experienced some generalized abdominal cramps with rigors which come and go. He is asthmatic and uses a salbutamol inhaler as required. He has no other medical history. On further questioning you find that he had eaten at a Chinese restaurant 3 days ago and some of his friends are also having similar symptoms.

CASE 5

A 17 year old girl presented to A&E with severe nausea and vomiting occurring 2–3 times throughout the day for the last 10 days. She does not complain of any pain or changes in bowel habit. She usually takes the oral contraceptive pill but has not been very compliant recently. Her last menstrual period was 5 weeks ago.

CASE 6

A 38 year old desk clerk presents with 1 week history of nausea and vomiting associated with dizziness and ringing of the ears. She notes that she feels the whole room spinning around her and that these episodes last for about 30 minutes to an hour. On further questioning she mentions she has had a cough and coryzal symptoms for a week. There is no mention of any hearing loss.

CASE 7

A 21 year old female student complains of recurrent attacks of unilateral headaches. They can last for a number of hours and are beginning to interfere with her studies. She also states seeing flashing lights and zigzag lines as well as feeling nauseous during the episodes. She has recently been started by her GP on an OCP.

Chapter 1.7
Dysphagia

What to do . . .

- Introduce yourself to the patient – establish rapport
- Ask the patient's name, age and occupation
- Ask the patient relevant questions relating to their dysphagia, including site, onset and type
- Ask about associated symptoms such as pain, coughing, regurgitation or weight loss
- Ask about any past medical history, e.g. HIV, ulcers, rheumatological conditions
- Ask about any drug history and for any drug allergies
- Ask about any social history – ask if the patient smokes or drinks alcohol; take a brief diet history
- Ask about any family history, specifically for Barrett's oesophagus.
- Perform a brief systems review and sum up your findings
- Thank the patient and conclude the consultation

Dysphagia is the abnormality or dysfunction of the swallowing reflex. The normal swallowing mechanism requires a complex interaction between a number of different muscles to facilitate the passage of fluid or solid bolus from the oral cavity through the pharynx and down into the stomach. Normal deglutition is usually divided into three stages as per the locations where they take place:

- oral phase
- pharyngeal phase
- oesophageal phase

Dysphagia, or difficulty swallowing, is a fairly common symptom with around 8% of people complaining of it at some stage of their life. It is seen most frequently in the elderly, with the vast majority of patients in nursing homes having some degree of dysphagia.

Before a person eats, neurological and psychological factors cause saliva to fill the oral cavity. As food passes into this cavity the muscles of the tongue and of mastication are used in a co-ordinated manner (cranial nerves V, XII) to chew and break down the content into smaller pellets. These are mixed with saliva and propelled towards the back of the cavity and into the pharynx. As this occurs there is a reflex closure of the soft palate against the nasal pharynx to prevent food from entering the nasal cavity. The pharyngeal phase commences as soon as the bolus of food enters the pharynx. As the food passes down, an involuntary swallowing reflex is triggered which is controlled by the medulla (cranial nerves IX and X). This involves the temporary involuntary closure of the larynx by the epiglottis. This prevents the aspiration of food contents into the respiratory tract. The final phase of swallowing is the oesophageal phase which acts as a conduit to pass food into the stomach. The smooth muscle of the oesophagus wall contracts in a rhythmic manner (known as peristalsis) to push the bolus of food down. The lower oesophageal sphincter remains relaxed from the start of the swallow process until the food has passed into the stomach.

Dysphagia can be caused by a range of different conditions, from psychological through to neurological disease such as stroke. It is important to fully assess the patient who presents with dysphagia to prevent the possible life threatening complication of aspiration pneumonia.

1.7.1 **Taking the history**

Start your consultation by introducing yourself to the patient, stating your name and job title. Establish from the patient their full name, date of birth and occupation before commencing your dysphagia history.

1.7.2 **Ideas, concerns and expectations**

After appropriately introducing yourself and establishing rapport, try to establish whether the patient has any specific concerns or anxieties about their condition. Dysphagia can be quite a disturbing and frightening experience for the patient: sudden dysphagia may make the patient worry that they are having a stroke, whilst slowly worsening dysphagia may make the patient concerned about dying a slow death.

1.7.3 **History of the presenting complaint**

The patient's complaint of difficulty in swallowing may not correlate with the medical definition of dysphagia. Common symptoms may be confused with difficulty swallowing, such as:
- dry mouth (xerostomia) – this is a common complaint that can be caused by anxiety, drugs (tricyclic antidepressants) and dehydration, with the lack of saliva causing a degree of discomfort when swallowing
- feeling of a lump in the throat (globus pharyngeus) – this is often seen in women with chronic anxiety states; they complain of a fullness in the back of their throat which can occur at any time regardless of swallowing and is supported with normal investigation results
- sore throat

True dysphagia (see *Box 1.6*) is almost always indicative of underlying pathology and warrants some degree of investigation.

Site

Begin exploring the patient's symptoms of dysphagia by asking them to indicate the site at which the discomfort is felt. Most patients, if asked, may point either to their throat or chest area. Dysphagia occurring at the retrosternum corresponds well to an oesophageal lesion. However, if the patient feels that the difficulty in swallowing is at the level of the throat or pharynx, studies have shown that this has poor diagnostic value because oesophageal dysfunction may also present with throat symptoms.

Patients who present with difficulty in initiating swallowing are likely to have oropharyngeal dysphagia, typically due to neurological conditions such as bulbar palsy. This is because there is dysfunction of the cranial nerves that

> **TOP TIP!**
>
> Achalasia, scleroderma and diffuse oesophageal spasm are the most common causes of neuromuscular motility disorders.

> **TOP TIP!**
>
> Risk factors for oesophageal cancer include smoking, alcohol, weight loss, Barrett's oesophagus. Although all forms of dysphagia may cause some degree of weight loss, profound weight loss is a red flag symptom of cancer.

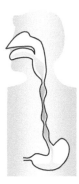

Oesophageal spasm

Abnormal contraction of the oesophageal muscles. It may be triggered by hot or cold foods in some people causing dysphagia, odynophagia and pain in the chest. This can easily be confused with acute coronary syndrome.

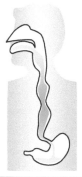

Achalasia

Dysphagia to both solids and liquids. Gradual process with regurgitation of food. Associated with heartburn and common in middle-aged women.

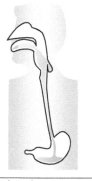

Pharyngeal pouch

This is a herniation of the posterior wall of the pharynx and is seen particularly in the elderly. Presents with regurgitation and halitosis. Patients may report a lump in the neck that gurgles on palpation.

Fig 1.9 Common causes of dysphagia.

BOX 1.6 **Causes of dysphagia**

Luminal lesion
- Stricture (benign, malignant)
- Oesophageal web
- Foreign body
- Pharyngeal pouch

Extraluminal lesion
- Thyroid goitre
- Lymph nodes

Motility disorder
- Achalasia
- CREST syndrome
- Oesophageal spasm

Neuromuscular disorder
- Bulbar palsy
- Myasthenia gravis

---

supply the surrounding muscle groups. Patients typically complain of a cough on swallowing caused by aspiration into the respiratory tract.

Onset

Try to find out when the patient first noticed the dysphagia. Did it occur suddenly or was there a slow gradual deterioration? Have the symptoms remained constant since its onset or is the dysphagia episodic? Sudden onset of acute constant dysphagia should alert you to the possibility of a stroke, particularly if it is associated with other neurological features such as hemiparesis or spasticity. A slow progressive dysphagia is often caused by a peptic stricture, particularly if there is a background history of long term acid reflux and mild weight loss. In contrast to this, a more rapid worsening dysphagia, associated with marked weight loss, should raise the suspicion of oesophageal malignancy. An insidious onset of difficult swallowing is likely to be caused by neuromuscular disease such as myasthenia gravis or progressive bulbar palsy seen in motor neurone disease. A long standing dysphagia that presents intermittently is likely to be due to oesophageal spasm or web.

Type

Next ask the patient how the dysphagia has affected their ability to eat or drink foods. Oesophageal disorders that obstruct the lumen initially present with dysphagia to solids only. Examples include foreign body ingestion, mediastinal lymphadenopathy or oesophageal web. In oesophageal cancer, as the malignancy spreads to affect the whole oesophagus, the dysphagia will change over time from only solids to include both solids and liquids. Motility disorders, such as achalasia, cause both solids and liquids dysphagia from the outset, due to the lack of organized muscular contraction of the oesophagus.

Associated symptoms

Pain (odynophagia) is a common feature associated with dysphagia. It can occur with swallowing itself or present shortly afterwards. Pain that comes in waves and varies in intensity may be due to achalasia or oesophageal spasm. Pain that is expressed as a burning sensation and worsened with hot fluids, like coffee, is suggestive of oesophagitis or reflux disease. If the pain occurs at a specific level this may be suggestive of oesophageal cancer; this is because the bolus of food is impacting against the tumour causing the discomfort.

A cough is another common symptom that may present along with difficulty swallowing. It may be seen immediately on swallowing or shortly afterwards. Coughing that presents early on may point towards an oropharyngeal cause such as a stroke or pseudobulbar palsy. In such cases, damage to the vagus or glossopharyngeal nerve affects epiglottal function, allowing food to trickle into the larynx. Coughing seen shortly after swallowing is most commonly due to an oesophageal disorder such as achalasia, oesophagitis or reflux disease.

Some patients may note that food, which they had swallowed earlier, is brought back up and regurgitated. This may be caused by oropharyngeal or oesophageal problems. The most common oropharyngeal cause is a pharyngeal pouch, which is a herniation or out-pouching of the posterior wall of the pharynx just superior to the entrance of the oesophagus. Typically, food is initially swallowed without incident and collects within the pouch. However, on subsequent ingestion swallowing becomes more troublesome, with regurgitation of food and halitosis noted.

Oesophageal causes may include achalasia or reflux. Achalasia occurs when there is failure of the lower oesophageal sphincter to relax, thereby causing food to build up superiorly in the oesophagus. This is believed to be caused by a loss of ganglia at the Auerbach's plexus. Regurgitation may occur between meals and the vomit lacks the distinct acidic taste (acid brash) seen in reflux disease.

It is also important to ask about symptoms of anxiety because anxious patients sometimes describe the feeling of a 'lump in their throat' preventing them from swallowing. This is known as globus hystericus and is a diagnosis of exclusion. It is commonly, but not always, seen in young females. Classically, patients complain of symptoms even when they are not eating.

1.7.4 **Past medical history**

Take a detailed past medical history including any previous medical illnesses and hospital admissions. Ask specifically about any previous investigations including endoscopies, pH manometry or barium swallow. Ask whether the patient has previously suffered from iron deficiency anaemia as this can be associated with an oesophageal web; seen in Plummer–Vinson syndrome. You should also establish if the patient has had previous episodes of dyspepsia, ulcers or GORD as these may all be associated with reflux. Patients diagnosed with HIV are at risk of oral candida which may present with painful dysphagia. Eliciting a history of rheumatoid arthritis or Raynaud's disease may alert you to the possibility of CREST syndrome.

Drug history

Ask the patient what medication they are currently taking. There are a number of medications that can produce side effects causing dysphagia, such as:
- non-steroidal anti-inflammatory drugs (NSAIDs) that inhibit the COX-1 enzyme that protects the lining of the stomach causing reflux and dyspepsia

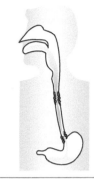

Oesophageal carcinoma

The most common is squamous cell carcinoma. Leads to dysphagia of solids and odynophagia at a particular level. Weight loss is characteristic. Smoking, alcohol and reflux disease are known risk factors.

Fig 1.9 (*cont.*)

- SSRIs, alendronate and certain antibiotics, including erythromycin, can also cause oesophagitis
- antihistamines, anticholinergic inhibitors as well as tricyclic antidepressants can cause xerostomia (dry mouth), which can be a cause of dysphagia.

Social history

Enquire about the patient's alcohol and smoking habits as these have been implicated in oesophagitis. Spend some time taking a dietary history because a number of foods such as chilli, spicy and fatty meals may worsen reflux symptoms.

Family history

You should enquire whether the patient has any first-degree relatives who suffer or have suffered from dysphagia. Establish if anyone in the family has had cancer of the oesophagus or its pre-malignant form, Barrett's oesophagus.

1.7.5 Systems review

Complete your history with a brief systems review. Ask the patient about relevant symptoms such as problems with nausea and vomiting or loss of appetite. You may also wish to enquire more generally about common symptoms such as changes in bowel habit, chest pain, palpitations or neurological symptoms or any muscle or joint pain in order to check the patient's health and wellbeing.

1.7.6 Summing up

Summarize your findings back to the patient and ask if they would like to add anything that you may have missed. End the interview by thanking the patient. In an exam situation, provide an appropriate summary to the examiner.

1.7.7 Common clinical scenarios

The following are a list of common dysphagia cases which you may encounter. For each one, consider:
- what the possible differential diagnosis of each could be
- what key features you would look for
- what questions you would ask to refine or confirm your diagnosis

You could use role play with a friend, using the histories in the cases below as a framework.

CASE 1 A 47 year old farmer presents to his GP complaining of episodic difficulty in swallowing over the last 5 months. He mentions that when he eats he feels that food 'sticks' and does not go down. He is drinking more water to wash the food down. He has been diagnosed with swallowing syncope by his cardiologist. He drinks 8 units per week and does not smoke.

CASE 2

A 70 year old retired painter presents with a 7 week history of problems with her swallowing and lump in her neck when eating. She also complains of bad breath and occasionally regurgitation. When she presses on her neck she can sometimes make the lump 'go away'. She has no past medical history of note. She claims not to smoke or drink.

CASE 3

A 38 year old nurse presents with a gradual onset of difficult swallowing and vomiting. She describes a feeling of food getting stuck in her throat and can also feel pain in her chest. She has previously been diagnosed with iron deficiency anaemia but is poorly compliant with her treatment. She drinks 12 units of alcohol per week on average and does not smoke. On examination she has spoon-shaped nails (koilonychias).

CASE 4

A 32 year old chemical engineer presents with an 8 month history of gradually worsening dysphagia to both liquids and solids. He often wakes up at night coughing, but denies a bitter taste in his mouth following regurgitation. He has been told by his friends that he looks thinner. He drinks 20 units of alcohol per week on average and smokes 10 cigarettes a day. Barium swallow shows a dilated column of contrast tapering to a fine point (bird's beak deformity).

CASE 5

A 58 year old woman presents with a 2 week history of gradually worsening dysphagia. She also complains of pain in her hands when she goes out in the cold. She appears to have tight skin with a beak-shaped nose and furrowing of her lips.

Chapter 1.8
Jaundice

What to do . . .

- Introduce yourself to the patient – establish rapport
- Ask the patient's name, age and occupation
- Ask the patient relevant questions relating to their jaundice including onset and associated symptoms (pain, pruritus, darkened urine, pale stools, anorexia, weight loss, fever)
- Specifically ask about the risk factors of hepatitis
- Ask about any past medical history, e.g. gallstones, cirrhosis, hepatitis
- Ask about any drug history and for any drug allergies
- Ask about any social history – establish if the patient smokes or drinks alcohol; note for any IV drug abuse
- Ask about any family history and specifically for Gilbert's syndrome or G6PD deficiency
- Perform a brief systems review and sum up your findings
- Thank the patient and conclude the consultation

Jaundice (icterus) is the term given to the yellowish hue seen on the skin, mucous membranes or sclerae due to the abnormal increase of serum bilirubin above 35 µmol/l. Bilirubin is created as a by-product of haemoglobin breakdown in the spleen which occurs at the end of the natural lifespan of red blood cells at around 120 days:

- the breakdown products are transported to the liver via the bloodstream as unconjugated bilirubin that is bound to the serum albumin
- at the liver, the bilirubin is conjugated by glucuronyl transferase to become conjugated bilirubin that is water soluble
- the conjugated bilirubin is then excreted from the liver into the biliary system as bile
- as the bile is secreted into the small intestine the bilirubin is converted, by bacterial action, into urobilinogen
- at this point the majority of the urobilinogen is reabsorbed by intestinal cells with the remainder passing out into the faeces as stercobilinogen – oxidation of the stercobilinogen provides the brown colouration to the faeces
- the reabsorbed urobilinogen can either be recycled to the liver via the enterohepatic circulation or excreted into the urine through the kidneys

Each stage along the production and excretion of bilirubin is open to dysfunction by a pathological process. This can result in an abnormally elevated bilirubin level within the blood or urine which is subsequently deposited in the extracellular fluids and can manifest as jaundice. Depending on which part of the physiological mechanism the pathology affects, jaundice can be categorized as pre-hepatic, hepatocellular or post-hepatic (see *Fig 1.10*).

Pre-hepatic jaundice represents dysfunction resulting in excessive production of unconjugated bilirubin. This may happen outside the liver due to increased rates of haemolysis, as seen in haemolytic anaemia including sickle cell anaemia or hereditary spherocytosis. It may also occur at the cellular level in the liver due a hereditary defect of enzyme conversion that prevents conjugation as seen in Gilbert's syndrome and Crigler–Najjar syndrome.

Hepatocellular jaundice is most commonly caused by liver disease such as hepatitis, alcoholic liver disease and cirrhosis. The damaged hepatocytes reduce the liver's ability to metabolize and excrete bilirubin, resulting in hyperbilirubinaemia. Other causes to consider include liver metastases, abscess or Wilson's disease.

Post-hepatic jaundice, also known as obstructive jaundice, is usually caused by an obstruction of the common bile duct preventing drainage of bile. The conjugated bilirubin therefore overspills into the bloodstream and is excreted predominantly via the kidneys into the urine. As there is reduced excretion into the faeces and increased clearance of bilirubin into the urine, a common presenting feature of obstructive jaundice is dark urine and pale stools. The most common cause of this is impacted gallstones in the common bile duct. Other causes include carcinoma of the head of the pancreas, strictures of the common bile duct, biliary atresia, cholangiocarcinoma and drugs.

1.8.1 Taking the history

Begin the history by introducing yourself to the patient, giving your full name and job title. Ask the patient their name, date of birth and occupation before taking a jaundice history. The patient's occupation may play a key role in the development of jaundice. Patients who are farmers or sewage workers are at increased risk of leptospirosis that may lead to jaundice. Healthcare professionals who are in contact with patients' bodily fluids may be at risk of contracting hepatitis B and C. Similarly sex workers are at risk of hepatitis B infection.

1.8.2 Ideas, concerns and expectations

After appropriately introducing yourself and establishing rapport, try to find out the patient's own beliefs and ideas about their symptoms. You should also try to determine if they have any concerns about their jaundice. Patients may be fearful that they have contracted an infectious disease, such as hepatitis, on their travels, or be worried about a potential hepatocellular carcinoma.

Spend some time establishing how the symptoms have affected the patient's life. Jaundice can be particularly striking because of the way in which it overtly manifests itself, and so the patient may be facing constant undue attention from passers-by or unwanted questions from friends and family. These may all add to and heighten the patient's anxiety levels, making it all the more important to be sensitive to their concerns.

1.8.3 History of the presenting complaint

Taking a jaundice history can be quite tricky as the causes of jaundice can be quite diverse. Begin by taking a relatively broad history of the presenting complaint before using questions to narrow your list of differentials.

TOP TIP!

Keep in mind that jaundice itself is not a disease, but rather a symptom of an underlying pathological process that can occur at any point along the normal physiological pathway of the metabolism of bilirubin.

TOP TIP!

Pre-hepatic jaundice often shows signs of haemolysis: low Hb, increased MCV, increased reticulocyte count associated with normal ALP and liver function tests. There is an elevated level of serum unconjugated bilirubin.

TOP TIP!

Hepatocellular jaundice often shows signs of liver dysfunction on the blood tests, i.e. significantly raised AST and ALT.

TOP TIP!

Post-hepatic (obstructive) jaundice often reveals significantly raised ALP with abnormal GGT.

TOP TIP!

Leptospirosis, also known as Weil's disease, can be contracted by direct exposure of broken skin to contaminated rat urine.

PRE-HEPATIC

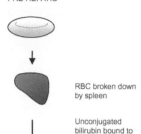

RBC broken down
by spleen

Unconjugated
bilirubin bound to
albumin transported
to the liver

Bilirubin conjugated
with glucuronic acid
by hepatocytes
(water soluble)

HEPATOCELLULAR

POST-HEPATIC

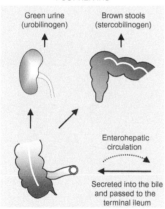

Green urine
(urobilinogen)

Brown stools
(stercobilinogen)

Enterohepatic
circulation

Secreted into the bile
and passed to the
terminal ileum

Conjugated bilirubin converted into
urobilinogen by gut bacteria.

Fig 1.10 Categories of jaundice.

Onset

Start by asking the patient when their jaundice was first noticed and how long it has been present. It is also useful to ask who noticed it first: was it a friend or family member, or were suspicions raised following a recent blood test? An acute rapid onset of jaundice, for example over a few weeks, often suggests a viral aetiology. Insidious onset of jaundice over a few months may be due to liver cancer. A more protracted history of jaundice over several years is likely to be due to liver cirrhosis.

Associated symptoms

Eliciting the associated symptoms that arise with jaundice will give vital clues towards the underlying diagnosis. It may be useful to group the associated symptoms into the three categories described above: pre-hepatic, hepatocellular and post-hepatic jaundice.

Pre-hepatic jaundice

Pre-hepatic jaundice is largely caused by haemolytic anaemia. In such conditions the jaundice may not be particularly marked. In addition, because the raised bilirubin is unconjugated and is not soluble in water it produces normal coloured faeces and urine. Patients usually complain of symptoms associated with anaemia such as weakness, fatiguability, dizziness and possibly shortness of breath. Other causes of pre-hepatic jaundice, such as Gilbert's syndrome, usually do not present with any concurrent symptoms. However, their jaundice may be revealed after a recent bout of illness, medication or surgery.

Hepatocellular jaundice

Ask the patient if they have noticed any fever, malaise, myalgia in addition to nausea and vomiting in the week or two leading up to their jaundice. Prodromal symptoms are often encountered in acute hepatic infection and indicate high infectivity. Establish if they have experienced any abdominal pain. A dull ache in the right upper quadrant may also be experienced in hepatitis.

Post-hepatic jaundice

Cholestatic or obstructive jaundice (as post-hepatic jaundice is often known) is most commonly caused by gallstones impacting on the common bile duct. Patients usually present with either severe right upper quadrant pain or epigastric pain that is worsened after consuming fatty foods. There may also be an associated fever and tenderness over the affected area which can be caused by acute cholangitis. Patients often describe an intense itch (pruritus) throughout their body that can be persistent and intense. It is believed that an overflow of bile salts and acids that later deposit into the skin causes this phenomenon. Dark urine and pale stools may precede the jaundice by a few weeks.

In patients with cancer of the head of the pancreas, the most common distinguishing features after painless jaundice would be weight loss and steatorrhoea (this is the presence of excess fat in the stools giving an oily appearance and foul smell). Steatorrhoea occurs because the obstruction prevents bile acids from entering the bowel leading to fat malabsorption. Patients usually complain of difficulty flushing away their stools.

1.8.4 **Past medical history**

Take a detailed medical history including any previous medical illness and hospital admissions. Enquire about previous investigations, such as ultrasound scans and endoscopic retrograde cholangio-pancreotography (ERCP). Also ask about any previous operations, particularly on the biliary tract. Surgical strictures from such operations may present with obstructive jaundice. Ask whether the patient has undergone recent general anaesthesia as there is evidence that halothane exposure is implicated in both hepatitis and jaundice.

Establish whether the patient has suffered with previous gallstones, hepatitis, cirrhosis or haemolytic anaemia. Patients who suffer from ulcerative colitis are at increased risk of developing sclerosing cholangitis. A presentation of jaundice in a patient known to have sickle cell anaemia would lead you to consider it as a possible cause. Finally, establish if the patient has previously been diagnosed with any form of cancer as the liver is a common site for secondary metastases.

Drug history

Ask the patient what medication they are currently taking or have taken in the past. Do not forget to also ask about any OTC medications or herbal remedies that the patient has tried. Recent commencement of a new drug may suggest the possible implication of drug-induced jaundice (*Box 1.7*). Drugs such as statins, taken for cholesterol, have been shown to cause hepatitis occasionally, as has the oral contraceptive pill. Antibiotics such as flucloxacillin, fusidic acid and co-amoxiclav can also cause jaundice. Do not forget to ask about drug allergies or intolerances.

Social history

Establish whether the patient smokes and if so, determine the number of pack years. Ask if they drink alcohol and, if so, note the type of alcohol and how many units a week they drink. A patient who drinks above the recommended limits may be at risk of alcoholic liver disease. Alcohol is associated with a number of conditions, including alcoholic hepatitis, cirrhosis, pancreatitis, and pancreatic cancer, that can cause jaundice directly.

Discreetly ask about illicit drug use. Patients who are intravenous drug users are at an increased risk of developing hepatitis B and C, particularly if the patient shares needles with others.

Ask the patient about recent travel abroad, particularly to areas known to be endemic for hepatitis A, malaria and yellow fever such as subtropical Africa

---

TOP TIP!

Painless jaundice seen in the elderly should immediately be investigated for cancer of the head of the pancreas.

QUESTIONS TO ASK . . .

To assess risk of hepatitis
- Have you recently travelled abroad to an endemic area?
- Have you had any tattoos or body piercings?
- Have you ever had a blood transfusion?
- Have you ever used intravenous drugs or shared needles?
- Have you engaged in any unprotected sex with a person of the same sex?

TOP TIP!

In the UK, patients who received a blood transfusion prior to 1991, or plasma products before 1985, are at risk of contracting blood borne disease such as hepatitis B and C and HIV as they were not routinely screened for at that time.

TOP TIP!

Jaundice, fever with rigors and pain is known as Charcot's triad, and is commonly associated with ascending cholangitis.

BOX 1.7 **Common causes of drug-induced jaundice**	
Drugs	**Mechanism**
Paracetamol overdose, methyldopa, erythromycin, statins	Hepatocellular dysfunction
Amiodarone, anti-TB (isoniazid)	
Flucloxacillin, co-amoxiclav, nitrofurantoin	Post-hepatic dysfunction
Oral contraceptive pill	(cholestasis)
Sulfonylurea, gold, anabolic steroids, chlorpromazine	

and South America. In addition, try to establish whether the patient has had unprotected sexual intercourse whilst abroad, especially if they have travelled to South East Asia because there is a high incidence of hepatitis B.

Family history

Liver disease may run in families: Wilson's disease and Gilbert's syndrome may be inherited. It is also important to ask if any first-degree relatives suffer from glucose-6-phosphate dehydrogenase (G6PD) deficiency which is X-linked and can cause jaundice in the presence of infections or after medication use (such as anti-malaria drugs or quinolone).

1.8.5 Systems review

Complete your jaundice history with a brief systems review. Ask the patient about relevant symptoms such as nausea and vomiting, anorexia or change in bowel habits.

1.8.6 Summing up

Summarize your findings back to the patient and ask if they would like to add anything that you may have missed. Reassure your patient by coming to an agreement with them about what the next step will be, checking to make sure they understand what is going on. Ask them if they have any questions they would like you to answer. In addition, offer the patient information leaflets and discuss when you (or another health professional) will see them next. End the interview by thanking the patient. In an exam situation, deliver an appropriate summary to the examiner.

1.8.7 Common clinical scenarios

The following are a list of common jaundice cases which you may encounter. For each one, consider:
- what the possible differential diagnosis of each could be
- what key features you would look for
- what questions you would ask to refine or confirm your diagnosis

You could use role play with a friend, using the histories in the cases below as a framework.

CASE 1   A 40 year old businessman presents to his GP after his wife noticed a yellowish tinge to his eyes. He has also suffered with pain in the right upper quadrant which has worsened over the last 2 days. He complains of feeling generally unwell for the past 3 weeks, including bouts of diarrhoea and fever. He has also noticed that his stools are pale. He has no past medical history of note. He regularly travels to the Indian subcontinent and parts of Africa on business and was away a month ago. He doesn't drink.

CASE 2

A 19 year old medical student presents to his GP complaining of flu-like illness for the last few days. He noticed that he has been tired and complains of productive cough and runny nose. His friends have commented on his yellow appearance frequently during this time. He notices that he has had similar episodes in the past whenever he catches a cold. Things have been noticeably worse since puberty. He does not drink, does not use any drugs and has not travelled abroad.

CASE 3

A 68 year old publican presents with a 3 month history of fatigue, nausea and vomiting. Sometimes the vomit is mixed with blood. He has noticed a yellowish tinge to his skin and a distended abdomen. He also mentions that at times he feels confused. He has previously attended for help with alcoholism with mixed results. He drinks 40 units per week on average and smokes 25–30 cigarettes a day.

CASE 4

A 42 year old obese fast food worker presents with acute onset of swinging fever, jaundice and right upper quadrant pain. She has a past history of gallstones and is on a waiting list for a cholecystectomy.

CASE 5

A 62 year old known alcoholic presents with a 6 month history of weight loss, anorexia and painless jaundice. He also mentions that he is embarrassed by his foul smelling stools that are difficult to flush away. His past medical history includes diabetes and chronic pancreatitis. He smokes 20 cigarettes a day and drinks more than 50 units of alcohol a week.

Chapter 1.9
Haematuria

What to do . . .

- Introduce yourself to the patient – establish rapport
- Ask the patient's name, age and occupation
- Ask the patient relevant questions relating to their haematuria, including onset, duration, nature and timing
- Ask about any associated symptoms such as pain, fever, weight loss, frequency, urgency, poor stream
- Ask about any past medical history, e.g. sickle cell anaemia
- Ask about any drug history and for any drug allergies, e.g. warfarin and aspirin
- Ask about any social history – ask if the patient smokes and about recent travel to areas affected by schistosomiasis
- Ask about any family history, specifically for CKD, polycystic kidneys and Alport's syndrome
- Perform a brief systems review and sum up your findings
- Thank the patient and conclude the consultation

The word haematuria literally means blood in the urine. In medicine it represents the detection of erythrocytes or red blood cells in a urine sample from a patient. Blood found in the urine may be frank, clearly visible to the eye, or seen as a brown or pinkish tinge to the urine – this is known as macroscopic haematuria. Blood that is not visible but is detectable on a urine dipstick is known as microscopic haematuria. Whilst frank haematuria may be an alarming symptom, the amount of blood passed in the urine does not necessarily correlate to the seriousness of the underlying illness.

The presence of blood in the urine is often regarded as signifying renal disease, because the kidney plays a vital role in preventing red blood cells from crossing through the glomerular basement membrane within the glomeruli, and any dysfunction would lead to haematuria. Whilst this may be true, this represents only one of the possible causes: haematuria can arise from any site along the urinary system, including the kidneys, ureters, bladder, prostate (if present) and urethra. The majority of cases of haematuria are due to stones, infections, cancers or trauma affecting any site along this tract. However, there are also non-renal causes (see *Fig 1.11*) of haematuria that should be considered, such as sickle cell anaemia, bleeding disorders, anticoagulants or abdominal trauma.

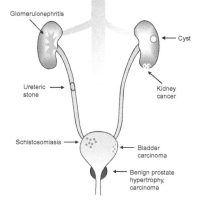

Fig 1.11 Causes of haematuria.

1.9.1 **Taking the history**

Begin your history by introducing yourself to the patient, stating your name and job title. Ask the patient some background questions such as their name, age and occupation before enquiring about their haematuria. The patient's age and gender can play a role in the consideration of an appropriate differential diagnosis. For example, urinary tract infections (UTIs) commonly cause haematuria in young women, whereas tumours become more prevalent in the elderly. Nephritis (inflammation of the kidneys) is the most common cause of blood in the urine in children and young adults but can also be seen at any age. The patient's occupation may also be relevant in cases of haematuria, because patients working in the rubber or dyes industries may be exposed to chemicals or carcinogens that may lead to bladder cancer. Other risk factors for bladder cancer include smoking (about 50%), aromatic amines (from textiles and rubber), and chronic urinary tract infections.

1.9.2 **Ideas, concerns and expectations**

Ensure that you ask questions to try to elicit the patient's own ideas as to what is going on. You should also try to explore whether they have any concerns about their symptoms; as described above, frank haematuria can be quite a startling symptom and the patient may reveal concerns about cancer or a sexually transmitted infection as possible causes. Spend some time enquiring about how the symptom has affected the patient's life and establish whether it has hindered them from performing a particular activity.

1.9.3 **History of the presenting complaint**

First establish what the patient means when they claim that they have blood in the urine. Is there true blood in the urine or could it originate from another site? For example, in a menstruating lady sometimes the beginning of a heavy period can be confused with haematuria. Similarly, in an elderly incontinent patient, blood seen on the continence pads may actually be from bleeding haemorrhoids rather than a urinary source.

Onset and duration

Establish when the episode of haematuria started and for how long they have noticed blood in their urine. A short period of haematuria may point towards an infective cause such as a UTI, whereas persisting haematuria may suggest a more sinister cause.

Nature

Try and gauge the severity of the haematuria (see *Box 1.8*). The intensity of the discolouration of the urine is often a useful indicator. The urine may be described as being slightly tinged, pink in colour, bright red or even deep brown like cola. In heavy bleeds, patients may even report the passing of clots. However, be

> **TOP TIP!**
>
> In patients who work in the textile or dye industry it is easy to jump to conclusions and assume that an episode of haematuria may be due to an underlying bladder cancer. Whilst these patients are at risk it is more likely that another common cause of haematuria is involved.

> **TOP TIP!**
>
> Microscopic haematuria usually indicates an upper urinary tract pathology whilst macroscopic haematuria suggests lower urinary tract lesion – however, this is not always true in every case.

> **TOP TIP!**
>
> A thin worm-shaped clot suggests an upper urinary tract disorder.

BOX 1.8 **Red flags for haematuria**

- Frank haematuria at any age
- Painless haematuria in a patient older than 50 years
- Unexplained persistent microscopic haematuria in a patient older than 50 years
- Persistent UTIs with haematuria in a patient older than 40 years
- Weight loss and night sweats

careful not to base all your findings on the urinary colour because a number of foods, such as beetroot or berries, and medications (such as Rifampicin) can also discolour the urine.

Timing

The period at which the haematuria is noticed within the stream may provide a clue to the possible site of bleeding. Blood in the urine noticed at the beginning of the stream usually indicates a lower urinary tract lesion, particularly within the urethra. Continuous or midstream haematuria suggests possible bladder involvement or suprabladder pathology (ureter or renal). Terminal stream bleeding could arise from the neck of the bladder, posterior urethra or schistosomiasis.

Associated symptoms

Spend some time eliciting any symptoms that present along with the haematuria; symptoms such as pain on micturition, fever, urgency and weight loss may direct you towards the correct diagnosis.

Pain is an important associated symptom that can indicate a number of pathologies. First, establish where the pain is felt: is it over the flank, loin area, suprapubic, or the tip of the urethra? Does the pain move anywhere, i.e. to the groin or is it fixed at one site? Does it come and go or is it persistent in nature? A patient presenting with severe colicky loin pain radiating down to the groin may be suffering from a renal stone, whereas a patient complaining of burning pain, particularly when passing urine, frequency and cloudy urine may be suffering from a UTI.

Sweating or fevers is another typical feature of concurrent infection and can be seen in UTIs, prostatitis and pyelonephritis. Patients with pyelonephritis are often exquisitely tender over the loin area from an ascending UTI that has begun to affect the kidney. Night sweats may be suggestive of renal TB. If a young patient had a recent sore throat and fever with the subsequent development of haematuria, this should make you consider glomerulonephritis caused by a group A β-haemolytic streptococcus bacterial infection.

Patients may notice changes to their urinary stream or the number of times they pass urine. Obstructive symptoms such as poor stream, hesitancy, terminal dribbling and incomplete emptying may be seen in benign prostatic hyperplasia or cancer. Irritative symptoms may also been seen that include urgency, frequency, incontinence and nocturia.

Weight loss is a less common symptom associated with haematuria; however, if present it should lead you swiftly to the diagnosis of renal cell carcinoma. In an elderly patient with painless frank haematuria and weight loss you should exclude transitional cell carcinoma of the bladder.

1.9.4 Past medical history

Take a detailed past medical history including any previous medical illness and hospital admissions. Check whether the patient has suffered from recurrent UTIs or a kidney stone. Has the patient had any recent operations or procedures such as TURPs or cystoscopies or catheters? Check that the patient does not suffer from sickle cell anaemia or any inherited blood clotting disorders.

Drug history

Take a detailed drug history about the current medication they are taking or for any OTC medication. Aspirin and warfarin can cause thinning of the blood leading to painless haematuria. Cyclophosphamide, a drug commonly used in transplants, has been linked with causing carcinoma of the bladder as well as haemorrhagic cystitis.

Social history

Ask whether the patient smokes and, if so, how many cigarettes a day and for how long; smoking is the largest risk factor in bladder cancer. Establish whether they drink alcohol and if they do, note the type of alcohol and how many units a week. Also ask if they have recently travelled abroad; certain countries in Africa, including Egypt, have increased prevalence of schistosomiasis which may be a cause of haematuria.

Family history

It is important when taking a haematuria history to ask whether the patient has any first-degree relatives who suffer or have suffered from similar symptoms. Polycystic kidney disease can be inherited in an autosomal dominant manner and is associated with strokes and end-stage renal disease. Alport's syndrome is an X-linked condition that presents with blood in the urine, end-stage renal disease and hearing loss.

1.9.5 Systems review

Complete your haematuria history with a brief systems review enquiring about bone pain, tiredness, rashes and joint pains.

1.9.6 Summing up

Summarize your findings back to the patient and ask if they would like to add anything that you may have missed. It may be useful to summarize once you have completed the history of the presenting complaint as this may give you some time to reflect upon the information gathered so far. Thank the patient and, in an exam situation, summarize your findings to the examiner.

1.9.7 Common clinical scenarios

The following are a list of common haematuria cases which you may encounter. For each one, consider:
• what the possible differential diagnosis could be
• what key features you would look for
• what questions you would ask to refine or confirm your diagnosis

You could use role play with a friend, using the histories in the cases below as a framework.

CASE 1

A 22 year old office clerk presents with a 2 day history of burning sensation whenever she passes urine. She has noticed that her urine is dark and smelly and that she is going to the toilet more often. She also mentions that she has a dull suprapubic pain whenever she voids. She denies any nausea or vomiting and has not felt feverish. Past history includes previous UTI. She is currently on the combined oral contraceptive pill and is allergic to penicillin.

CASE 2

A 25 year old female presents with recurrent urinary symptoms which have been ongoing for the last 5 years. She has had multiple UTIs, blood in her urine, and more recently pain in her lower back. Over the last year she has had recurrent headaches and visual disturbances. Her mother and grandmother both had kidney disease and her mother died of a bleed inside the brain.

CASE 3

A 26 year old male student normally fit and well presents to A&E with severe left-sided pain in his lower back. The pain started 8 hours ago and it has gradually increased in intensity and is now unbearable. The pain comes and goes in waves and radiates down to the groin. He has had two similar episodes in the past. He denies any fever or rigors or pain on passing urine. He smokes five cigarettes a day and occasionally drinks alcohol.

CASE 4

A 53 year old bank manager who has been fit and well until 5 months ago. Initially he noticed occasional episodes of blood mixed with his urine but, more recently, he has had severe episodes of passing blood. This is associated with a dull pain in his left loin and slight swelling in the area too. He has lost several kilograms in weight and has poor appetite. He has no energy to do anything and feels continually tired. In the last few weeks he has also had a fever at night and has woken on many occasions drenched in sweat. He does not smoke, and drinks about 15 pints of beer each week. He is worried that something serious may be wrong.

CASE 5

A 63 year old retired teacher presents with worsening urinary symptoms. He has had frequency and nocturia for some time, but over the last few months he is now complaining of poor stream and dribbling a few drops of urine after he has voided. There is no history of weight loss or fevers.

Chapter 1.10
Headache

What to do . . .

- Introduce yourself to the patient – establish rapport
- Ask the patient's name, age and occupation
- Ask the patient relevant questions about their headaches, such as site, onset, character, radiation, aggravating and relieving factors, and timing
- Ask about any associated symptoms, e.g. nausea, vomiting, photophobia, phonophobia, neck stiffness, flashing lights, scalp tenderness/jaw claudication
- Establish any precipitants for migraines, such as red wine, chocolate, cheese
- Ask about any past medical history including migraine and epidurals
- Ask about any drug history and elicit any drug allergies
- Take a social history – establish if the patient smokes or drinks alcohol
- Ask about any family history, specifically for migraines and brain tumours
- Perform a brief systems review and sum up your findings
- Thank the patient and conclude the consultation

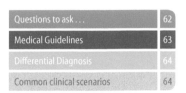
Headache is one of the most common neurological symptoms with which patients present. Its description and intensity may differ from patient to patient, often making it difficult to differentiate the most urgent cases from the more benign. Although the majority of headaches are benign, they may be the first sign to suggest more sinister underlying pathology, such as a brain tumour, subarachnoid haemorrhage or temporal arteritis. Its presentation can vary from a simple tension headache to the more severe debilitating migranous headache with an associated aura.

Taking a headache history follows a similar structure to taking a general pain history. However, it is important to tailor your history to include specific symptoms commonly associated with headaches and to screen for any serious underlying pathology.

1.10.1 **Taking the history**

Introduce yourself to the patient, mentioning your name, job title and the reason for interviewing the patient. Ask the patient some background questions such as their name, age and occupation before enquiring about the headaches. The patient's age and gender can play a role in the consideration of an appropriate differential diagnosis. Young women, for example, are more likely to suffer from migraines, whilst men are more likely to suffer with head injuries. Headaches due to an intracranial bleed are more likely to be seen in the elderly or alcoholics.

Occupational history plays a fairly limited role in headache diagnosis, but you should consider contact with solvents, vapours, carbon monoxide or other chemicals if relevant to the patient's profession.

> **TOP TIP!**
>
> Temporal arteritis is associated with blindness. In a patient with suspected temporal arteritis, do not wait for the ESR (erythrocyte sedimentation rate) result. Give the patient prednisolone as soon as possible and seek the help of a senior doctor.

Establish rapport with the patient by asking open questions regarding their symptoms before asking more focused questions regarding their headache. This may help the patient relax and be put at ease, hopefully leading to them answering your questions more openly.

1.10.2 **Ideas, concerns and expectations**

After appropriately introducing yourself and establishing rapport, ask the patient what they think may be the cause of their headaches. By allowing the patient to express their own views of their complaint, their symptom will be put into context and you will be able to address any misconceptions or worries they may hold. A common fear that patients hold is that their headache is caused by a brain tumour, or they are worried about dying, mental incapacity, and loss of work.

Spend some time enquiring about how the symptom has affected the patient's life and elicit whether their headaches have hindered them from performing any particular activity.

1.10.3 **History of the presenting complaint**

As with any pain history, you must elicit as much information as possible about the headache itself. This will help you to categorize the headache and filter out improbable diagnoses.

Site

Ask the patient where the pain is located and request them to point to it if necessary – the site of the headache may give you a clue as to the root cause. Unilateral headaches may be due to migraines or cluster headaches, while bilateral headaches are commonly due to stress (tension headaches). Pain in a dermatomal distribution is likely to be neuralgic pain whereas a sudden severe pain in the back of the head may be due to a subarachnoid haemorrhage.

Onset

It is important to elicit when the headache started and whether it is chronic or acute in nature. Knowledge about the time of onset of the headache is often crucial in distinguishing between potential causes: sudden onset should alert you to the possibility of a subarachnoid haemorrhage (see *Box 1.9*), especially if there are also signs of meningeal irritation. A more insidious onset with progressive worsening of symptoms, especially with associated signs of raised intracranial pressure, should alert you to the possibility of a tumour.

Character

Try to establish the character of the pain and ensure that you allow the patient to freely describe their symptoms in their own words. If the patient is unable to

> **TOP TIP!**
>
> In clinical exams, patients are often concerned that their headaches are caused by a brain tumour. It is important not to be dismissive of this concern but instead you should try to allay this fear through the course of the consultation.

BOX 1.9 **Subarachnoid haemorrhage**

A sudden onset headache is felt as if being 'hit by a bat'. It is usually accompanied by neck stiffness and photophobia. It often has a familial distribution and can be associated with berry aneurysms.

express the exact nature of their pain, consider offering a number of descriptions for them to choose from: ask the patient whether the pain they are experiencing is dull, sharp, continuous or throbbing in nature. If it has a sharp, shooting component, often described as an electric shock, then it is known as lancinating pain and this is usually due to nerve root irritation or neuralgia.

Dull throbbing headaches are often described by patients with migraines, whereas sharp stabbing headaches may be caused by trigeminal neuralgia. A pressure or band-like headache around the head is often described in tension headaches.

Radiation

It can be useful to establish whether the pain radiates away from initial site of presentation. Pain that starts at the corner of the eye and spreads to encompass the ipsilateral side of the head is common in cluster headaches. A headache that starts in the frontal area of the head, radiating to the occipital region is likely to be a tension headache.

Associated symptoms

Headache can often present in conjunction with other symptoms and eliciting these will help to narrow down the list of possible differentials. Enquire specifically about nausea, vomiting and photophobia which are implicated in both migraine (see *Box 1.10*) and headaches due to meningeal irritation. You should ask if the pain is worsened by loud noises (phonophobia), strong smells or head movement. Also check if the patient is experiencing a visual defect or suffering from any neurological deficit.

- Fever in the presence of headache should raise the suspicion of an intracranial infection, primarily meningitis, which often presents along with a non-blanching rash and neck stiffness. It may also present in sinusitis if it is throbbing in nature, worsened by leaning forwards and associated with localized pain and tenderness over the sinus areas.
- Headache associated with a fluctuating level of consciousness following trauma to the head, especially in an alcoholic or elderly person, may be due to a subdural haematoma.
- Headache associated with nausea and vomiting along with a focal neurological deficit is likely to be caused by a space-occupying lesion.
- Premonitory or warning symptoms are common in people who suffer with migraines and include feelings of being detached, energized or even high. Some sufferers also have sensory illusions before developing a headache. This includes colours appearing brighter or sounds being heard more sharply. Auras are symptoms that occur just prior to a migraine and tend to follow a fixed pattern. Initially, they consist of positive neurological symptoms followed by a deficit. Those who suffer from visual auras classically describe a wave of moving lights in the form of zigzag lines that

---

BOX 1.10 **Migraine headaches**

These are unilateral recurrent headaches that occur over days or weeks with periods of freedom. Usually described as a dull throbbing ache with nausea and vomiting, and photophobia. May occur with prodromal symptoms which precede the headache by an hour.

QUESTIONS TO ASK . . .

- Do you ever feel sick or vomit with your headaches?
- Do they ever wake you up from sleep?
- Have you had any fever, neck stiffness or intolerance to light?
- Are your headaches worsened by loud sounds (phonophobia)?
- Do you have any blurring of vision or flashing lights along with the headaches?
- Are the headaches worse on eating/chewing?

TOP TIP!

It can be useful to perform a quick visual acuity test in the consultation to exclude poor eyesight instantly. In the young, a useful question may be to ask if they sit near the front of the class or the back, i.e. try to assess the distance from the board.

TOP TIP!

'Red flags' for underlying pathology include:

- a sudden onset of headache
- an onset after 50 years of age
- new onset of headache with an underlying medical condition (HIV, cancer, TB)
- headache subsequent to head trauma
- headache in association with fluctuating consciousness or personality
- increased frequency or severity of headache
- focal neurological signs or symptoms and papilloedema

is followed by a scotoma or a localized area of visual impairment. Whilst visual auras are the most common, auras can also present with tinnitus, paraesthesia, weakness, or aphasia.

- In the elderly, pain associated with chewing food (jaw claudication) and combing hair necessitates the exclusion of temporal arteries immediately.
- In the young, a headache associated with a red watery eye is likely to be due to cluster headaches.

Timing

Establish when the headaches occur and how long they last for. Note whether the headaches occur at a particular time of day or whether there is a notable pattern to them. Headaches due to intracranial pressure are normally worse in the mornings and may awaken a patient prematurely from their slumber, whereas tension headaches (see *Box 1.11*) start first thing in the morning and worsen towards the end of the day.

Cluster headaches are recurrent headaches that last for up to an hour and occur intensely over several weeks. The attacks are followed by symptom-free periods often lasting several months.

BOX 1.11 **Tension headaches**

Often reported as pressure or tightened bands around the head. May present bilaterally over the occipito–frontal area. There is often a stressful event that has precipitated the headaches and they can recur daily. Chronic tension headaches can last for months to years.

Headaches occurring after sexual intercourse are known as postcoital headaches. They are usually severe, throbbing or explosive in nature and can be confused with subarachnoid haemorrhage.

In women, it is important to establish whether the headaches occur in association with their periods. Menstrual headaches tend to be migranous in nature and may occur shortly before, during or after their regular periods. Occasionally they may occur in mid-cycle due to ovulation.

A commonly overlooked cause of headaches is a headache caused by eye straining due to poor eyesight. The headache is typically frontal or over the temporal areas and may be made worse after long periods of computer usage. Symptoms will resolve with appropriate glasses or contact lenses.

Exacerbating and relieving factors

It is imperative to enquire about the factors that make the headache better or worse. You may wish to establish whether there are any obvious factors that precipitate and bring on the headache. Some of these may include foods or drinks such as red wine, caffeine, ice cream, mature cheeses, activities such as exercise, sex, sun exposure or reading or a feeling of hunger. Patients often recall a particular food that precipitates a migranous attack, with the most common offenders being cheese, red wine, chocolate, caffeine and foods containing monosodium glutamate (MSG).

Ask whether a change in posture such as lying down, bending, coughing or straining has a bearing on the intensity of the headache. In headaches caused by raised intracranial pressure, such postures would worsen the headache, whereas standing or sitting up would tend to lessen it.

In trigeminal neuralgia, the headaches are often precipitated by shaving, washing the face or brushing teeth. The headaches are sharp, lancinating in nature and found within the trigeminal nerve (5th cranial nerve) distribution. They are brought about by the activation of 'trigger zones' often by touch or rubbing and are short-lived (typically lasting for up to a minute).

Severity

Gauging the severity of the headache can give vital clues as to both the seriousness of the headache and its possible cause. Grading the headache also helps to assess the efficacy of initiated therapy at future consultations. A useful tool by which you can measure subjectively the intensity of the headache is by requesting the patient to rank the pain on a scale of one to ten, one being minimal pain and ten being the worst pain ever experienced.

Subarachnoid headaches are often described by patients as the worst headache that they have ever experienced. They may describe it as if someone had hit them on the back of the head with a baseball bat (see *Box 1.9*). This description holds two of the key components of a subarachnoid haemorrhage, the first being sudden onset and the second being the intensity. In addition, other symptoms may corroborate this diagnosis, such as vomiting, confusion and neck stiffness.

1.10.4 Past medical history

Take a detailed past medical history including any previous medical illnesses and hospital admissions. Enquire about previous investigations, such as a lumbar puncture or CT head scan, or any neurosurgical operations. Also ask about any recent epidural or spinal anaesthesia as these may cause a post-procedural headache.

Specifically ask about previous migraine, meningitis, epilepsy or any other neurological disorder. You may also wish to ask the patient whether they have suffered with either low or high blood pressure as both of these may cause headaches.

Drug history

Elicit what medications the patient is currently on or has taken in the past. Do not forget to also ask about any OTC or herbal remedies. If the patient has tried any analgesia, ask about its effectiveness and duration of activity. Try to establish if the patient is over-using common analgesics, such as codeine, which may cause rebound headaches. A number of drugs that have been implicated in causing headaches include the oral contraceptive pill, nitrates and indometacin. Do not forget to ask about drug allergies or intolerances.

Social history

Enquire whether the patient has ever smoked and if so, how many cigarettes a day and for how long. Establish whether they drink alcohol and, if they do, note the type of alcohol and how many units a week. Discreetly ask about illicit drug use.

Medical Guidelines
Diagnosing migraine without aura

A At least 5 attacks fulfilling criteria B–D

B Headache attacks lasting 4–72 hours

C Headache has at least two of the following characteristics: unilateral location, pulsating quality, moderate or severe pain intensity, aggravation by or causing avoidance of routine physical activity (e.g. walking or climbing stairs)

D During headache at least one of the following: nausea and/or vomiting, photophobia and phonophobia, not caused by any other condition

International Headache Society – www.ihs-headache.org

It is important in the headache history to enquire how the headache is affecting the patient's life and particularly their work or studies. Ask how many sick days off they have had to take. This not only gives you an indication as to the severity of the headache but also helps you tailor your treatment towards the patient. In a patient who suffers from migraines more than twice a month, leading them to take significant time off work, you may wish to commence prophylactic therapy.

Family history

It is helpful to enquire whether the patient has any first-degree relatives who suffer or have suffered from similar symptoms. The familial incidence of migraine is almost 60%, supporting the theory of a genetic aetiology. A family history of brain tumour in a patient presenting with signs of raised intracranial pressure may point towards this as a cause, but it is important not to jump to any conclusions, especially with regard to prematurely mentioning cancer as a possible cause; you may inadvertently create undue anxiety in the patient.

1.10.5 Systems review

Complete your headache history with a brief systems review. Ask the patient about any relevant neurological symptoms such as experiencing any fits or faints, weakness in arms or legs, any problems with their vision or hearing, or problems in swallowing. You may also wish to enquire more generally about common symptoms such as chest pain, palpitations or change in bowel habits, or any muscle or joint pains, which are good indicators of the patient's health and wellbeing.

1.10.6 Summing up

Summarize your findings back to the patient and ask if they would like to add anything that you may have missed. It may be useful to summarize once you have completed the history of the presenting complaint as this may give you some time to reflect upon the information gathered so far.

Reassure your patient by coming to an agreement with them about what the next steps will be, checking to make sure they understand what is going on. Ask them if they have any questions they would like you to answer. In addition, offer the patient information leaflets and discuss when you (or another health professional) will next see them, if appropriate. End the interview by thanking the patient. In an exam situation, deliver a relevant summary to the examiner.

1.10.7 Common clinical scenarios

The following are a list of common headache cases which you may encounter. For each one, consider:
- what the possible differential diagnosis could be
- what key features you would look for
- what questions you would ask to refine or confirm your diagnosis

You could use role play with a friend, using the histories in the cases below as a framework.

CASE 1

A 30 year old housewife presents complaining of a frontal headache for 2 weeks. She describes it as a pressure-like pain between and around her eyes. The headache is worse in the morning and when she leans forward. It is also associated with a mild fever and nasal congestion. She has been indoors for the last 2 days because of a 'cold' and has no past medical history of note.

CASE 2

A 28 year old newly qualified lawyer complains of a recent history of recurrent headaches for the last 3 weeks. The headache is described as a tight band around her head, worsening when she returns home in the evening from work. She does not get any headaches on weekends or whilst on holidays. The pain does not move anywhere. She recalls having similar headaches as a student during exam periods, but has no other medical or family history of note. She is not currently on the contraceptive pill.

CASE 3

A 38 year old gentleman presents complaining of a 3-week history of right-sided headache. The pain starts at the corner of his eye feeling like a 'red hot poker' and lasts for half an hour. During attacks, he also complains of a watery red 'drooping' right eye. He had a similar 4-week episode last year and is now worried this may be something serious. He is otherwise fit and well.

CASE 4

An 18 year old college student presents with a 1-week history of recurrent left-sided headache. She describes the pain as throbbing and severe, with a score of 7/10. She states that she has not been sleeping well because she has been drinking several cans of caffeinated fizzy drinks. She also complains of feeling nauseous and notes visual disturbances prior to the attacks. The attacks last for approximately 8 hours and she locks herself in a dark quiet room until they pass. She was recently started on the oral contraceptive pill. She is a non-smoker and drinks a glass of wine a day. She mentions that her brother and paternal uncle suffered with similar symptoms.

CASE 5

A 46 year old man complains of a 6-month history of a gradually worsening frontal headache. He notes that the pain is worst first thing in the morning but improves when he sits up or stands. He has been feeling nauseous for a while but has only recently started to vomit. He also states that he has problems with his vision, particularly in his peripheral area. He notes that his skin has become more greasy and his wife thinks that his appearance has changed somewhat. His wedding ring is too tight and no longer fits his finger.

CASE 6

A 64 year old housewife presents with a 3-week, progressively worsening history of left-sided headache located over the peri-orbital area associated with visual problems. She describes tenderness along the hairline where her hat sits. The pain is worse on eating or when she combs her hair in the morning. On systems review she states that she has been suffering with generalized muscle aches and tiredness.

CASE 7

A 50 year old car mechanic presents suffering with a sudden onset severe headache over the occipital area. He describes it as if he has just been hit over his head. He complains of feeling nauseous but has only vomited once. Previous medical history includes polycystic kidney disease and poorly controlled hypertension. He mentions that his uncle passed away unexpectedly.

CASE 8

A 35 year old unkempt man complains of sudden onset of 'electric shock' pain when he washes his face in the morning. It has been going on for a few weeks with each attack lasting for only a few seconds. He mentions that shaving his face or brushing his teeth triggers the headaches. There is no other relevant past medical or social history.

CASE 9

A 68 year old man complains of a 3-month history of gradually worsening headache. The pain worsens as the day goes on and is exacerbated by movement. He sometimes also experiences earache and pain in the neck. He believes the neck pain may have actually begun 6–8 months ago, but recently he noticed tingling in his arms and a worsening of the pain. He suffers from osteoarthritis.

Chapter 1.11
Loss of consciousness

What to do . . .

- Introduce yourself to the patient – establish rapport
- Ask the patient's name, age and occupation
- Ask the patient relevant questions relating to their blackout, including pre-syncope (chest pain, shortness of breath, palpitations, pallor), syncope (seizure, tongue biting, urinary incontinence) and post-syncope (post-ictal sleepiness, amnesia)
- Ask about any past medical history, e.g. DM, epilepsy
- Ask about any drug history and for any drug allergies
- Ask about any social history – establish if the patient smokes or drinks alcohol
- Ask about any family history and specifically for premature sudden death
- Perform a brief systems review and sum up your findings
- Thank the patient and conclude the consultation

Syncope, or a blackout episode, is due to transient impairment of cerebral perfusion resulting in temporary loss of consciousness. It is usually preceded by a feeling of dizziness which is the initial stage of cerebral hypo-perfusion. When the patient has truly lost consciousness they lack their responsiveness to the environment or external stimuli (see *Box 1.12*). A syncope episode is usually sudden, temporary and short-lived with patients eventually recovering to full consciousness. Causes may vary from a simple faint to postural hypotension, cardiac arrhythmias and hypoglycaemia. Patients who remain in a prolonged state of unconsciousness and cannot be aroused are considered to be in a coma.

Syncope and dizziness should be distinguished from vertigo where the patient may describe dizziness that is sudden and rotary in nature. Vestibular disorders and disease of the inner ear do not usually cause loss of consciousness. Patients who present complaining of loss of consciousness should have a thorough history taken including events leading up to the episode, their symptoms at the time and in the post-syncopal phase. Although a good history should guide to a possible list of differentials, most patients are likely to need further investigations to confirm or negate any serious pathology.

TOP TIP!

Syncope accounts for up to 5% of all elderly A&E attendances; half of which are admitted for further investigation.

1.11.1 Taking the history

Introduce yourself to the patient, giving your name and job title. Confirm the patient's name and date of birth before asking about their occupation. Having some knowledge about the patient's occupation is of relevance when taking a syncope history since the symptom can affect the patient's level of functioning. Jobs that require the use of heavy machinery or being underwater may be particularly inappropriate for a patient who has been recently diagnosed with

Medical Guidelines
Management of transient loss of consciousness

Assess and record:

- Details of any previous transient loss of consciousness, including number and frequency
- The person's medical history and any family history of cardiac disease (for example, personal history of heart disease and family history of sudden cardiac death)
- Current medication that may have contributed to transient loss of consciousness (for example, diuretics)
- Vital signs (for example, pulse rate, respiratory rate and temperature) – repeat if clinically indicated
- Lying and standing blood pressure if clinically appropriate
- Other cardiovascular and neurological signs

NICE Guidelines: Transient loss of consciousness ('blackouts') management in adults and young people (2010)

BOX 1.12 **Glasgow Coma Scale**

The Glasgow Coma Scale (GCS) is a widely used and recognized scale to rapidly assess the level of consciousness in a patient. It is an assessment of three areas: eye, verbal and motor responses. The maximum score is 15 which is considered normal, whilst the lowest score is 3 and this is seen in patients in a deep coma.

Best eye response (E). There are 4 grades starting with the most severe:
1. No eye opening
2. Eye opening in response to pain
3. Eye opening to speech
4. Eyes opening spontaneously

Best verbal response (V). There are 5 grades starting with the most severe:
1. No verbal response
2. Incomprehensible sounds
3. Inappropriate words
4. Confused
5. Oriented

Best motor response (M). There are 6 grades starting with the most severe:
1. No motor response
2. Extension to pain
3. Abnormal flexion to pain
4. Flexion/withdrawal to pain
5. Localizes to pain
6. Obeys commands

---

epilepsy. In addition, occupations that involve driving may require a period of abstinence because the possibility of having an episode whilst at the wheel, losing control and causing harm to oneself as well as others is extremely high. This is particularly important for jobs such as taxi, bus or HGV drivers as the risk of harm from any incident is greater. As a clinician it is a statutory requirement to inform patients that they must contact the DVLA if they suffer from syncope attacks or epilepsy.

1.11.2 **Ideas, concerns and expectations**

Establish what the patient believes is causing their blackouts and what particularly concerns them about their symptoms. Patients may reveal that they are worried about an underlying brain tumour, being diagnosed with a stroke or the possibility of losing their licence or livelihood as a driver. Such concerns should be acknowledged and every effort should be made to address and reassure the patient if relevant.

1.11.3 **History of presenting complaint**

When a patient presents with loss of consciousness it is important not only to take a history from the patient themselves but also try to establish whether there were any witnesses to the incident. A collateral history may give you vital information that the patient was not aware of during the episode, such as the length of the blackout or any abnormal posturing.

Clarify with the patient what they mean by the term they use to describe the blackout. Patients may incorrectly use the word blackout to mean a wide variety of symptoms such as dizziness, light-headedness, vertigo and faints. Explore

TOP TIP!

An altered level of consciousness must not be confused with altered states of consciousness, such as delirium.

Medical Guidelines
DVLA restrictions to driving

	Group 1 (cars, motorbikes)	Group 2 (large lorries and buses)
Simple faint - definite provocation factors with associated prodromal symptoms and unlikely to occur whilst sitting or lying	No driving restrictions	No driving restrictions
Unexplained syncope and low risk of re-occurrence	Can drive 4 weeks after the event	Can drive 3 months after the event
Unexplained syncope and high risk of re-occurrence	Can drive 4 weeks after the event if the cause has been identified and treated. If no cause identified, then 6 months off	Can drive after 3 months if the cause has been identified and treated. If no cause, then licence refused/revoked for one year

Factors indicating high risk of re-occurrence include an abnormal ECG, clinical evidence of structural heart disease, syncope causing injury, occurring at the wheel or whilst sitting or lying, more than one episode in previous six months.

DVLA: At a glance guide to the current medical standards of fitness to drive (2011) – www.dft.gov.uk

TOP TIP!

An effective way of eliciting a syncope history is to consider the symptoms in the order in which they occurred to create a timeline of events.

their understanding and determine whether they are actually describing a syncopal event or not.

Pre-event

Enquire carefully about the events leading up to the loss of consciousness, and establish what the patient was doing just prior to the attack.

- Did they suffer with any chest pain, shortness of breath or palpitations, or did it occur whilst exercising? Answers to these questions may indicate possible cardiac aetiology such as arrhythmias or, in the case of exercise, valve disease such as aortic stenosis or cardiomyopathy.
- Had they been standing for a prolonged period of time or did they experience severe pain or anxiety? This type of history would suggest a simple faint or a vasovagal response whereby there is splanchnic and peripheral vasodilatation along with bradycardia.
- Did the patient suffer from a coughing fit or were they micturating at the time? These two may also point towards a vasovagal type of attack. Coughing may increase intra-thoracic pressure thereby inhibiting venous return, whilst micturition stimulates the vagus nerve that causes bradycardia and hypotension.
- Had the patient been lying down and just got up or did they suddenly tilt their head upwards just prior to their dizzy spell? An elderly patient feeling dizzy and light-headed upon standing may be suffering with postural hypotension and should have their medications reviewed. Syncope related to head movements may be caused by carotid sinus hypersensitivity or vertebrobasilar insufficiency where there is temporary restriction to the posterior circulation of the brain.
- Did they begin to slur their words or notice any other problems before the episode? This may indicate a transient ischaemic attack, or mini stroke.

TOP TIP!

Patients may report combing their hair just prior to their loss of consciousness in vertebrobasilar insufficiency, because tilting the head back may lead to a compromise of the blood supply to the brain.

TOP TIP!

Fainting rarely occurs in the laid back or lying position.

QUESTIONS TO ASK . . .

Pre-event
- Did you have any warning signs before you passed out?
- What where you doing at the time (exercising, micturating, combing your hair)?

Event
- How long did you lose consciousness for? Were there any witnesses?
- Did your body go stiff and shake? Did you wet yourself or bite your tongue?
- Did you experience any symptoms such as chest pain or palpitations?

Post-event
- When you came around did you feel confused or did you recover quickly?
- Did you have any recollection of the episode?

- Finally try to establish whether the patient had abnormal changes to their taste or smell. These may be the prodromal symptoms of an ensuing epileptic fit.

The event

Move on to take a more detailed history about the loss of consciousness. If the patient truly blacked out it is unlikely that they would have much recollection of the event itself. In such situations a witness statement or description of events would be ideal. However, in the absence of a witness, with some investigative questioning it may still be possible to paint a picture of what happened.

Enquire about how long the patient was unconscious. Was this their first blackout or have they had similar episodes in the past? Try and establish whether the patient had a seizure or not. If they did, note whether their whole body went stiff and shook (tonic-clonic) or whether there was a gradual spread of seizure activity (Jacksonian march). Also ask if the patient had bitten their tongue or had an involuntary episode of urinary incontinence as this may confirm a diagnosis of epilepsy.

The manner in which the patient loses consciousness may direct you towards possible differentials. For example, in a patient who unexpectedly collapses and sustains a head injury one must first exclude a cardiac syncopal attack. Such episodes are not affected by posture and can occur even in sleep. Patients with aortic stenosis may experience a similar collapse after a period of exertion. Patients with a complete heart block may become alarmingly pale, black out for around half a minute before rapidly recovering and appearing flushed (Stokes–Adams attack).

Post-event

The patient's state after their episode should also be investigated in detail. Ask the patient how they felt on recovery and how long it took for them to return to normal. Delayed recovery with disorientation and tiredness may be suggestive of the post-ictal phase of an epileptic fit. Rapid regaining of consciousness points more towards a syncopal cause.

If the patient awakes with little recall of events preceding the blackout, as well as shortly after, it is essential to examine the patient and exclude a head injury. Although transient amnesia has been noted in epilepsy, retrograde amnesia, whereby all events are poorly recollected, is typically found in head injury cases.

1.11.4 Past medical history

Take a detailed past medical history including any previous medical illnesses and hospital admissions. Ask about previous investigations including EEGs, CT scans of the head, and lumbar punctures. Check whether the patient has ever had a pacemaker inserted and when it was last checked. Does the patient suffer from diabetes and if so are they taking any hypoglycaemic agents?

Drug history

Ask the patient what medication they are currently on. Diabetic patients on insulin or sulphonylurea oral agents can suffer from hypoglycaemic attacks and these may present with pallor, sweating, palpitations, increase in anxiety and hunger as well as disorientation and confusion. Cardiac agents such as anti-arrhythmic drugs, β-blockers, digoxin, diltiazem or amiodarone may cause arrhythmias in their own right. Drugs used in hypertension (anti-hypertensives) may cause postural hypotension – causing the patient to feel dizzy upon standing quickly from a prone position. Finally, tricyclic antidepressants (TCAs) can cause fitting in overdose.

Social history

Enquire whether the patient has ever smoked and, if so, how many cigarettes a day and for how long. Establish whether they drink alcohol and if they do, note the type of alcohol and how many units a week. Alcohol can cause hepatic encephalopathy which may cause fitting. It may also predispose them to hypoglycaemic attacks as well as head injuries.

Family history

Take a brief family history from the patient focusing on any first-degree relatives suffering from epilepsy, brain tumour or whether there have been any unexplained premature sudden deaths. Long QT syndrome is a genetic disorder that has been associated with unexplained syncope or sudden death in young people.

1.11.5 Systems review

Complete your history with a brief systems review. Ask the patient about relevant neurological symptoms, such as limb weakness, loss of sensation or paraesthesia. You may also wish to enquire about cardiac symptoms such as chest pain, shortness of breath and palpitations.

1.11.6 Summing up

Summarize your findings back to the patient and ask if they would like to add anything that you may have missed. Reassure your patient by coming to an agreement with them about what the next steps will be, checking to make sure they understand what is going on. Ask them if they have any questions they would like you to answer. In addition, offer the patient information leaflets and discuss when you (or another health professional) will see them next. End the interview by thanking the patient and, in an exam situation, deliver an appropriate summary to the examiner.

1.11.7 Common clinical scenarios

The following are a list of common loss of consciousness cases which you may encounter. For each one, consider:
- what the possible differential diagnosis could be
- what key features you would look for
- what questions you would ask to refine or confirm your diagnosis

You could use role play with a friend, using the histories in the cases below as a framework.

DIFFERENTIAL DIAGNOSIS

Cardiac
- Aortic stenosis/HOCM
- Arrhythmias
- Long QT syndrome

Vasovagal
- Coughing
- Micturition
- Situational

Postural hypotension
- Antihypertensives
- Anti-arrhythmic agents
- TCAs

Neurological
- Epilepsy
- TIAs
- Brain tumours
- Head injury

TOP TIP!

Alcohol withdrawal syndrome may also present with seizures and confusion.

CASE 1

A 15 year old girl presents to her GP after falling unconscious at a rock concert. She had been standing in line for a long time and started feeling nauseated, slightly sweaty and weak. Her friend states that she fell limp to the ground and lay there for 10 seconds before rising again. She has no past medical history of note and is not on any medication. Her recent sugar level is normal.

CASE 2

A 67 year old recently diagnosed hypertensive presents with multiple episodes of fainting over the last 3 months. It normally occurs in the morning when she gets out of bed, though it happened yesterday when she got out of the car. She suffered a myocardial infarction last year and is currently on atenolol, ramipril, ISMN, nicorandil and aspirin. She claims not to smoke or drink.

CASE 3

A 68 year old retired Asian postman presents with an episode of loss of consciousness. He was out with his grandchildren looking up at the firework display during New Year celebrations. He began to feel faint and slightly dizzy. His 13 year old granddaughter relates that he fell to the ground and lay there for a minute before waking up. He drinks 18 units of alcohol per week on average and smokes 10 cigarettes a day.

CASE 4

A 17 year old girl is brought in to A&E by ambulance with her mother. The girl states that she was out shopping when she started to smell a strange odour. Her mother then tearfully describes her daughter falling limp to the ground, before going rigid with her arms flexed to her chest. This was followed by a rhythmic jerking of her arms and legs which lasted about 3 minutes. She lay there slightly confused for about 10 minutes afterwards, by which time the ambulance had arrived. She found blood in her mouth when she fully roused. She does not drink or smoke.

CASE 5

A 25 year old solicitor presents to A&E after having been found unconscious by his girlfriend. He had been out jogging and suddenly complained of chest pain and palpitations before immediately collapsing. He was brought into A&E with bruises to his face. He had full recollection of the events.

CASE 6

A 47 year old former bus driver presents with a 1-month history of light-headedness and dizziness. Last week the symptoms were worse in the morning and evenings following taking his medication. He is a known diabetic with poorly controlled sugar results on his finger prick test. His GP had recently referred him for insulin initiation.

CASE 7

A 71 year old man complains of loss of consciousness that occurs episodically. He notices his dizzy spells are usually worse first thing in the morning after attempting to shave.

Chapter 1.12
Loss of vision

What to do . . .

- Introduce yourself to the patient – establish rapport
- Ask the patient's name, age and occupation
- Ask the patient relevant questions relating to their visual loss including onset, type and whether it is temporary or permanent
- Ask about any associated symptoms such as pain, floaters, headache, scalp tenderness, jaw claudication
- Ask about any past medical history, such as diabetes, AF, hypertension
- Take an ocular history, asking about glasses or contact lenses, previous surgery or recent trauma
- Ask about any drug history and for any drug allergies, e.g. amiodarone, steroids, chloroquine
- Ask about any social history – establish if the patient smokes
- Ask about any family history and specifically for close angle glaucoma and cataracts
- Perform a brief systems review and sum up your findings
- Thank the patient and conclude the consultation

Loss of vision describes the complete or partial loss of sight. It may occur suddenly or progress slowly over time and affect just one eye or involve both eyes simultaneously. It can be an alarming symptom to experience, not least because vision is an important part of daily life.

In the UK, there are approximately 300 000 people who are registered blind or partially sighted. The majority of these are elderly people with reduced activities of daily living who are unable to read, write or mobilize independently. As such, there are a number of financial benefits available, the levels of which depend on the degree of visual loss. Blindness is defined as a person having visual acuity of less than 3/60 whilst partial sightedness is between 3/60 and 6/60.

Loss of vision is broadly divided into two categories:
- visual loss that occurs suddenly – acute sudden loss of vision usually indicates a vascular aetiology such as a retinal artery or vein occlusion, stroke or vitreous haemorrhage; however, non-vascular causes such as retinal detachment, optic neuritis and glaucoma may be implicated
- gradual loss of vision over a period of time – gradual deterioration of vision is usually suggestive of a degenerative disease such as macular degeneration, diabetic retinopathy, cataracts or chronic glaucoma.

TOP TIP!

Only a consultant ophthalmologist can register a patient as blind or partially sighted.

1.12.1 **Taking the history**

As with any history, it is essential to begin by introducing yourself. Give your full name, job title and the reason for interviewing the patient. Ask the patient their name, age and occupation before enquiring specifically about their visual loss. Elderly patients have a higher prevalence of visual loss and this is primarily caused by age-related macular degeneration or glaucoma. Chronic visual loss in younger people may be caused by a congenital cataract or a retinoblastoma.

Knowing the patient's occupation may allow you to put into perspective the possible implications their loss of vision may have on their employment. Drivers are particularly affected by loss of vision and there are strict DVLA criteria as to who may drive or not.

Medical Guidelines
DVLA rules for visual loss

Visual disorders	Group I Drivers of motor cars and motorbikes	Group 2 Drivers of goods vehicles
Decreased visual acuity	Visual acuity of at least between 6/9 and 6/12	Corrected visual acuity must be at least less than 6/9 in the better eye. Uncorrected acuity cannot be worse than 3/60
Monocular vision	Need not notify DVLA	Barred from holding a Group 2 licence
Visual field defects	A field of vision of at least 120° on the horizontal with no defect in the binocular field within 20° of the meridian	Normal binocular field of vision is required

DVLA: At a glance guide to the current medical standards of fitness to drive (2011) – www.dft.gov.uk

Patients who are blind or partially sighted may enter the consultation room using a walking cane or a guide dog. It is courteous to stand up and assist or guide the patient to a chair to be seated. Be careful not to be overzealous as this may make the patient feel uncomfortable or patronized. In addition, it is useful to bear in mind that because they have poor vision they may be unable to pick up your non-verbal forms of communication such as body language, facial expression or other visual cues. Hence, extra attention and effort should be placed on your verbal communication.

1.12.2 **Ideas, concerns and expectations**

After appropriately introducing yourself and establishing rapport, it is useful to find out what the patient believes and what worries them about their visual loss. Common patient concerns include the implication their loss of vision may have on their occupation or whether their symptom may worsen or re-occur. Patients may be particularly concerned that they are suffering from or have experienced a stroke.

1.12.3 **History of presenting complaint**

Take a detailed history about the patient's loss of vision, establishing which eye is affected, when it started and how long it has been a problem. Also elicit any concurrent ocular symptoms such as pain, photophobia, blurry vision, discharge or systemic associations, e.g. headaches, nausea, rash and joint pain.

TOP TIP!

'Dry' AMD tends to cause a gradual fading of reading vision.

Onset

First it is appropriate to ask about the onset of the patient's symptoms. Did the visual loss occur suddenly or has it been gradually worsening over time? Did the patient wake up with loss of vision? Sudden visual loss is mostly vascular in origin, either by vascular occlusion or vitreous haemorrhage. For example, venous occlusion can present with sudden development of blurred vision in one eye, commonly on waking. A gradual deterioration of vision can be attributed to chronic processes such as dry AMD (age-related macular degeneration), diabetic retinopathy or cataracts.

Next try to establish whether the patient's visual loss was permanent or, if temporary, establish the speed of recovery. Sudden onset of temporary painless visual loss that lasts for a day, taking an appearance of a curtain falling down over the field of vision of one eye, is strongly suggestive of an amaurosis fugax seen in a transient ischaemic attack. Patients are at a high risk of a stroke in the following days and may encounter recurrent symptoms.

Migraines present similarly and can easily be confused with an ischaemic event. The visual loss occurs in the early aura phase of the migraine and typically lasts for less than an hour. Visual loss can vary from scotomas, hemianopia to monocular blindness. Optic neuritis may also cause rapid temporary loss of vision but classically presents with severe pain affecting one eye. It usually lasts for several hours to a couple of days and patients report reduced colour vision, specifically with red desaturation.

Type

It is very important to ascertain the degree and type of visual loss, as this can often give you a strong clue as to the underlying cause. Ascertain if the loss of vision affects the whole eye, half the eye (hemianopia), or a partial segment, i.e. quadrant or an ill-defined area (scotoma). For example, unilateral monocular visual loss can be caused by damage to, or inflammation of the retina or optic nerve as seen in retinal detachment or retinal artery occlusion. Bitemporal hemianopia presents with loss of the outer vision in both eyes and usually indicates compression at the optic chiasm due to a pituitary tumour or aneurysm.

Patients may report poor central vision and describe an inability to recognize faces or read text. This is usually caused by macular degeneration or damage to the optic nerve. Patients with AMD can awaken with a dark patch in the centre of their vision that rapidly fades soon afterwards. It can easily be misconstrued as a ghost or a 'shadowy figure' and this can be a frightening experience.

Conversely, loss of peripheral vision, otherwise known as tunnel vision, can be caused by glaucoma or retinal disorders such as retinitis pigmentosa. Retinitis pigmentosa is an autosomal dominant condition that begins in adolescence and usually presents with gradual visual loss with night blindness.

Small, patchy visual loss can occur due to localized damage to the retina; this is found in diabetic retinopathy and retinal detachment.

Associated symptoms

Try to establish any other symptoms that occur in conjunction with the loss of vision. If the patient mentions pain, clarify whether the pain is within or around the eye, or occurs with eye movements. Optic neuritis presents with ophthalmoplegia (pain on eye movements), whereas pain within the eye with halos around lights at night, and nausea and vomiting, should raise the suspicion of an acute glaucoma.

Elderly patients complaining of a persistent headache, pain on combing their hair (scalp tenderness) or with chewing foods (jaw claudication) may require high dose steroids and a temporal artery biopsy to exclude giant cell arteritis.

Another condition that requires urgent attention is a retinal detachment. This presents with painless unilateral visual loss. However, patients may report early warning symptoms such as flashing lights and the appearance of a number of floaters that move despite the eye coming to a halt.

1.12.4 Past medical history

Take a detailed past medical history including any previous medical illness and any hospital admissions. Enquire about previous investigations and any operations the patient may have undergone, including eye surgery or the removal of cataracts. Establish whether the patient wears glasses or contact lenses and whether they are short- or long-sighted. Enquire specifically about diabetes, hypertension, atrial fibrillation and migraines.

Drug history

Ask the patient what medication they are currently on or have taken in the past. Do not forget also to ask about any OTC medications or herbal remedies that the patient has tried. Patients taking high-dose steroids may be at risk of developing glaucoma. There is also a theoretical risk of developing closed angle glaucoma after using agents such as tropicamide to cause mydriasis for an eye examination. Amiodarone has been shown to cause optic neuritis.

Social history

Enquire whether the patient has ever smoked and, if so, how many cigarettes a day and for how long. Smoking is an independent risk factor for ocular disease including AMD, glaucoma and the development of cataracts. It is also a cardiovascular risk factor and increases the risk of cerebrovascular events.

Family history

You should ask whether the patient has any first-degree relatives who suffer or have suffered from blindness or any type of visual impairment. Family history is a risk factor in acute angle glaucoma, retinitis pigmentosa and cataracts.

1.12.5 **Systems review**

Complete your history with a brief systems review. Ask the patient about relevant symptoms including red eye, nausea and vomiting, loss of appetite, changes in bowel habit, palpitations or neurological symptoms, or any muscle or joint pain, in order to check the patient's general health and wellbeing.

1.12.6 **Summing up**

Summarize your findings back to the patient and ask if they would like to add anything that you may have missed. Reassure your patient by coming to an agreement with them about what the next step will be, checking to make sure they understand what is going on. Ask them if they have any questions they would like you to answer. In addition, offer the patient information leaflets and discuss when you (or another health professional) will see them next. End the interview by thanking the patient. In an exam situation, deliver an appropriate summary to the examiner.

1.12.7 **Common clinical scenarios**

The following are a list of common loss of vision cases which you may encounter. For each one, consider:
- what the possible differential diagnosis could be
- what key features you would look for
- what questions you would ask to refine or confirm your diagnosis

You could use role play with a friend, using the histories in the cases below as a framework.

CASE 1
A 49 year old architect presents to A&E with severe eye pain which came on over the last hour. He has also been feeling sick and has vomited twice. He claims to see rainbow rings around lights and complains that his eyesight is failing. He is known to be long-sighted. His eye appears very red and angry looking. He has previously been diagnosed with essential hypertension.

CASE 2
A 54 year old shop-keeper presents to his GP complaining of sudden visual loss. He said that he noticed his vision was blurry and reduced on waking in the morning, especially centrally. He does not complain of any pain in the eye. He suffers from hypertension, high cholesterol and diabetes. He smokes 40 cigarettes a day and drinks 16 units of alcohol per week. Fundoscopy shows dilated, tortuous veins, cotton wool spots and flame-shaped haemorrhages.

CASE 3
A 21 year old fine arts student presents with a 1-day history of deteriorating visual loss preceded by severe eye pain of 3 days in her right eye. The pain was especially bad when she was drawing, and she complained that pale colours did not seem as bright. She has been diagnosed with multiple sclerosis and is taking the oral contraceptive pill.

CASE 4

A 78 year old woman presents with a 6-month history of gradually worsening vision particularly when reading. She states that she has noticed dark spots in the middle of her vision, especially when trying to knit. She often finds herself looking at things out of the corner of her eyes. Recently, she claims that telephone poles along the road appear slightly wavy to her. She does not drink or smoke.

CASE 5

A 41 year old complains of a 2-week history of noticing floaters and flashing lights. Today he described sudden onset of a loss of the lower segment of his vision. He is otherwise well and is short-sighted. He stated that 1 month ago he had been playing squash and was hit in his eye with the ball.

Chapter 1.13
Red eye

What to do . . .

- Introduce yourself to the patient – establish rapport
- Ask the patient's name, age and occupation
- Ask the patient relevant questions relating to their red eye including site, onset, visual acuity
- Ask about any associated symptoms such as pain, photophobia, itchiness, discharge
- Ask about any past medical history such as connective tissue or systemic diseases, e.g. rheumatoid arthritis, ankylosing spondylitis, inflammatory bowel disease
- Take an ocular history, asking about contact lens use, previous surgery, or recent trauma
- Ask about any drug history and for any drug allergies, e.g. atropine, warfarin
- Ask about any social history – ask if the patient smokes and about alcohol intake
- Ask about any family history and specifically for close angle glaucoma
- Perform a brief systems review and sum up your findings
- Thank the patient and conclude the consultation

Red eye describes an abnormal reddish appearance to the eye; it is a fairly common problem that usually presents in primary care or A&E. Although the majority of cases are often simple and non-life threatening, more serious conditions may occasionally be implicated. Red eyes generate much fear in the hearts of patients and doctors alike due to the potentially devastating complication of blindness if the wrong diagnosis is made (see *Box 1.13*).

A red eye may be caused by infection, inflammation or allergies affecting a number of structures within the eye, including the conjunctiva, sclera, episclera or uveal tract. It may present suddenly or gradually build up over time. Red eyes commonly present with pain and this is often a useful symptom to help discriminate between benign and more serious conditions.

TOP TIP!

The most common causes of red eye include infectious or allergic conjunctivitis.

TOP TIP!

Change in visual acuity with a red eye should warrant immediate investigation.

BOX 1.13 **Red flags in red eye**

- Sudden, severe pain and vomiting
- Zoster skin rash
- Decreased visual acuity
- Corneal crater
- Branching, dendritic corneal lesion
- Ocular pressure >40 mmHg

1.13.1 **Taking the history**

Begin by introducing yourself to the patient, stating your name and job title. Confirm the patient's name, age and occupation. Knowing the patient's age may narrow down the potential list of differentials; for example, in young people the most common cause of a red eye is conjunctivitis. However, in the elderly you should always consider acute glaucoma as a possible cause due to its increased prevalence in this group.

Occupation can also be relevant. Patients who use power tools or are welders may suffer from corneal abrasions or an arc eye. Gardeners and domestic cleaners can be exposed to chemicals such as pesticides or detergents that can trigger allergic conjunctivitis.

1.13.2 **Ideas, concerns and expectations**

Establish the patient's own thoughts and perceptions as to what may be causing their symptoms. This may prompt them to reveal any recent history of trauma or possible allergen exposure that may be implicated. Patients may have heightened concerns about their red eye because people value the importance of their vision to maintain a good quality of life, and so most patients are likely to be very concerned about becoming partially sighted or even completely blind. Such concerns may make the patient request or expect an urgent specialist referral to see an ophthalmologist.

Spend some time enquiring about how the eye symptoms have affected the patient's life and whether they are interfering with their normal daily activities. Are they able to read a newspaper or watch the television as normal?

1.13.3 **History of presenting complaint**

Take a detailed history about their red eye establishing which eye is affected, when it started and how long it has been a problem. Also elicit any concurrent ocular symptoms such as pain, photophobia, blurry vision, discharge or systemic associations such as headaches, nausea, rash and joint pain.

Site

Do not immediately assume from observing the patient's appearance that only one eye is affected. Asking the patient directly may reveal symptoms in the other eye that may have otherwise been overlooked. Unilateral redness may be due to a subconjunctival haemorrhage which is usually painless and resolves spontaneously. It often presents as a blood-shot eye with no visual disturbances and it can be associated with raised blood pressure or clotting disorders. However, a subconjunctival haemorrhage following even minor trauma may warrant further investigation to exclude orbital haematoma or penetrating injury. If both eyes are affected this is usually due to conjunctivitis.

Onset

Find out when the red eye first started: did it occur suddenly or has it been gradually worsening? Did the red eye start in one eye before affecting the other? Infective conjunctivitis, such as through viral or bacterial infection, can present in one eye before spreading to the other. This may be caused by the patient inadvertently rubbing the eye and contaminating the unaffected one. Patients

BOX 1.14 **Distinguishing features of the common causes of red eye**

	Conjunctivitis	Anterior uveitis	Acute glaucoma
Pain	+/− (gritty)	++ (boring)	++ to +++ (ache)
Photophobia	+	+++	+
Acuity	Normal	Reduced	Reduced
Cornea	Normal	Normal	Steamy/hazy
Pupil	Normal	Small irregular	Fixed dilated oval
Intraocular pressure	Normal	Normal	Raised

TOP TIP!

Acute presentations of a red eye are often more serious than chronic cases. If preceded by other symptoms such as blurred vision and halos at night, consider a classical presentation of acute glaucoma. Other conditions such as anterior uveitis often present with an acute painful red eye.

mention a gritty sensation and a watery discharge with sticky eyes first thing in the morning (see *Box 1.14*).

Nature

It is very important to ascertain the degree and characteristics of the red eye, as this can often give you a strong clue as to the underlying cause. A red eye can be monocular or binocular and the redness may occur in different parts of the eye. For example, in episcleritis the inflammation is often seen beneath the conjunctiva and the sclera may look blue beneath the engorged vessels. This is unlike scleritis where the engorged vessels are deeper. Both conditions, however, may be associated with connective tissue disorders.

Visual acuity

In patients with red eye, it is important to check whether there is any evidence of a decrease in their visual acuity, as this can often be a poor prognostic indicator and may be associated with severe pathology. Decreased visual acuity is commonly seen in acute closed angle glaucoma (see *Box 1.15*) whereby the patients complain of severe ocular pain, moderate photophobia and nausea and vomiting. Symptoms are made worse with mydriasis, such as watching TV in a dark room and improved by going to sleep because the pupil constricts, thus relieving the attack. Patients may report halos being seen around lights and they may have a fixed dilated pupil.

Other causes of reduced visual acuity include anterior uveitis. The patient complains of ocular pain, and there is a marked degree of associated photophobia. Patients may also have an element of ciliary flushing and may even have an irregular small pupil.

TOP TIP!

Patients who are short-sighted (myopic) are at risk of primary open angle glaucoma whilst long-sighted (hypermetropic) people are at risk of acute closed angle glaucoma.

TOP TIP!

Visual loss is one of the most important symptoms to enquire about with an acute red eye because any deterioration in vision may become irreversible and could potentially affect the other eye. Pupillary reflexes or shapes may also give a clue to the diagnosis such as the small irregular pupil associated with anterior uveitis.

BOX 1.15 **Features of acute closed angle glaucoma**

- Acute pain, hazy corneal appearance
- Halos seen around bright lights, particularly in those over the age of 50 years
- Reduced visual acuity, nausea and vomiting
- Fixed dilated pupil, hard tense eye on palpation

Associated symptoms

These have a very important role in distinguishing between the causes of red eye. Ask the patient if they have noticed any other symptoms with their red eye, particularly with regard to the presence or absence of pain.

Pain, as described before, is a useful measure of the severity of a red eye. Pain can be described as boring, burning, a dull ache or as a gritty irritation. An insidious onset of severe, boring pain that is associated with gradual photophobia and possible visual impairment should make you consider scleritis. A burning itchy eye that occurs seasonally and is associated with nasal congestion and sneezing should make you think of allergic conjunctivitis.

Corneal ulcers are another cause of a severely painful red eye and, due to their ability to cause perforations, they are considered an ophthalmic emergency. Most ulcers are associated with viral or bacterial infections that are introduced following a break within the corneal epithelium. They may start as a result of previous damage to the cornea from a corneal abrasion or by poorly fitted contact lenses.

Discharge may be present with a red eye, such as with conjunctivitis. The consistency of the discharge may give you a clue as to whether the conjunctivitis is bacterial (more purulent), viral (more watery) or allergic (where the duration of symptoms may be more prolonged). It is important to take swabs, particularly in the newborn, to rule out bacterial or venereal infection.

1.13.4 Past medical history

Take a detailed past medical history including any previous medical illness and hospital admissions. Enquire about previous investigations and any operations the patient may have undergone, including any eye surgery. Do they see an optometrist regularly? Ask whether they have a history of connective tissue disease or systemic diseases such as ankylosing spondylitis, rheumatoid arthritis, Behçet's disease, sarcoidosis or inflammatory bowel disease. These can all have serious ophthalmic complications leading to a loss of vision. In patients with prolonged conjunctivitis chlamydial infection should be considered and so it is important to ask about sexual history.

Past ocular history

Take a brief ocular history asking specifically about previous episodes of red eye, any recent trauma or contact lens use. Prolonged use of contact lenses can put you at risk of developing keratitis. If left in overnight and not replaced this may increase the risk of forming corneal ulcers.

Specifically enquire about trauma, however minor it may appear to have been. If there is trauma, you must elicit whether the patient has a foreign body sensation as this may lead to scarring if not removed promptly.

Drug history

Ask the patient what medication they are currently taking or have taken in the past. Do not forget to also ask about any OTC medications or herbal remedies that the patient has tried. Atropine and other parasympathetic drugs can often worsen the pain of acute glaucoma because they cause the pupils to dilate and block drainage of aqueous humour from the anterior chamber via the canal of Schlemm. Patients on anticoagulation therapy may be predisposed to having subconjunctival haemorrhages. Do not forget to ask about drug allergies or intolerances.

Social history

Enquire if the patient has ever smoked and, if so, how many cigarettes a day and for how long. Establish whether they drink alcohol and, if so, note the type of alcohol and how many units a week. Discreetly ask about illicit drug use. Also ask about contacts with similar symptoms of red eye.

Family history

You should enquire whether the patient has any first-degree relatives who suffer or have suffered from visual impairment resulting from red eye. Closed angle glaucoma can run in families.

1.13.5 Systems review

Complete your history with a brief systems review. Ask the patient about relevant symptoms, including eye pain or visual loss. You may also wish to enquire more generally about common symptoms such as nausea and vomiting, loss of appetite, changes in bowel habit, neurological symptoms or any muscle or joint pain, in order to check the patient's general health and wellbeing and establish if there is a possible connective tissue disease.

1.13.6 Summing up

Summarize your findings back to the patient and ask if they would like to add anything that you may have missed. Reassure your patient by coming to an agreement with them about what the next step will be, checking to make sure they understand what is going on. Ask them if they have any questions they would like you to answer. In addition, offer the patient information leaflets and discuss when you (or another health professional) will see them next. End the interview by thanking the patient. In an exam situation, deliver an appropriate summary to the examiner.

1.13.7 Common clinical scenarios

The following are a list of common red eye cases which you may encounter. For each one, consider:
• what the possible differential diagnosis could be
• what key features you would look for
• what questions you would ask to refine or confirm your diagnosis

You could use role play with a friend, using the histories in the cases below as a framework.

CASE 1

A 42 year old salesman presents to A&E with severe eye pain that came on over the last hour. He has been feeling quite unwell and has vomited in the waiting room. He claims to see circular rings around lights and cries that he has gone blind. It initially started when watching TV in a dark room.

CASE 2

A 4 year old boy presents with a 2-day history of redness and irritation initially in the left eye which also now affects the right eye. He complains that both eyes feel itchy and burning and are sticky and closed in the morning. There is also a thin watery discharge. He has recently recovered from a viral upper respiratory tract infection. He had a normal birth at full term and did not require any special care. There is no relevant family history. He lives at home with his parents and is an only child.

CASE 3

A 46 year old cab driver of Turkish origin presents to his GP complaining of sore, red eyes. He said that he noticed his vision was blurry and that the pain worsened in light. He also complains of mouth ulcers as well as generalized joint pain. He has a past medical history of genital ulcers and arthritis. He smokes 20 cigarettes a day and does not drink.

CASE 4

A 36 year old ward clerk presents with an intermittent history of mild dull ache and red eyes over the last year. It affects her every 6–8 weeks for 2–3 weeks at a time. She has been told it may be conjunctivitis in the past, though she has never experienced any discharge. She currently suffers with Crohn's disease and has no relevant family history. She does not smoke and drinks 16 units of alcohol per week.

CASE 5

A 41 year old metal-shop worker presents with a 2-day history of redness in his left eye. His eye has become extremely painful and his vision has become affected. On further questioning he describes focal irritation especially when blinking.

Chapter 1.14
Hearing loss

What to do . . .

- Introduce yourself to the patient – establish rapport
- Ask the patient's name, age and occupation
- Ask the patient relevant questions relating to their hearing loss including site, onset and nature
- Ask about any associated symptoms, such as pain, fever, vertigo, tinnitus and discharge
- Enquire about how their symptoms have affected their life
- Ask about any past medical history, such as previous ear infection or grommets
- Ask about any drug history and for any drug allergies, e.g. gentamicin, furosemide, aspirin
- Ask about any social history – establish if the patient smokes and ask about alcohol intake
- Ask about any family history and specifically for osteogenesis imperfecta, otosclerosis
- Perform a brief systems review and sum up your findings
- Thank the patient and conclude the consultation

Hearing loss is a problem that may be experienced at any age; however, it is more commonly seen in the elderly. It is usually categorized as mild, moderate or severe (see *Box 1.16*) and can lead to a reduced quality of life, as hearing plays an integral part in communication and social interaction. Patients often live an isolated life as they can be acutely embarrassed when repeatedly asking people to speak up. They may even try and mask their disability by lip reading or gaining clues from the speaker's gestures.

The ear auricle, canal and ear drum constitute the outer ear and help capture and amplify environmental sounds before passing it into the middle ear. The middle ear runs from the ear drum to the inner ear and contains, amongst other things, three small bones called the malleus, the incus, and stapes. These act to convert

BOX 1.16 **Degrees of hearing loss**	
Normal hearing	0–20 dB
Mild hearing impairment	21–40 dB
Moderate hearing impairment	41–55 dB
Moderately severe impairment	56–70 dB
Severe hearing impairment	71–95 dB
Profound hearing impairment	≥95 dB

audible sounds into tiny vibrations that are modified and conducted into the inner ear. The inner ear consists of the bony labyrinth that encompasses both the cochlear and vestibular systems and is responsible for receiving sound, and also for controlling balance and orientation. Vibrations are then converted into electrical impulses that are fed into the brain.

Depending on which part of the ear is affected, hearing loss may be classified as:
- conductive – may be caused by impaction of the external canal with wax or a foreign body, damage to the ear drum by perforation or infection, collection of fluid behind the tympanic membrane by a middle ear effusion or otosclerosis
- sensorineural – can be congenital, caused by old age (presbycusis), ototoxic drugs, acoustic neuroma and infections such as meningitis, mumps or measles.

1.14.1 Taking the history

Introduce yourself to the patient by mentioning your name and job title. Establish the patient's name, age and occupation. The patient's age may provide a clue as to what the potential cause of hearing loss may be, for example, in an elderly patient bilateral gradually worsening hearing loss may be due to presbycusis, whereas in a young child with acute hearing loss, ear pain and fever the most likely cause is otitis media.

Finding out about the patient's current or previous occupations may reveal a possible cause. Exposure to regular loud sounds greater than 80 dB can cause permanent hearing damage. Jobs such as DJs, road-workers, process or factory workers and infantry may expose the patient to unhealthy levels of excessive sounds.

Begin by asking open questions regarding their symptoms before asking more directed questions related to the nature of their hearing loss. It is often useful when dealing with patients with severe hearing loss to ask them how they usually communicate – some patients are happy to lip read whilst others may prefer things written down.

1.14.2 Ideas, concerns and expectations

After appropriately introducing yourself and establishing rapport, try to establish what the patient themselves believes is the cause of their hearing loss. Patients may recall a specific event or episode that they feel is implicated in the cause of their symptoms, e.g. attendance at a rock concert or scuba diving. Patients may reveal underlying anxieties and concerns about their hearing loss; common concerns include the need to use hearing aids for the rest of their life, or parental concern about language development in a younger child.

1.14.3 History of presenting complaint

Site

Begin by establishing whether the patient's hearing loss affects both ears (bilateral) or only one ear (unilateral). Patients with bilateral hearing loss are likely to be suffering from presbycusis or environmentally induced hearing loss.

TOP TIP!

Employers are legally bound to provide ear protector equipment. People who have suffered from occupational hearing loss are eligible for compensation.

TOP TIP!

Just because the patient is hard of hearing does not mean they have a low IQ. Do not act in a condescending manner towards them.

Bilateral hearing loss may also be due to ototoxic drugs or otosclerosis. Unilateral deafness may be caused by trauma, acoustic neuroma or cholesteatoma.

Onset

Ask the patient when they first noticed the hearing loss. Did it start suddenly or has it been gradually getting worse? Sudden onset hearing loss may be due to an acute head injury, ear drum perforation, barotrauma or Ménière's disease. Gradual onset hearing loss with a more insidious onset can occur with age (presbycusis), otosclerosis and ototoxic drugs. Patients who have suffered from hearing loss since childhood may have been exposed to an *in utero* infection such as measles, mumps or rubella.

Character

Ask the patient to describe the nature of the hearing loss – are they unable to hear high pitched sounds or low volume soft whispers?

In high pitched hearing loss, patients lose the ability to hear certain consonant letters such as 'c', 'd', 'k', 'p', 's' and 't'. People's speech may become more difficult to follow and understand, appearing mumbled even if the volume is maintained. Patients may find it difficult to follow a conversation particularly in a crowd where the sound is drowned out by background noise – this is commonly seen in presbycusis.

Low frequency hearing loss is often asymptomatic unless profound and is usually picked up on audiometry studies. It can be seen in glue ear where the effusion behind the ear drum dampens down the degree of vibrations.

Associated symptoms

Go on to establish whether the patient has noticed any other symptoms along with their hearing loss. A painful ear can signify an infective or traumatic process. Occasionally, impacted wax can cause significant discomfort in the ear and cause conductive hearing loss. Fever is a good indicator of infection and may confirm the presence of otitis media or externa as a possible cause.

Ask specifically about ringing in the ear (tinnitus), dizziness/vertigo, discharge or any neurological symptoms such as facial weakness. Severe attacks of vertigo combined with fluctuating deafness, tinnitus and a feeling of pressure in the affected ear are characteristic of Ménière's disease. This commonly affects middle-aged people with episodes lasting from minutes to hours and with vertigo being the most prominent feature. If the hearing loss presents with vertigo, tinnitus and café au lait (milky coffee-coloured) patches, an acoustic neuroma secondary to neurofibromatosis must be excluded. Cerumen build-up can result in partial hearing loss associated with earache, a sensation of fullness and tinnitus.

Impact

It is important to assess the impact the hearing loss has on the patient's life. Are they still able to understand speech or locate the source of a sound? Are they able to communicate with friends and family? Can they still perform their duties at work? If the impact on the patient's life is significant, consider performing a brief depression screen.

DIFFERENTIAL DIAGNOSIS

Conductive
- Ear wax
- Otitis media
- Otitis externa
- Ear drum perforation
- Foreign body
- Otosclerosis
- Cholesteatoma

Sensorineural
- Presbycusis
- Ototoxic drugs
- Noise exposure
- Ménière's disease
- *In utero* infections
- Acoustic neuroma

1.14.4 **Past medical history**

Take a detailed past medical history including any previous medical illness, investigations or previous procedures such as grommet insertions, tympanectomy or myringoplasty. Enquire about any recent operations the patient may have undergone because there is an association with general anaesthesia as a cause of sensorineural hearing loss. Specifically enquire about recurrent ear infections and possible ear injury that can be caused by air travel, strenuous exercise, weight lifting, or diving.

Drug history

Ask the patient what medication they are currently on or have taken in the past. Do not forget to also ask about any OTC medications or herbal remedies that the patient has tried. A common cause of hearing loss is ototoxicity and is suggested by the recent initiation of a new drug. Although there are a wide variety of ototoxic drugs, the most commonly used include gentamicin, furosemide, NSAIDs, salicylates and chemotherapy such as cisplatin and vincristine.

Social history

Enquire whether the patient has smoked and if so, how many cigarettes a day and for how long. Also establish whether they drink alcohol and, if so, note the type of alcohol and how many units a week.

Family history

Find out if there are any first-degree relatives who have suffered with hearing loss. Hearing loss can be inherited in both a dominant and autosomal recessive manner. Osteogenesis imperfecta is an autosomal dominant bone disorder that affects the ability to make connective tissue or collagen. There are eight types differing in their severity; however, they broadly present with brittle bones, blue sclera and hearing loss. Otosclerosis is another autosomal dominant condition that affects the stapes. The bone is replaced by vascular spongy bone which has reduced ability to transmit sound and results in conductive hearing loss. It affects younger adults and is usually bilateral. Patients paradoxically report an improvement in hearing when in a noisy environment.

1.14.5 **Systems review**

Complete your history with a brief systems review. Ask the patient about relevant symptoms such as problems with nausea and vomiting. You may also wish to ask more generally about common symptoms such as changes in bowel habit, chest pain, palpitations or neurological symptoms, or any muscle or joint pain, in order to check the patient's general health and wellbeing.

1.14.6 **Summing up**

Summarize your findings back to the patient and ask if they would like to add anything that you may have missed. Reassure your patient by coming to an agreement with them about what the next step will be, checking to make sure they understand what is going on. Ask them if they have any questions they would like you to answer. In addition, offer the patient information leaflets and discuss when you (or another health professional) will see them next. End the interview by thanking the patient and, in an exam situation, deliver an appropriate summary to the examiner.

1.14.7 **Common clinical scenarios**

The following are a list of common hearing loss cases which you may encounter.
For each one, consider:
- what the possible differential diagnosis could be
- what key features you would look for
- what questions you would ask to refine or confirm your diagnosis

You could use role play with a friend, using the histories in the cases below as a framework.

CASE 1
A 7 year old presents to his GP with a 3-day history of difficulty hearing out of his left ear. He also complains of severe pain inside his left ear that resolved after noticing a watery discharge on his pillow in the mornings. He was suffering from a minor cold last week.

CASE 2
A 21 year old medical student presents to his GP complaining of difficulty hearing his consultant during ward rounds. He says that it has gradually become more and more difficult to hear though surprisingly it improves in noisy areas. He also at times notices a ringing in his ears. His parents have complained that he never listens. He has no past medical history of note but his uncle is known to suffer from deafness.

CASE 3
A 17 year old cheerleader presents with a 2-week history of problems with her hearing, balance and vision. She also complains of a ringing noise in her ears and occasional headache. She also noticed some numbness and weakness to the left side of the face after applying some makeup. She has no past medical history of note and is currently taking the oral contraceptive pill. Her uncle died from a brain tumour. She claims not to smoke or drink.

CASE 4
A 28 year old ward clerk presents to A&E with a 4 hour history of dizziness, nausea and vomiting and fluctuating hearing loss in the right ear. She also complains of some tinnitus as well as fullness to the same ear. She has no past medical history of note. She drinks 10 units of alcohol per week on average and does not smoke.

CASE 5
A 62 year old retired civil engineer presents with a 3-month history of gradually worsening hearing loss. He first noticed it when he struggled to hear people speak, and has particular difficulty with his hearing in a noisy room. He has no sensation of vertigo and does not report any tinnitus. He drinks 20 units of alcohol per week on average and smokes 15 cigarettes a day.

CASE 6

A 12 year old boy presents with a 2-week history of gradually worsening hearing loss. He has no other associated symptoms. His mum is also concerned about his height, claiming he is the shortest in his class. He has previously been to A&E for a fractured wrist and arm within the last year. His father was diagnosed with a 'bone problem' as a child.

Chapter 1.15
Depression

What to do . . .

- Introduce yourself to the patient – establish rapport
- Ask the patient's name, age and occupation
- Ask the patient relevant questions relating to their depression including onset and triggers
- Ask about core symptoms including low mood, anhedonia and fatiguability
- Ask about cognitive symptoms such as hopelessness, helplessness, poor concentration, guilt
- Ask about biological symptoms such as insomnia, early morning waking, poor appetite, loss of libido
- Check for evidence of psychosis or bipolar disorder
- Ask if the patient has any suicidal ideation
- Ask about past medical history, e.g. chronic disease
- Ask about any past psychiatric history, e.g. schizophrenia, depression
- Ask about any drug history and for any drug allergies
- Ask about any social history – establish if the patient is in a relationship or has children; establish if the patient smokes or drinks alcohol
- Ask about any family history and specifically for suicide or depression
- Perform a risk assessment and sum up your findings
- Thank the patient and conclude the consultation

Depression is a mental disorder characterized by persistent low mood and lack of pleasure in performing normally pleasurable activities (anhedonia). It is the most common mental disorder encountered by GPs with up to two-thirds of adults having a bout of depression significant enough to affect their life. The exact aetiology of depression is unknown, although it is believed that there is an interaction between a number of different factors including genetic, psychosocial and environmental.

Whilst many patients may have low mood it does not necessarily mean that they are clinically depressed. The diagnosis of depression is made by eliciting the presence of two core depressive symptoms that the patient has suffered from over the last 2 weeks. These include having low mood, lack of energy or fatiguability (anergia), and anhedonia. The presence of two out of these three features makes the diagnosis of depression highly likely and should prompt further enquiry about the presence of other biological or cognitive symptoms. The absence of core symptoms reduces the likelihood of a depressive disorder.

Depression can vary in intensity and can range from a mild single episode to a severe recurrent lifelong disorder. People who have experienced an episode

TOP TIP!

Always consider the differential of a bipolar disorder in a patient with depression, particularly if they have periods of elation between bouts of depression.

of depression are at risk of developing another in the future. Patients may also present predominantly with biological symptoms also known as 'somatic depression'. Patients with severe depression may also harbour delusion or even auditory hallucinations.

Depression can be a serious and often disabling disorder that may negatively affect a patient's social life, work and relationships. In approximately 4% of cases the depression will be severe enough to lead them to take their own life. It is therefore essential that when taking a depression history the physician obtains enough information to make a diagnosis and classify its severity, whilst also assessing suicidal risk and intent. Based upon these findings, appropriate management, treatment and support care can be arranged.

1.15.1 Taking the history

Begin your depression history by introducing yourself to the patient by telling them your name and job title. Ask the patient their name, age, and occupation. Depression occurs most commonly in adolescence and peaks again in middle age. The patient's gender is also important, with depression affecting men more than twice as frequently as women. However, major depressive episodes are four times more common in women than men.

Knowing whether a patient is in employment is also relevant when taking a depression history. The unemployed experience depression twice as often compared to people in full-time employment. However, do not forget to consider that stressors experienced in employment, such as being threatened with redundancy, failure to be promoted or being in a mundane or repetitive job can be also source of low mood and dissatisfaction.

Establishing rapport in a depression history is extremely important. Depressed patients are usually withdrawn and so display little eye contact and spontaneity. The clinician must work hard to try to establish rapport and gain the patient's trust and respect.

- Use pauses appropriately and reflect back to the patient at regular intervals. Pitch the tone and speed of your voice at a similar level to that set by the patient – this will create a favourable environment in which the consultation can flow.
- Ensure that you show empathy throughout and respond appropriately to any verbal or non-verbal cues. A patient may state that they feel 'all right' whilst their facial expression and body demeanour may indicate otherwise. This is an important non-verbal cue that should be pursued.
- Be ready for the patient to possibly break into tears because of their emotional instability – keep a box of tissues to hand.

> **TOP TIP!**
>
> Make use of reflection because it shows you are listening and opens up new discussions.

1.15.2 Ideas, concerns and expectations

After appropriately introducing yourself and establishing rapport, it is important to establish what the patient believes may be the cause of their depression. This will allow the patient to contextualize their symptoms and may provide you with key information that you may have otherwise missed. Spend some time exploring the patient's concerns about their problem and how they have been coping.

> **Medical Guidelines**
> *Depression definitions (taken from DSM-IV)*
>
> ---
>
> **Symptoms of depression:**
>
> Key symptoms: persistent sadness or low mood and/or marked loss of interest or pleasure; at least one of these, most days, most of the time for at least 2 weeks
> If any of above present, ask about associated symptoms:
>
> * disturbed sleep (decreased or increased compared to usual)
> * decreased or increased appetite and/or weight
> * fatigue or loss of energy
> * agitation or slowing of movements
> * poor concentration or indecisiveness
> * feelings of worthlessness or excessive or inappropriate guilt
> * suicidal thoughts or acts
>
> **Sub-threshold depressive symptoms:** fewer than five of the associated symptoms of depression.
>
> **Mild depression:** few, if any, symptoms in excess of the five required to make the diagnosis, and symptoms result in only minor functional impairment.
>
> **Moderate depression:** symptoms or functional impairment are between 'mild' and 'severe'.
>
> **Severe depression:** most symptoms, and the symptoms markedly interfere with functioning – can occur with or without psychotic symptoms.
>
> *NICE Guidelines: Depression, the treatment and management of depression in adults (2009)*

1.15.3 **History of presenting complaint**

Begin your depression history by establishing when the patient's symptoms first started. Ask open questions to allow the patient to fully express themselves using their own words. Try to elicit any triggers that may have precipitated the depressive episode such as relationship breakdowns, loss of a job, or death of a loved one. Try to gain enough background information to get an insight into how the patient has been coping up until now.

Next go on to ask specific questions to try to establish the core biological and cognitive symptoms.

Core symptoms

Once you have established the background information, assess for the presence of the diagnostic symptoms of depression:

* check whether the patient has been feeling low for at least the past 2 weeks
* does the patient still enjoy undertaking or performing activities that they would normally consider pleasurable (anhedonia)?
* does the patient feel constantly tired and easily fatigued for no apparent reason?

If two of these symptoms are present then the patient can be formally diagnosed with an episode of depression.

Cognitive symptoms

The cognitive theory of depression (a theory postulated by Beck) states that the symptoms of depression are often a direct result of harbouring negative thoughts. These thoughts then create negative feeling that spirals downwards into depression. Such thoughts may be directed against oneself, the immediate environment or may even be about the future.

Ask the patient about their ability to concentrate: are they able to follow a news broadcast or a newspaper article or are they easily distracted? Ask how they perceive themselves: do they lack self-esteem and self-belief? Do they feel worthless? Do they feel a sense of disproportionate guilt about simple minor failings that may have occurred? Are they preoccupied and consumed by it? How does the patient feel about their current predicament: do they feel helpless and hopeless for the future?

Depressed patients usually suffer from poor concentration and weakened memory. They often feel a sense of guilt and responsibility for their situation with poor self-belief. They may feel alone and helpless with a negative and pessimistic view of their future outlook.

Biological symptoms

Depression can affect the mind as well as the body. Enquire about the patient's sleep habits. Have they changed recently; do they have trouble going to sleep? Do they find themselves waking up early in the morning with difficulty returning to sleep (early morning waking)? How is their mood first thing in the morning and does it improve throughout the remainder of the day (diurnal variation)? Patients suffering from depression may experience a range of biological symptoms including early morning waking, whereby they wake from sleep several hours before they intended and struggle to return to sleep thereafter. Patients may also find difficulty in getting to sleep and instead lie in bed ruminating about minor failings in their life. Upon waking their mood is at its lowest point but it usually gradually improves as the day progresses.

Move on now to ask about the patient's appetite and eating habits. Have they gone off food and noticed a reduction in their weight and appetite or conversely do they comfort eat and unexpectedly put weight on? These are atypical depressive features. Depressed patients often experience a loss of interest in eating food which may be severe enough to cause significant weight loss.

Ask the patient whether friends or family have noticed or commented that their actions, appearance, as well as train of thought appear to be slow and lethargic (psychomotor retardation).

If the patient is currently in a relationship ask whether they have noticed a lack of interest in sex (loss of libido) – this is common in depression.

Associated symptoms

Depression on occasions can be severe enough to cause a range of psychotic symptoms such as experiencing auditory or tactile hallucinations or complex fixed delusions. Ask the patient if they have ever seen or heard anything that others have not noticed. If they hear voices ask what they say and whether they were praising or accusatory in nature.

Severely depressed patients may experience second person auditory hallucinations that are negative in nature and are critical of their patient. They may also experience mood congruent delusions whereby the intensity of the delusion is directly linked to their mood. Patients may even believe that they have died or that their internal organs are rotting (Cotard's syndrome).

Check whether the patient displays other symptoms that may indicate other diagnoses such as bipolar disorder. Has the patient ever felt disproportionately

BOX 1.17 **Psychiatric conditions that may present with depression**

Psychiatric	Bipolar disorder (manic depression), generalized anxiety disorder (GAD), bereavement disorder, somatization disorder, post-traumatic stress disorder (PTSD)
Organic mental disorders	Delirium (acute confusional state), subcortical dementias, frontal lobe dysfunction, neuroleptic-induced parkinsonism

elated or undertaken acts such as spending excessively or engaged in promiscuous activity?

Suicidal ideation

Depressed patients may feel so low that they are preoccupied with death and even taking their own life. As there is clear evidence that shows that depressed patients have an increased risk of attempted suicide, all patients whom you suspect to be depressed should have a formal suicide risk assessment; ask the patient:

- have you ever thought about taking your own life?
- how often do you get these thoughts?
- have you taken them seriously and made any plans or do you resist them?

Past psychiatric history

Ask the patient if they suffer from any other psychiatric illnesses (see *Box 1.17*). Schizophrenia may present with depression and is known as schizoaffective disorder. If the patient has suffered from any previous psychiatric illness, take a more detailed history enquiring about its onset, episodes, treatments, any admissions or sectioning, or whether they have seen a psychiatrist.

1.15.4 Past medical history

Take a detailed past medical history including any previous medical illness and any hospital admissions. A patient with a history of thyroid disease, particularly hypothyroidism, may present with low mood and depression. Studies have shown that patients suffering with two or more chronic diseases are at a higher risk of being depressed.

Drug history

Ask the patient what medication they are currently on or have taken in the past. Do not forget to also ask about any OTC medications or herbal remedies that the patient has tried. It is important to be thorough because many drugs including corticosteroids, the contraceptive pill, ranitidine, indomethacin and vincristine may cause depression.

Social history

Enquire whether the patient has ever smoked and, if so, how many cigarettes a day and for how long. Establish whether they drink alcohol and, if so, note the type of alcohol and how many units a week they drink. Discreetly ask about illict drug use. Drugs and alcohol are common causes of depression, and drugs such as heroin or cannabis in particular have a depressant effect on the patient's mood.

Ask the patient whether they are currently in employment and, if so, check what type of employment it is. Next establish if the patient is single or in a relationship. Confirm if they have any children or not. Finally, ask about any support systems they may have in place such as friends or family. Patients with extended support networks usually have better prognosis with their depression.

Family history

It is important to enquire whether the patient has any first-degree relatives who have seen a psychiatrist or suffered from any mental illness. You should ask specifically about a family history of depression.

Insight

Try to establish whether the patient has insight into their condition. Does the patient believe they have a problem and do they feel they need help for it? Patients who have insight and are aware of their mental illness tend to fare better.

1.15.5 Summing up

Summarize your findings back to the patient and ask if they would like to add anything that you may have missed. Having taken a detailed history, you must try to determine the severity of the patient's depression, because this will help determine whether the patient needs inpatient admission, outpatient follow-up or simple medication. Those patients who you deem to be high risk, i.e. have evidence of psychosis or suicidal ideation, are likely to need inpatient admission, whereas those who have good support networks and display a few of the classical features of depression may only need medication review and outpatient follow-up. End the interview by thanking the patient. In an exam situation deliver an appropriate summary to the examiner.

1.15.6 Common clinical scenarios

The following are a list of common depression cases which you may encounter. For each one, consider:
• what the severity of depression could be
• what key features you would look for
• what questions you would ask to refine or confirm your diagnosis

You could use role play with a friend, using the histories in the cases below as a framework.

CASE 1

A 32 year old unemployed lady presents complaining of low mood and tearfulness for the past 2 months since losing her job as an office secretary. Previously an outgoing person, she has found herself lying in bed feeling tired all the time. She has no interest in watching television or reading novels. She wakes at 5am when her mood is at its lowest. She has no previous medical or psychiatric illness. She feels guilty because she is no longer bringing any money into the household and has lost interest in sex. She has had no thoughts of harming herself. She denies any hallucinations or abnormal delusions or episodes of mania.

CASE 2

A 27 year old mailroom clerk has been brought into hospital by his wife. He has recently been behaving very oddly. He has lost interest in reading, which was previously something he enjoyed. Instead he has been building car models which he only half finishes before moving on to the next. He often awakes around 6 am and demands sex from his wife, being aggressive if it is refused. He has been spending excessively in the last few days and has exceeded his credit card limit. He has previously been diagnosed with depression and has attempted to harm himself.

CASE 3

A 68 year old lady presents with a history of low mood which has not improved since her husband passed away 5 months ago. She has no interest in any of the activities which she formerly enjoyed. She sometimes feels like she is moving in slow motion. She blames herself for not looking after her husband properly and feels that she has nothing left to give to the world. She has no previous medical or psychiatric illness. She wishes to join her husband and is tired of life, though she has not made any suicide attempts so far. She denies any hallucinations or abnormal delusions or episodes of mania.

CASE 4

A 36 year old dentist presents complaining of low mood for the past 3 months. He has lost interest in most things and has stopped going in to work. He has difficulty falling asleep and wakes up around 5am or 6am feeling agitated and especially low. He claims he feels low because everyone at work hates him and his patients are plotting to harm him. He even states that his partners at his practice have bugged his phone and are desperate to sack him. He has thought about harming himself but has not actually made an attempt. He denies any episodes of mania. He has experienced similar episodes in the past and has had to take time off work.

Chapter 1.16
Suicide risk assessment

What to do . . .

- Introduce yourself to the patient – establish rapport
- Ask the patient's name, age and occupation
- Ask the patient relevant questions relating to their suicide attempt, including the planning (spontaneous or planned, did they make a will or leave a note?)
- Enquire specifically about the event and the method used
- Ask questions related to the period after the attempt (how did they feel, who discovered them?)
- Ask about any past medical history, e.g. MS, cancer, epilepsy
- Ask about any past psychiatric history, e.g. schizophrenia, obsessive–compulsive disorder, panic attacks
- Ask about any drug history and for any drug allergies
- Ask about any social history – establish if the patient is in a relationship or has children; enquire if the patient smokes or drinks alcohol
- Ask about any family history and specifically for suicide or depression
- Perform a risk assessment and sum up your findings
- Thank the patient and conclude the consultation

Suicide is defined as the final act of self-harm that was intended to end one's life prematurely. Parasuicide refers to the unsuccessful attempt at taking one's life. Both of these are subsets of deliberate self-harm where the individual undertakes or carries out an intentional act of self-mutilation.

There are fewer than 5000 recorded acts of suicide in the UK every year, although it is believed that this grossly underestimates real attempts at suicide by up to 50%. It is widely perceived that an act of suicide is an unplanned event made spontaneously following an acute adverse experience (see *Box 1.18*). However, on closer inspection studies have revealed that up to two-thirds of suicide attempts are in fact premeditated and planned in advance. It has also been found that up to 90% of people who had attempted suicide had some sort of suicide ideation or thoughts in the year prior to the attempt. It is therefore vital that a patient who displays suicidal intent is appropriately risk-assessed and referred to the relevant specialities based upon their degree of risk.

Deliberate self-harm can involve self-injury in the form of cutting one's wrists or taking an overdose of medication or another substance. Deliberate self-harm is extremely common, with several hundred thousand cases reported each year, particularly amongst young females. It is distinct from attempted suicide in that the patient does not intend to die but rather seeks to use this act to air their emotional grievances. Recent studies have shown that people who self-harm have a 10% chance of committing suicide, with the greatest risk occurring in the following year.

BOX 1.18 **Statistics about suicide**

- 90% of patients committing suicide have an underlying mental health disorder
- 70% of patients who have completed suicide suffered from depression
- Patients with personality disorder have a 7 times greater risk of suicide compared with the general population
- The lifetime risk of suicide in patients suffering from schizophrenia is approximately 9%

TOP TIP!

Clinicians often shy away from asking the obvious question: 'Have you thought about ending your life?' in fear of offending the patient or instilling this thought into their head. On the contrary, patients are often relieved to answer this question and are hopeful that their doctor will address this need.

Assessing the patient's suicide risk is not an exact science but depends on a number of epidemiological, environmental and clinical factors. You should attempt to elicit from the patient certain risk factors that would make them more likely to commit suicide, such as being unemployed, separated, suffering from mental health disorders, or previous suicide attempts. These risk factors should be balanced against any protective factors that may reduce the likelihood of the patient acting upon their ideations, such as being married, having children and strong moral or religious beliefs. To complete your assessment, perform a mental state examination and take into account the patient's current level of social support.

Having completed this you should now be in a position to state whether the patient has a low, medium or high risk of suicide and plan your management accordingly.

1.16.1 **Taking the history**

Begin your suicide assessment by introducing yourself to the patient, mentioning your name and job title. Establish the patient's name, age and whether they are in employment. The patient's gender, age and lack of employment are all risk factors for suicide. Elderly patients are more likely to commit suicide than young people, whilst suicide rates for men outnumber those for women by 3 to 1. Employment is considered to be a protective factor against suicide whilst unemployment or being retired increases one's risk. However, not all forms of employment lower the risk of suicide. Doctors, people in the armed forces, veterinary surgeons and farmers have a higher suicide rate compared with the general population.

Establishing rapport in a suicide risk assessment is extremely important because the lines of questioning clearly cover sensitive issues. By gaining the patient's trust they should feel more relaxed and more likely to discuss their innermost thoughts and plans. Assure the patient that what you discuss will be kept confidential and not shared with their relatives or work colleagues.

Try to show empathy and display active listening to the patient. Encourage them by using non-verbal forms of communication such as silence, nodding, pauses and reflection. Unfortunately there is no definitive test to determine exactly the probability of a patient attempting suicide; however, a thorough risk assessment hinges upon a good history.

1.16.2 **Suicide intent**

Having created rapport with the patient move on to try to elicit as much information as possible about the patient's intent to commit suicide. An effective way of doing this is to divide the attempt into stages, by considering the events leading up to the attempt, the attempt itself, and the state of mind of the patient after the attempt.

Before the attempt (planning)

Having knowledge about the degree of planning employed by the patient prior to attempting to end their life is a good indicator of future suicide risk. The more intricate and considered the plan is, the greater the chance the patient will attempt suicide again. Establish whether the patient planned their suicide attempt in advance or did they act spontaneously on a spur-of-the-moment impulse? Did the patient make a will, leave a suicide note or close any bank accounts? A young person who has just split up with their partner and tried to end their life is less likely to repeat the attempt compared to an individual who meticulously planned their suicide for several months in advance and left a will and a suicide note.

Did the patient tell anyone about their plans or did they make efforts to avoid being caught? A patient who had informed friends and family about their ideation is often less likely to perform the final act compared to a person who has driven some distance to be isolated from loved ones.

Ask the patient about their mood prior to the attempt. Had they been suffering from low mood or depression for a long time, or were there any recent grievances such as relationship breakdowns, bereavements or loss of a job? Patients who suffer from severe depression are at a very high risk of suicide and parasuicide attempts.

The attempt

Once you have a thorough understanding of the patient's state of mind prior to the attempt, and how well they had planned the attempt, you should begin to ask the patient about the suicide attempt itself. Establish the method used by the patient to try to take their own life. Did they use a weapon, try to take an overdose, jump from a height or even attempt to hang themselves? Research suggests that the more violent the mode of suicide attempted the stronger the intent to die is, and there is a higher risk of further attempts from these patients. For example, a person who went out and purchased an illegal firearm would be deemed a greater risk than an individual who overdosed with OTC medication.

> **TOP TIP!**
>
> In overdoses, try to establish what medication was taken and in what quantities. It is easy to assume that taking a low quantity of an easily obtainable medication (such as paracetamol) equates to a low risk and represents more of a 'cry for help'. However, you should determine whether the patient believed such a dose was sufficient to be fatal before making any assumptions.

After the attempt

Ask the patient how they were found after the attempt. Did someone chance upon them or did they seek help immediately afterwards? A person discovered by chance by a passer-by is more at risk than an individual who rang 999 immediately after consuming a number of tablets.

Establish how the patient currently feels about their suicide attempt. Are they remorseful of the event or are they unhappy that it was unsuccessful?

1.16.3 Past psychiatric history

Establish from the patient whether they suffer from any mental health disorders including depression, schizophrenia, obsessive–compulsive disorder, panic

> **Medical Guidelines**
> *Risk factors for suicide*
>
> A useful acronym or tool to assess suicide risk was developed by Patterson *et al.* (1983) and is known as the SAD PERSONS scale, and the following represents an adapted version. Each letter of the acronym represents a risk factor as follows:
>
> *Sex:* males are three times more likely to commit suicide than females
>
> *Age:* there is bimodal distribution for suicide risk; highest in young adults between 15 and 24 years and in the elderly above 65 years old
>
> *Depression:* patients who are severely depressed are at much higher risk of suicide compared to the general population
>
> *Previous attempt:* prior suicide attempt by any method represents one of the highest risk factors for a repeat attempt
>
> *Ethanol abuse:* alcoholics have a lifetime risk of suicide of 3–4%
>
> *Rational thinking loss:* schizophrenics have a 10% lifetime risk of suicide
>
> *Social supports lacking:* the suicidal patient often lacks significant others, employment at a meaningful job and religious supports.
>
> *Organized plan:* patients who have meticulously planned their suicide or leave a note or will are at higher risk
>
> *No spouse:* those not in a relationship have a higher risk of suicide than married patients
>
> *Sickness:* patients suffering from chronic and debilitating conditions, such as MS, AIDS, epilepsy and cancer, are at a higher risk of suicide
>
> *Patterson et al. (1983) Psychosomatics, 24: 343–349.*

attacks or personality disorder. Patients with psychiatric illness have an elevated risk of suicide, with eating disorders and major depression leading the pack.

If the patient has suffered from any mental health disorder take a more detailed history enquiring about its onset, episodes, treatments, any admissions or sectioning, and whether they have seen a psychiatrist. Ask if they have attempted suicide or harmed themselves in the past? Have they previously suffered from depression or any other psychiatric illnesses? It is important to delineate which illness, when it was diagnosed, the duration of care, if there were any precipitants, what the treatment was, and the outcome.

1.16.4 Past medical history

Take a detailed past medical history including any previous medical illness and hospital admissions. Enquire about previous investigations or operations the patient may have undergone. Ask particularly about any chronic illnesses. Patients who suffer from epilepsy, AIDS and MS are approximately 3–6 times more likely to commit suicide than the general population. Chronic disabling diseases or disabilities raise the risk of suicide because it may appear to be the only way for the patient to escape their predicament.

Drug history

Ask the patient what medication they are currently on or have taken in the past. Do not forget to also ask about any OTC medications or herbal remedies that the patient has tried. Take a detailed history asking specifically about corticosteroids, oral contraceptives and β-blockers as these medications can cause depression (see *Box 1.19*). Champix, as used in smoking cessation, and sibutramine, recently used for weight loss, have been shown to increase the risk of suicide. Be cautious

---

BOX 1.19 **Drugs that can cause depression**

- Propranolol
- Oral contraceptives
- Cimetidine
- Steroids
- Levadopa
- Metronidazole
- Phenytoin

---

with patients who have recently been started on an SSRI for severe depression because for the first few weeks they may experience increased levels of anxiety and therefore are at a higher risk of suicide.

It is important to take a thorough drug history to try and establish if there are any medications that the patient is taking that may be lethal in an overdose. Drugs such as amitriptyline should be discontinued if the patient is at risk of suicide due to its cardiotoxic side effects.

Social history

Enquire whether the patient has ever smoked and if so, how many cigarettes a day and for how long. Also establish whether they drink alcohol, noting the type of alcohol and how many units a week. Patients suffering from alcoholism are at an increased risk of depression and suicide and alcohol is often consumed at the time of the suicide attempt. Discreetly ask about illicit drug use. Find out which ones and quantify how much and for how long.

Establish whether the patient is in a relationship and has any children. Single males have been found to have an increased risk compared to their married counterparts, whilst children can act as a protective factor.

Family history

It is important to enquire whether the patient has any first-degree relatives who suffer from mental illness. Specifically ask about family history of suicide, alcoholism and depression.

Insight

This is fundamental in any psychiatric history and a very good indicator of prognosis. Does the patient believe they have a problem and do they feel that they need help? Patients who have insight into their problem often have better prognosis.

Follow-up

Provide an appropriate patient risk assessment and discuss the management with the patient. It is important to decide whether the patient needs inpatient admission or outpatient follow-up. Those patients whom you deem to be high risk, for example those that do not regret the attempt or would attempt suicide again if allowed home, need admission. Do not forget to consult a senior colleague if in doubt.

TOP TIP!

Suicide risk assessment should distinguish between acute and chronic risk. Acute risk can be due to recent changes in the person's circumstances or mental state, while chronic risk is determined by a diagnosis of a mental illness and social and demographic factors.

1.16.5 **Summing up**

Summarize your findings back to the patient and ask if they would like to add anything that you may have missed. It is vital that you make an appropriate suicide risk assessment to help you decide how to manage the patient. As we have mentioned previously, making an assessment about the patient's risk is not an exact science, but is instead based upon their current mental state, the severity of the attempted suicide, and factors such as previous attempts. Based upon this information you should categorize patients into low, medium and high risk. Patients who are deemed to be at a high risk of suicide should be admitted to a psychiatric unit to mitigate any potential harm they may cause themselves. Those who have low or moderate risk may still require outpatient psychiatric assessment.

End the interview by thanking the patient. In an exam situation, deliver an appropriate summary to the examiner.

1.16.6 **Common clinical scenarios**

The following are a list of common suicide cases which you may encounter. For each one, consider:
- what the level of risk could be
- what key features you would look for
- what questions you would ask to refine or confirm your diagnosis

You could use role play with a friend, using the histories in the cases below as a framework.

CASE 1	A 67 year old retired dentist was admitted yesterday after attempting to hang himself. He was discovered by his son who had paid an unplanned visit to his father's house. This was the first time he had tried to take his life. On questioning, he mentions that he was tired of life and did not see the point of going on. He has been suffering from bouts of depression since the death of his wife last year. His son mentions that his father has used his savings to pay off his mortgage and closed his bank accounts. He was initially very upset with his son for discovering him. He lives on his own. He does not have any positive psychiatric family history. He denies hallucination, low mood or delusions. He is a non-smoker and has not tried any recreational drugs. He has become a heavy drinker this last year, consuming around 45 units of alcohol per week.

CASE 2

A 22 year old university student presented to A&E yesterday after slitting her wrists. She cut herself after having an argument with her boyfriend who she discovered had cheated on her. This was the first time she had tried to harm herself or take her life and she denies planning the attempt. She mentions that she was angry and wanted to make her boyfriend 'feel guilty'. She feels remorseful for what she has done and does not wish to carry it out again. She is glad that she is well and was discovered. She lives with her parents and two siblings. She has no previous psychiatric history nor is there any positive psychiatric family history. She denies hallucinations, low mood or delusions. She is a non-smoker, a social drinker and has not tried any recreational drugs. She is happy to seek help and is willing to attend outpatient follow-up clinics.

Chapter 1.17
Alcohol

What to do . . .

- Introduce yourself to the patient – establish rapport
- Ask the patient's name, age and occupation
- Ask the patient relevant questions about their drinking habits, such as the amount, type, place and time of drinking
- Ask when they first started drinking
- Ask about any reasons behind their current level of use: triggers/stressors/life events
- Ask about any features of alcohol dependence, such as drinking compulsions, drinking primacy over other tasks, narrowing of drinking repertoire, tolerance, withdrawal symptoms, relief drinking, reinstatement after abstinence
- Elicit patient beliefs about drinking and use despite harm
- CAGE questionnaire
- Ask about any social history, e.g. smoking, stress, family/employment/financial/legal issues
- Ask about any past medical history, e.g. medical complications of alcohol abuse, depression and substance abuse
- Ask about any drug history and for any drug allergies
- Ask about any family history
- Perform a brief systems review
- Give advice on cutting down and support groups, e.g. Alcoholics Anonymous
- Summarize your findings
- Thank the patient and conclude the consultation

Alcohol is widely available and commonly consumed in Western societies. It contains ethanol which has a psychoactive effect, leading people to feel elated, disinhibited and euphoric. In moderation, alcohol is believed not to cause direct harm; however, in excess it can have a number of different toxic effects on the body. Problems such as oesophagitis (and oesophageal varices), gastritis, hepatitis, liver cirrhosis, pancreatitis, hypertension, hypoglycaemia, peripheral neuropathy and sexual health problems are all physical consequences of alcohol abuse. Excessive drinking is also associated with psychiatric problems such as depression, hallucinations and anxiety disorders. Socially, alcohol dependence can lead to financial, legal, employment, marital, and housing problems. All of these factors need to be considered when managing patients with a history of alcohol abuse (see *Box 1.20*).

Alcoholic drinks are available in three basic types: beers, wines and spirits, each of which has a different alcohol content. When trying to assess a patient's typical consumption it is important that you ask direct questions about their drinking habits, such as frequency of drinking, types of alcohol consumed, and

TOP TIP!

One unit is equivalent to 10 ml of alcohol. To calculate the 'strength' of a particular alcoholic beverage you should use 'alcohol by volume' (ABV) which is usually found on the label. Multiply the ABV by the millilitres drunk and divide by 1000 to arrive at the units. For example, one bottle of wine typically has an ABV of 12% in 750 ml (12 x 750) / 1000 = 9 units.

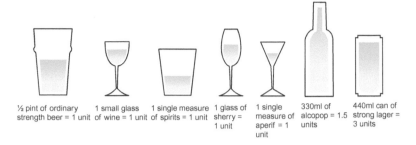

½ pint of ordinary strength beer = 1 unit

1 small glass of wine = 1 unit

1 single measure of spirits = 1 unit

1 glass of sherry = 1 unit

1 single measure of aperif = 1 unit

330ml of alcopop = 1.5 units

440ml can of strong lager = 3 units

Fig 1.12 Typical units in alcoholic drinks.

volumes. This is because patients have a tendency to underestimate their total alcohol consumption. Because of the varying strengths, quantities and types of alcohol, there is a universally accepted standardized unit of alcohol which should be employed to help provide an objective measure of a patient's alcohol consumption.

The UK government recommends that men should not drink more than 3 units a day (21 units a week) and women no more than 2 units a day (14 units a week). It has been shown that males who regularly drink more than 50 units a week and females drinking more than 35 units a week expose themselves to the highest risk of developing alcohol cirrhosis. In women who are pregnant, alcohol abstinence is advised due to the risk of foetal alcohol syndrome in the neonate. If women choose to drink, NICE recommend that they should not drink in the first trimester and thereafter that they drink no more than one to two units once or twice a week.

When taking an alcohol history it is important to determine whether or not the patient is alcohol dependent. There are a number of different accredited screening questionnaires that can be employed to facilitate this:

- the CAGE questionnaire is the most frequently used screening tool covering four questions (see below for full details)
- the FAST test
- the five-shot tool
- AUDIT-C

The FAST, five-shot and AUDIT-C tools are more sensitive and specific to alcohol misuse compared to CAGE questions alone. One should always adopt a sensitive

---

Medical Guidelines
The FAST test

This is a four item questionnaire with each question scored from 0 to 4 depending on the response. If the patient scores 0 for question one (by answering "never") then they are not misusing alcohol. Scores of 3 or more in total over the four questions indicate hazardous drinking.

1 *MEN: How often do you have EIGHT or more drinks on one occasion?*
WOMEN: How often do you have SIX or more drinks on one occasion?

2 *How often during the last year have you been unable to remember what happened the night before because you had been drinking?*

3 *How often during the last year have you failed to do what was normally expected of you because of drinking?*

4 *In the last year has a relative or friend, or a doctor or other health worker been concerned about your drinking or suggested you cut down?*

Health Development Agency: Manual for the Fast Alcohol Screening Test (2002).

BOX 1.20 **Alcohol dependency**

The ICD-10 definition of alcohol dependency requires three or more features for diagnosis:

- Compulsion to drink
- Difficulties controlling alcohol consumption
- Physiological withdrawal (*Box 1.21*)
- Tolerance to alcohol
- Neglect of alternative activities to drinking
- Persistent use of alcohol despite evidence of harm

BOX 1.21 **Alcohol withdrawal**

Features of alcohol withdrawal include anxiety, shakiness, headaches, nausea and vomiting. These symptoms usually present at 6–12 hours after alcohol cessation. Seizures occur approximately 36 hours after alcohol cessation, whilst features of delirium tremens (hallucinations, acute confusion, tremors) appear after 72 hours.

and empathetic approach when taking an alcohol history as this will make the patient feel more relaxed and forthcoming and this should help to provide more accurate responses.

1.17.1 Taking the history

Start your alcohol history by introducing yourself to the patient by stating your full name and job title before proceeding to ask the patient's full name, age and occupation. Knowing the age of the patient may have legal implications. For example, in the UK it is illegal for a child under the age of 18 to purchase alcohol over the counter. However, minors at the age of 5 and above are permitted to consume some amount of alcohol in a private setting. At the age of 16 an adolescent is able to drink alcohol with a meal in public but must be accompanied by an adult.

Certain occupations have a higher incidence of alcohol-related diseases and death, including jobs such as publicans, sailors and senior civil servants, according to the Office for National Statistics (ONS).

It is essential to establish rapport with the patient by asking open questions regarding their symptoms. You should also listen attentively to the patient, watching out for any verbal or non-verbal cues which may reveal a hidden agenda. Trying to address alcohol dependence can be quite difficult as it is a sensitive topic to broach. Certain cultures and religions prohibit the consumption of alcohol and an inappropriate line of questioning may hinder the consultation. Attempt to establish rapport by being tactful and non-judgemental before delving deeper into the history.

1.17.2 Ideas, concerns and expectations

Once you feel that the patient has settled and you have gained their trust, try to elicit the patient's own views about their problem. Patients may have varying health beliefs and attitudes towards their alcohol habit. Some may show an active interest in what you say whilst others can be quite dismissive and will not accept any advice you may offer. By gaining an understanding of the patient's own health beliefs, you will be able to tailor your lifestyle advice accordingly. Some people may believe that their level of alcohol consumption is normal and not harmful, whilst others are more realistic and are amenable to changing their habits. Some patients may be concerned about the potential loss of their job, possible breakdown in their relationships or developing end-stage liver disease such as cirrhosis.

1.17.3 History of the presenting complaint

Now take a more detailed history of the patient's presenting complaint. It may be an idea to split your history into three areas.

Medical Guidelines
The AUDIT-C screening questionnaire

AUDIT-C consists of three questions, with each question scored out of four. An overall score of 5 or above indicates higher risk drinking and warrants the use of the more detailed full AUDIT questionnaire of 10 questions.

1 *How often do you have a drink containing alcohol?*
Never = 0, four or more times a week = 4

2 *How many units of alcohol do you drink on a typical day when you are drinking?*
1 or 2 drinks = 0
10 or more drinks = 4

3 *How often have you had 6 or more units (if female), or 8 or more (if male), on a single occasion in the last year?*
Never = 0, daily or almost daily = 4

World Health Organization: The Alcohol Use Disorders Identification Test (2001).

Medical Guidelines
DVLA guidance

Persistent alcohol misuse, confirmed by medical enquiry and/or by evidence of otherwise unexplained abnormal blood markers, requires licence revocation or refusal until a minimum 6 month period of controlled drinking or abstinence has been attained, with normalization of blood parameters. For alcohol dependency the period is for 1 year.

DVLA: At a glance guide to the current medical standards of fitness to drive (2011).

TOP TIP!

Empathy is very important when taking an alcohol history. Even quiet or depressed patients may feel more comfortable discussing their problems if a caring attitude is demonstrated.

- Begin by asking about the patient's drinking habit including the amount, types and frequency.
- Then concentrate more on symptoms of alcohol dependence to get an overall idea of the degree of addiction.
- Finish off by employing an alcohol questionnaire to objectively score or rate their degree of dependence.

Although you can use any of the questionnaires mentioned above, in an OSCE examination you will usually be expected to use the CAGE questionnaire.

Drinking habits

TOP TIP!

Establish the patient's insight into their alcohol consumption by asking: *"Do you believe alcohol is bad for you?"* and *"Do you know the effects of alcohol on your body?"* If the patient is familiar with the toxic effects of alcohol on the body but still unable to cut down their habit then this may be an early pointer to dependency behaviour.

Start by asking the patient whether they drink alcohol or not – it may be embarrassing to proceed to take a thorough alcohol history in a non-drinker. Next try to establish the type of drink consumed, i.e. whether beer, wine and/ or spirits. Try to find out how often they drink alcohol and whether they drink regularly during the week or binge at the weekends.

Sometimes patients may give vague or inaccurate responses to your questions. In such situations try to simplify your line of questioning by asking: *"What's the most you have had to drink on any one day in the past month?"* Patients tend not to count heavy drinking episodes in their estimate of average weekly consumption, even if these episodes occur frequently. If the patient fails to respond to this prompt, an alternative strategy may be to offer a wide range of options describing different volumes of alcohol drunk. For example: *"Would you say that you drink around 1–2 beers per night or is it closer to 8–10 beers per night?"*

TOP TIP!

New evidence has suggested that binge drinking can be more harmful than consistent consumption over a few days. If the patient drinks regularly, try to get the patient to talk through and describe a typical drinking day to you.

It is equally important to ask about the alcohol content, and the size of glass used. For example, a bottle of whisky at 40% ABV has a significantly higher alcohol content than a can of normal strength beer (3.5–4.5% ABV). With this information you should be able to arrive at an accurate estimation of the total number of units the patient consumes in a week.

Reason for drinking

Briefly touch upon when the patient had their first taste of alcohol and what prompted them to start drinking. Was there influence from peers or was the habit adopted from their parents? Ask the patient when their alcohol consumption started to increase and what caused this to happen.

Alcohol dependence

TOP TIP!

It may be helpful to enquire about the social context in which the alcohol is consumed. Younger patients tend to binge drink in pubs, nightclubs or at parties, whereas elderly patients usually drink in solitude.

It is important to gauge the degree of dependence the patient has on alcohol because the greater the degree, the more likely it is that they will encounter alcohol-related sequelae.

The ICD-10 classification (see *Box 1.20*) has six different criteria, with three or more features required to make a formal diagnosis of alcohol dependency. Begin by trying to find out whether the patient craves or has a deep rooted urge to drink alcohol. If so, check whether their drinking is central to their life and is the number one priority over other activities. Have other responsibilities such as family and relationships taken a back seat due to their alcohol habit? Is the patient having difficulty controlling their alcohol consumption, or do they feel that they need to drink more to get the same effect? If the patient is unable to drink alcohol, do they experience symptoms such as palpitations, anxiety, tremors, hallucinations or episodes of fits and are they relieved with the reintroduction of it?

CAGE questionnaire

CAGE is a rapid easily performed questionnaire that can be employed in any consultation as a screening tool for alcohol dependency. It consists of four questions to be posed to the patient with two or more positive response considered clinically significant.

1. Have you ever tried to **C**ut down on your drinking?
2. Have other people's comments about your drinking ever **A**ngered you?
3. Have you ever felt **G**uilty about how much you drink?
4. Do you feel the need to drink first thing in the morning as an **E**ye-opener?

Attempts to seek help

Most patients who are alcohol dependent are aware of the harmful effects that alcohol has on their body. As a result many of them have tried and failed, on a number of occasions, to give up or reduce their consumption individually. Some may have gone the extra mile and tried to access self-help groups such as Alcoholics Anonymous to seek assistance. Try to establish from the patient whether they have sought help and with whom. Have they been successful in abstinence for any period of time previously and what went wrong?

Social history

In a normal history you would swiftly move on to ask the patient about their past medical history. However, when taking a history of alcoholism it may be more pertinent to try to elicit the effects alcohol has on the patient's social circumstances. Alcoholism has been associated with domestic violence, child abuse, crime, unemployment and family relationship breakdown. Hence, you should focus on these aspects and allow the patient freedom and space to express their feelings and inner thoughts at their own pace.

Ensure that you check whether the patient is in a relationship or not. Are they married? Do they have children? If they are in a relationship establish if their partner also has alcohol problems. If they have any children try to find out if there are any child protection issues or social worker involvement.

Ascertain whether the patient is currently in employment or not. If not, how do they support their habit financially? Are they on benefits or have they had to resort to crime? If they currently have an occupation are there any issues such as late attendance, increasing mistakes or problems with bosses and colleagues? Is the patient at risk of losing their job and if so what could the possible ramifications be?

Ask the patient if they have ever smoked and, if so, how many cigarettes a day and for how long. Discreetly ask about illicit drug use such as cocaine and marijuana, if you haven't already done so. Enquire about the patient's level of activity and whether they undertake a basic level of exercise.

1.17.4 Past medical history

Having completed taking a thorough history of the presenting complaint, you should now move on to ask about the patient's past medical history

> **QUESTIONS TO ASK . . .**
>
> - Do you ever get a craving/urge for alcohol when not drinking? (Compulsion)
> - Does drinking alcohol take priority over other activities in your life? (Primacy)
> - Do you feel that you have difficulty controlling how much alcohol you drink? (Difficulty controlling consumption)
> - Do you have to drink more alcohol each time to get the same effect? (Tolerance)
> - Do you find that you neglect other responsibilities because of your alcohol habit? (Neglect)
> - When you stop drinking for a while do you ever feel anxious, sweaty, shaky, sick? Have you ever heard or seen things that aren't there? Have you ever had any fits/faints or funny turns? (Withdrawal symptoms)

> **TOP TIP!**
>
> Always ask about substance abuse and symptoms of depression in an alcoholic patient because they often co-exist.

BOX 1.22 **Alcohol withdrawal symptoms and chronic complications**

Withdrawal symptoms of alcohol	Complications of chronic alcohol abuse
Anxiety	Liver and heart disease
Tremors	Peptic ulceration
Sweating	Pancreatitis
Nausea and vomiting	Peripheral neuropathy
Delirium tremens	Oesophagitis/gastritis
Fits, faints, funny turns	Hypertension
	Impotence

including previous illnesses and any hospital admissions. Specifically enquire about common medical complications of alcohol abuse, such as peptic ulceration, pancreatitis, liver disease, heart disease, peripheral neuropathy, and hypertension. Ensure that you ask whether the patient has ever suffered from delirium tremens because this is associated with high morbidity and mortality. Also elicit whether the patient has had any fitting episodes after periods of abstinence from alcohol.

Remember to ask about features of depression because alcohol is implicated in low mood states. Symptoms such as tiredness/fatigue, low mood, loss of interest in activities, sleep disturbances, guilt and negative thoughts may point towards a concurrent diagnosis of depression. Note any suicidal tendency, particularly if there is evidence of recent social turmoil.

Drug history

Ask the patient what medication they are currently on or have taken in the past. Try to include any OTC medications as well as herbal remedies. Enquire specifically about the oral contraceptive pill, antibiotics, anticonvulsants and blood thinners such as warfarin and aspirin as these can be affected by alcohol.

Family history

Family history does not usually play a large role in alcoholism but you may wish to ask about excessive drinking in the family. Sometimes it is something that the patient has grown up around and they may think their intake is entirely normal.

1.17.5 **Systems review**

Complete your history with a brief systems review. This may give an insight into the patient's general health. You can also use this as a method of running through the systems from head to toe to ensure you have not missed anything. Ask the patient if they have experienced any headaches, visual disturbances, chest or abdominal pain, shortness of breath, change in their bowel habits or weight loss. Have they felt dizzy, lost consciousness or noted any swelling, stiffness or weakness in their limbs? Are they passing urine comfortably with no burning sensation?

Advice

After finishing your history taking, it's important to give the patient feedback and counsel them on their drinking habits. This advice should be in accordance

TOP TIP!

Alcohol both induces and inhibits the P450 enzyme system which regulates the metabolism of common medications in the liver:
- acute consumption inhibits the P450 system and prolongs or increases blood levels of medication
- chronic consumption induces the P450 system and reduces the concentration levels of medications, causing them to have shortened efficacy

---

BOX 1.23 **Practical steps to reduce alcohol intake**

- Try to avoid places that have alcohol readily available such as pubs, clubs and supermarkets
- Throw out any remaining alcoholic beverages or reminders of alcohol found in the house such as empty bottles or cans
- If going out with friends offer to buy others a round whilst missing yourself out
- If you are drinking in a group ensure that you are the slowest drinker and sip your drink instead of gulping it down
- Buy less concentrated forms of alcohol as you attempt to wean yourself off

---

with Department of Health guidelines as to what constitutes safe drinking levels. Use this information as a basis to explain to the patient what damage they are causing to their health and the long term consequences of chronic and consistent alcohol abuse. *Box 1.23* gives some useful advice that you can give to the patient to encourage them to reduce their intake.

You should be direct and realistic, accepting that the patient is unlikely to give up overnight; slow but steady steps are more likely to have a better outcome. You could say something along the lines of: *"Your current alcohol intake is unhealthy for your body and may also be affecting those around you. It is the reason you are developing these withdrawal symptoms and, if you continue to drink this much, you could damage your brain, heart and liver. I understand that it may be difficult to stop completely, but I recommend that you start to take it step-by-step. We can put you in touch with expert groups like Alcoholics Anonymous to help you deal with this. Are you willing to consider this?"*

1.17.6 **Summing up**

Summarize back your findings to the patient at relevant intervals as this will help you check that the information you have gained is correct and reassure your patient that you have been listening to what they have been telling you. End your consultation by agreeing a shared plan of action with clear steps as to what will happen next. Offer the patient any leaflets that will help to reinforce some of the key messages you have imparted and put them in touch with any relevant self-help or support groups. Thank the patient for their time and conclude the interview amicably.

1.17.7 **Common clinical scenarios**

The following are a list of common alcohol dependency cases which you may encounter. For each one, consider:
- what the level of the alcohol consumption is and whether it is in accordance with relevant guidelines
- what key features you would look for
- what questions you would ask to refine or confirm your diagnosis

You could use role play with a friend, using the histories in the cases below as a framework.

CASE 1

An 18 year old woman drinks a small glass of red wine with her dinner every night. On one night at the weekends she goes out with her friends and typically drinks 3 regular alcopop bottles at the night club. She began drinking when she was 16, and has never had any problems with the police. She is doing well in her studies and is in a stable relationship.

CASE 2

A 45 year old actor drinks 5 cans of strong beer daily. He began drinking when he was 14 years old and now needs more concentrated alcohol to get the same effect. He gets angry when people suggest he should stop drinking and finds that when he wakes up he has to drink a can of beer to calm his nerves. At weekends his friend comes over and he drinks around 10 cans of strong beer on both Saturday and Sunday. He has tried to give up his habit on two occasions around 3 years ago due to a relationship break-up; however, he was unable to do so. He still blames himself for the break-up and attributes it to his drinking problem.

CASE 3

A 28 year old banker has been drinking since she was 18 years old. She has a shot of vodka every weekday night before she sleeps as she feels it helps her relax her nerves before the morning. She does not drink any other alcohol during the week. On Friday nights she goes out and regularly downs 3 shots of vodka and 2 regular alcopop bottles. On Saturday she normally meets with her friends and goes out to the town, this time drinking 2 cans of regular strength beer. She denies any medical problems or psychiatric conditions.

Chapter 1.18
Psychosis

What to do . . .

- Introduce yourself to the patient – establish rapport
- Ask the patient's name, age and occupation
- Ask the patient relevant questions relating to their psychosis, including onset, duration and triggers
- Establish whether the patient has any hallucinations (visual, auditory, tactile, olfactory); if the patient reports any auditory hallucination establish type and content (first, second, or third person).
- Establish if the patient suffers with delusion and determine its type (persecutory, grandeur, perception, reference, control)
- Establish whether they suffer from thought disorder (insertion, withdrawal, broadcast)
- Check for evidence of depression or bipolar disorder
- Ask about any past psychiatric history, e.g. depression
- Ask about past medical history, e.g. chronic disease
- Ask about any drug history and for any drug allergies
- Ask about any social history – establish if the patient smokes (how many per day and for how long) or drinks alcohol (what type and how much) and ask discreetly if they have used any illicit drugs (what types and how often)
- Ask about any family history and specifically for schizophrenia
- Thank the patient and conclude the consultation

Psychosis describes the state a person is in when they are unable to distinguish between reality and their imagination; it may present as either a vivid hallucination or as a fixed unshakeable belief, i.e. a delusion. There are a variety of diseases that can cause psychosis, including brain tumour, severe depression, bipolar disorder and head injury; however, by far the most common cause is schizophrenia.

Schizophrenia is one of the most common serious mental health conditions, with a UK prevalence of just over 1%. Men and women are equally affected and, although there is no specific aetiology for schizophrenia, it is believed that a combination of genetic and environmental factors, such as drug use, living conditions or family disharmony, play a role.

Schizophrenia is a condition that leads to a variety of classic psychological symptoms (collectively known as Schneider's first-rank symptoms, see *Box 1.24*) including:

- hallucinations – these describe the process of seeing or hearing things that are not present; they are perceived through one of the patient's senses and hence are felt to be as real as any other stimuli

Medical Guidelines
Diagnostic criteria for schizophrenia

Both ICD-10 and DSM-IV agree on the symptom clusters that confirm a diagnosis of schizophrenia. There are three main domains, including:

- psychotic symptoms, such as certain types of auditory hallucinations (hearing voices), delusions ('paranoia' and 'telepathy') and thought disorder (incomprehensible speech)

- negative symptoms, such as poor self-care, reduced motivation, reduced ability to experience pleasure, alogia (reduced production of thought), affective blunting (lack of emotional expression) and reduced social functioning

- catatonia, which is much less common

ICD-10 requires that at least one such diagnostic symptom from one of the three domains should be clearly present for 1 month. ICD-10 also confirms the diagnosis if two of these symptoms have been present in a less clear way for 1 month.

The DSM-IV requires that two or more of the above symptoms are present in conjunction with social dysfunction and a prolonged presence of symptoms, usually for around 6 months.

International Statistical Classification of Diseases and Related Health Problems 10th Revision (ICD-10) (1992)

Diagnostic and statistical manual of mental disorders: DSM-IV-TR (2000)

BOX 1.24 **Schneider's first-rank symptoms for diagnosing schizophrenia**

- Auditory hallucinations:
    hearing thoughts spoken aloud
    hearing voices referring to himself/herself, made in the third person
    hearing a form of commentary
- Thought disorder: thought withdrawal, insertion and interruption, thought broadcasting
- Delusions of control: feelings or actions experienced as made or influenced by external agents
- Delusional perception: delusional meaning is attributed to a normal perception

- delusions – these relate to the patient holding a fixed firm belief that is unshakeable; it is also not in keeping with their cultural background or norms
- thought disorders – these include the feeling of the insertion or removal of ideas from the patient's mind by an external source; patients may also feel that their ideas are accessible and broadcasted to others.

Patients with schizophrenia often present with other concurrent mental health conditions such as depression or anxiety. In addition, such patients have an increased rate of drug and substance misuse and also have associated medical health problems, such as ischaemic heart disease, diabetes and hepatitis C. Due to their fragile mental state they commonly have numerous social problems such as homelessness, lack of employment and lack of social support.

Taking a psychosis history should allow you to formulate a working diagnosis of the potential cause of the psychosis, evaluate the severity of the symptoms and perform a mini risk assessment to determine whether the patient is a risk to themselves or others (see *Box 1.25*).

BOX 1.25 **Mental Health Act 1983**

The Mental Health Act (1983) was set up to help doctors to admit patients with mental health disorders that affect their insight. It covers patients who are over 16 years old, who are a danger to themselves and others and who have refused to be voluntarily admitted. Although there are a number of sections to this Act the most relevant ones related to patient admissions are highlighted below.

Section two: admission for assessment
Permits admission of a patient for assessment for up to 28 days. Medication and treatment can be given without formal consent.

Section three: admission for treatment
Admission for treatment for a period of up to 6 months. This is usually implemented whilst a formal diagnosis has been made and when section two has expired. This section can be extended initially for another 6 months and then yearly.

Section four: emergency admission
This is used for emergency admissions for a period of 72 hours and allows rapid assessment of the patient. It is indicated when an application for a section 2 would cause an undue delay.

1.18.1 Taking the history

Begin by introducing yourself by stating your name and job title. Ask the patient some background questions such as their name, age, and whether they are in employment before moving on to ask about their psychotic symptoms. The patient's age and gender at the point of presentation can provide supportive information about a possible diagnosis. Men suffering from schizophrenia often present between the ages of 15 and 30 years, whilst women tend to present later (typically between the ages of 25 and 30 years).

Try to establish rapport with the patient by adopting a warm welcoming posture and asking open questions that give the patient freedom to converse openly. It is important to appreciate that many schizophrenic patients may be reluctant to engage, particularly if you are meeting them for the first time. They may not trust you due to a lack of familiarity or even due to a paranoid delusion they may hold. Slowly gain their trust by being non-judgemental and non-dismissive of their beliefs regardless of how improbable they may sound.

1.18.2 Ideas, concerns and expectations

Try to elicit the patient's own ideas about what is going on and any concerns they may have. Note that most acutely psychotic patients lack any insight into their disorder and believe that they are perfectly well. Eliciting their ideas and concerns can therefore be a useful tool to gauge the degree of insight.

Patients recovering from schizophrenia may harbour concerns such as social exclusion, lack of employment or recurrence of their psychosis. Spend some time enquiring about how the problem has affected the patient's life and establish whether their symptoms have prevented them from performing a particular activity.

1.18.3 History of the presenting complaint

Start by asking the patient to describe the events leading up to their attendance to see a doctor today. It may have been that the patient was brought in by a concerned friend, relative or via a mental health section or restraining order.

Ask them if anything has happened recently and how long it has been going on for. Next move on to elicit the patient's psychotic symptoms. There are many possible symptoms that a schizophrenic patient may present with. However, to make a diagnosis of schizophrenia you should model your questions on Schneider's first-rank symptoms, looking for the presence of hallucinations, delusions, thought disorder and delusions of control.

Hallucinations

Although hallucinations may be tactile, visual or even olfactory, the most common seen in schizophrenia are auditory in nature. Patients may report hearing voices that are in the first, second or third person.
- In first person hallucinations the patient may complain of hearing their own thoughts repeated out loud like an echo (echo de la pensée).
- In second person hallucinations the patient reports voices talking directly to them. These voices may often be rude, unpleasant or commanding in nature, and as a result they are also known as derogatory hallucinations.

TOP TIP!

Young men who present with schizophrenia have on average suffered for 2.5 years before presenting to a medical professional

TOP TIP!

Visual hallucinations, whilst rare, usually point towards an organic cause or a drug-induced state. It can be useful to have the patient describe the hallucination and its frequency.

QUESTIONS TO ASK . . .

About hallucinations

Auditory
Do you hear voices when no-one else is there? How many voices do you hear?

Real/pseudo
Do you hear voices when no-one else is there? How many voices do you hear?

First person
Do you ever hear your own thoughts being repeated out loud like an echo (echo de la pensée)?

Second/third person
Are the voices talking to you directly (second person) or speaking about you (third person)?

Content
What do the voices say? Are they rude or supportive? Do they tell you to harm yourself or others?

Visual
Have you seen things with your own eyes that you could not explain?

Olfactory
Have you smelt anything that you could not explain or find the source of?

Tactile
Have you ever felt anything on your skin that you could not explain or felt bugs walking on your skin (formication – often from alcohol withdrawal, cocaine use)?

TOP TIP!

If a patient hears voices, clarify whether the content is praiseworthy or derogatory in nature. Try to establish if the patient is at risk of harming themselves or others.

TOP TIP!

Delusions of grandeur may emanate from the patient's own cultural or religious beliefs. For example, a Christian patient may hold a delusional belief that they are the chosen Messiah.

QUESTIONS TO ASK . . .

About the patient's delusion

Content
Establish the content of the delusion and use open questions:
- Tell me more about that?
- How long have you been feeling like that?

Fixed belief
How would you feel if I tell you that what you have said is wrong?

Persecutory
Have you felt that someone out there is trying to harm you?

Grandeur
Have you felt that you have any special powers that other people do not possess?

Nihilistic
Do you feel that everything around you or yourself is rotting or decaying?

Reference
Have you ever felt that the television or radio was speaking or communicating directly to you?

TOP TIP!

Never condemn or collude with a patient's delusion even if you feel that it may foster mutual trust and rapport; collusions tend to reinforce their delusional belief whilst condemnation can result in disengagement.

- In third person hallucinations the patient may report hearing one or more voices speaking about themselves and often providing a running commentary about their actions. It is essential to establish the content of such hallucinations and whether the patient poses a potential threat to themselves or others.

Delusions

Delusions are fixed false beliefs that a person holds firm even when challenged to the contrary. They are also not usually in keeping with the patient's own cultural or religious background. For example, a patient from the Tswana tribe of South Africa may believe that a witch doctor has cured them of their infertility; this belief conforms to the cultural norms of that tribe, but it may be interpreted incorrectly as a delusion by a doctor trained in the UK who does not appreciate such beliefs.

Whilst delusions may be diverse and can relate to almost anything, they usually follow common themes that allow them to be classified and distinguished from one another. Persecutory delusions are those in which the patient believes an individual (including friends and relatives) or organization is intending to cause harm to them – a patient may appear to be paranoid and actually fearful for their life. For example, a patient may claim that MI5 or the CIA want to assassinate him due to his occupation as a shopkeeper.

Delusions of grandeur pertain to those cases where the patient believes that they have special, often extraordinary powers that other people do not possess. They may even believe that they have been specifically chosen by a supernatural being for a specific purpose such as saving humanity.

Nihilistic delusions are when patients believe that they, or others, or the whole world is in a state of destruction, decay or death. Patients often say that their internal organs are rotting inside (Cotard's syndrome). Another similar delusion is the delusion of infestation (Ekbom's syndrome) whereby a person believes that their body has been infested with an organism; this may co-exist with tactile hallucinations such as formication.

Patients may attribute a false belief or meaning to a normal event or perception (delusions of perception). For example, a person may believe he is an assassin after seeing a traffic light turn red. This is comparable with delusions of reference, whereby the patient believes that events, activities or objects have a special and direct significance to themselves. For example, a patient may read a newspaper headline or watch TV and believe that it refers directly to them.

Delusions may be of the sort that can even lead the patient to believe that their actions, emotions or behaviour are controlled externally (delusions of control). Patients may deny instigating a particular activity and rather attribute them to an external source, i.e. a schizophrenic patient committing a murder and blaming aliens for having taken possession of his limbs.

Thought disorders

Thought disorders describe the process by which a patient's own thoughts are affected or interfered with. Patients may feel that their thoughts are not always their own and can be manipulated by an external source. They may believe that thoughts are being inserted and implanted into their head without their consent (thought insertion). Conversely, they may hold the belief that their thoughts are being removed (thought withdrawal) without their permission.

Thought insertion may be seen in conversation when a patient jumps from subject to subject without a plausible link or association between the topics. Thought withdrawal, on the other hand, may present with the patient pausing in mid-sentence and looking blank, as if they had lost their train of thought. Occasionally patients may believe that others around them are able to read their mind as if their thoughts were being broadcast out loud (thought broadcasting).

Associated symptoms

At times depression may be severe enough to cause a range of psychotic symptoms such as experiencing auditory or tactile hallucinations or complex fixed delusions that can be confused for schizophrenia. Delusions of mania and depression are often mood-congruent, i.e. their intensity is linked directly to the severity of the underlying condition.

Check whether the patient displays symptoms that may indicate other diagnoses such as bipolar disorder. Has the patient ever felt disproportionately elated or undertaken acts such as spending excessively or engaging in promiscuous activity?

1.18.4 Past medical history

Try to establish whether the patient has suffered from any other mental health illness such as depression, obsessive–compulsive disorder or personality disorder. Take a more detailed history enquiring about onset, episodes, treatments, any admissions or sectioning, or whether they have seen a psychiatrist.

Briefly enquire about any concurrent medical illnesses. Ask about ischaemic heart disease, diabetes, cancer and hepatitis C. Also enquire about other illnesses that may present with psychotic symptoms, such as brain tumours, HIV, TB, dementia, delirium, thyroid disorders, epilepsy (temporal lobe), and SLE.

Drug history

Try to take a full medication history including any OTC medications. There are a number of treatments that can cause or worsen psychosis, for example, steroids, anti-cholinergics and drugs for Parkinson's disease.

Family history

Ask the patient if any of their family suffer or have suffered from any psychiatric illness as hereditary factors are thought to be important in the development of schizophrenia. It is believed that first-degree relatives have a 10% chance of suffering with schizophrenia if a family member has been affected.

Social history

Ask whether the patient smokes and, if so, how many cigarettes a day and for how long. Determine if they drink alcohol and if so, attempt to work out the number of units a week. Schizophrenic patients tend to have greater incidence of alcoholism and three times the rate of smoking addiction. Also bear in mind

---

QUESTIONS TO ASK . . .

About thought disorders

Insertion
Do you ever feel that your thoughts are not your own and someone is inserting them into your head?

Withdrawal
Do you believe that someone is removing thoughts from your mind?

Broadcasting
Do you believe that others have access to your thoughts and hear what you are thinking?

TOP TIP!

When taking a history of psychotic symptoms from the patient you should observe them for any evidence of disorganized thought. Patients may display a number of altered thought processes throughout their speech. For example, loss of associations ('Knight's-move thinking') is when the person moves from one train of thought to another that has no apparent link to the first. In the extreme case, words and phrases may be totally incoherent and jumbled together with no apparent meaning, in a 'word salad.' This is in contrast with flight of ideas where the patient, under pressure of speech, jumps from one topic to another through a pun, clang or loose association. Patients may even engineer and create new words made up of sounds or syllables of other familiar words in their vocabulary (neologism).

TOP TIP!

Negative symptoms seen in a psychotic patient usually indicate poor prognosis and recovery. Patients may display signs of lack of motivation, poor concentration and blunted affect. They may stop mingling with their friends or family and socially isolate themselves.

TOP TIP!

Patients with psychosis may have had a number of brushes with the law or even spent time in prison and so it may be worth asking the patient about any criminal history. Ensure that you do this only once good rapport has been established.

that severe alcoholism may present with tactile hallucinations and delusions as seen in delirium tremens.

Establish whether the patient is single or in a relationship, whether they have children and, if so, who looks after them? Check whether they are currently in employment and also their accommodation status, i.e. whether they own their own house, live in rented accommodation or in a council house.

Also ask about any illicit drug use that may trigger their condition. For example, heavy cannabis users are six times more likely to develop schizophrenia than non-users. Many other drugs of abuse such as amphetamines, cocaine, ketamine, and lysergic acid diethylamide (LSD) can trigger a schizophrenia-like illness.

Insight

Try to establish whether the patient has insight into their condition. Does the patient believe they have a problem and do they feel they need help for it? Patients who have insight and are aware of their mental illness tend to fare better.

1.18.5 **Summing up**

Summarize your findings back to the patient and ask if they would like to add anything that you may have missed. Having taken a detailed history, you must try to determine the severity of the patient's psychosis, i.e. whether it is a mild, moderate or severe episode. Although this is not an exact science, taking into account all of the patient's symptoms, social circumstances and previous psychiatric history you may be able to make a decision about how bad the patient is. This will help determine whether the patient needs inpatient admission, outpatient follow-up or simple medication as an outpatient. Those patients whom you deem to be high risk, i.e. those with florid psychotic symptoms, are likely to need inpatient admission.

End the interview by thanking the patient. In an exam situation, deliver an appropriate summary to the examiner.

1.18.6 **Common clinical scenarios**

The following are a list of common psychosis cases which you may encounter. For each one, consider:
• what the severity of psychosis is
• what key features you would look for
• what questions you would ask to refine or confirm your diagnosis

You could use role play with a friend, using the histories in the cases below as a framework.

CASE 1

A 22 year old unemployed woman was referred by her parents who are concerned about her suspicious behaviour. She mentions that she believes people are following her wherever she goes and she is able to predict the future from messages she receives through her television. She mentions that she hears two voices inside her head which talk about her all the time, although they do not order her to harm herself or others. She denies any visual hallucinations. She has no previous medical or psychiatric illness and is not on any medications. She admits to 'experimenting' with different recreational drugs recently including cocaine and cannabis. She smokes 10 cigarettes a day and is an occasional drinker. She denies any mood disorders.

CASE 2

A 58 year old medically retired armed forces soldier presents as he is hearing screaming voices, and sounds of shooting and bombing. He states that he often goes to sleep and awakes after a few hours seeing nightmares of previous events when he was serving in the army. He also states that at times he is anxious, sweaty and suffering with palpitations, particularly when watching the news. He feels that he is hallucinating because he can see images of war and death whenever he goes shopping. He has previously served in the First Gulf War.

CASE 3

A 21 year old student was admitted via the A&E department having been thrown out of a casino after a fight with an attendant. He is brought in by his girlfriend and appears dishevelled and irritable. On direct questioning he has not slept for 3 days and has been frequenting a number of different gambling outlets over the past month. He has spent over £2000 in the past week and is now having problems paying his rent and is threatened with eviction. His girlfriend mentions that he is staying up all night writing obscure articles and novels that bear no relation to his degree course. He thinks that he is being followed by armed gangs as he believes that he has been chosen to win over £10 million in a lottery. Past medical history includes severe depression 4 years earlier requiring admission.

Chapter 2.1
Cardiovascular examination

What to do . . .

- Introduce yourself to the patient – establish rapport and seek consent
- Appropriately position and expose the patient
- Inspection: look at the hands, face, neck and chest
- Palpation: feel the radial and carotid pulses and comment on the rate, rhythm, character and volume. Also feel for the apex beat, describing its character and note any heaves and thrills
- Auscultation: listen at all four areas of the heart: mitral, tricuspid, pulmonary and aortic in that order and also assess for radiation to the axilla and carotids. Comment on S1, S2 and murmurs
- Auscultate the carotid and lung bases
- Examine for oedema at the sacrum and in the legs
- Consider performing a full peripheral vascular examination
- Thank the patient and conclude the examination

The cardiovascular examination is one of the most fundamental skills that doctors are expected to perform. It supplements a thorough cardiac history and may reveal signs and sequelae of illnesses that help to narrow your list of potential diagnoses. For example, cardiac symptoms often have considerable overlap with those found in the respiratory system, such as a patient presenting with acute shortness of breath. A good cardiovascular examination should help to confirm your suspicions of a cardiac aetiology rather than a respiratory cause, perhaps by the finding of various signs for ischaemic heart disease.

It is often assumed that a cardiovascular examination focuses solely on the heart and listening for valvular dysfunction. Although this is an important part of the examination, always remember that cardiac signs and symptoms can present outside the praecordium, such as in the hands, face, neck, lungs and ankles.

Anatomy of the heart

The heart is a dense muscular organ (see *Fig 2.1*) that pumps blood around the closed circulatory system in the body. In a healthy adult it expands horizontally from the right sternal margin to the left mid-axillary line and vertically from the second to the fifth intercostal space. It is divided into four chambers: two atria and two ventricles.

Blood flows into the heart via the superior vena cava and delivers deoxygenated blood from the body into

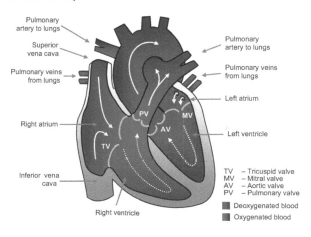

Fig 2.1 The internal structures of the heart.

the right atrium. From here it passes into the right ventricle through the tricuspid valve. As the ventricles contract, blood is pumped from the right ventricle and into the lungs through the pulmonary valve. The left atrium receives oxygenated blood from the lungs from where it is transported into the left ventricle through the mitral (bicuspid) valve. Finally, the left ventricle contracts, forcing blood into the aorta, and out to the rest of the body through the aortic valve.

2.1.1   Beginning the examination

Introduce yourself to the patient by stating your name and job title. Then ask the patient's name and age before establishing whether they are in any pain or discomfort.

It is important to explain clearly to the patient what you intend to do when examining the chest; for example, you may wish to say '*In view of the symptoms you have reported, I need to perform a cardiovascular examination. This will involve me examining and listening to your chest with a stethoscope, as well as looking at your hands, eyes and legs. Before I proceed can I ask if you are in any pain or discomfort?*'. Female patients may have to undress to their bra and so they should be offered the option of having a chaperone if they feel uncomfortable.

Check that the patient has understood what you have said and then seek their consent to proceed with the examination.

2.1.2   Patient exposure and position

Before beginning the examination and asking the patient to undress, ensure that adequate privacy is provided – you should draw curtains around the cubicle or close any doors that are open. Position the patient's bed or examination couch at a 45 degree angle and ask the patient to lie comfortably with their head resting on a pillow. This will help facilitate your examination of the JVP later on. Expose their chest and ensure that you have a clear view of their lower limbs so that you can assess for any evidence of pedal oedema.

Offer the patient a sheet or blanket to maintain their modesty. Ensure that there is good lighting to observe the patient as this will allow you to perform a proper inspection of the chest. Finally, you should always ensure that you have washed your hands thoroughly before commencing your examination.

2.1.3   Inspection

Start your inspection by taking a step back and observing the patient from the end of the bed. Look at the patient and see if they are grimacing with pain or lying comfortably. Look around the patient's bedside for any evidence of oxygen masks, heart monitors, IV cannula drips or GTN sprays. Observe the patient for any obvious difficulties such as laboured breathing or tachypnoea. Look at the general appearance of the patient, particularly at the face for any typical facies associated with Down, Marfan or Turner syndromes – these syndromes all have an effect on the cardiovascular system (see *Box 2.1*).

Observe the patient's skin for the presence of cyanosis (cyanotic congenital heart disease), pallor (anaemia) or bronze pigmentation (haemochromatosis cardiomyopathy). Stand back and listen for any clicking sounds from mechanical heart valves. Move closer to the patient and proceed, in a systematic way, to inspect the hands, face, neck, chest and legs in more detail.

BOX 2.1 **Typical features of common syndromes associated with cardiovascular dysfunction**

Down syndrome	Microgenia (abnormally small chin), oblique eye fissures with epicanthic skin folds on the inner corner of the eyes (mongoloid fold), a flat nasal bridge, a single palmar fold, a protruding tongue, macroglossia, short neck, short stature. Cardiac problems include aortic and ventricular septal defects.
Marfan syndrome	Arachnodactyly, scoliosis, pectus excavatum (abnormal indentation) or pectus carinatum (abnormal protrusion) of the sternum, a high palate, arm span greater than their height. Cardiac problems include aortic or mitral regurgitation, mitral prolapse, aortic dissection, and cardiac arrhythmias.
Turner syndrome	Short stature, low hairline with low set ears and a web neck, broad chest (shield chest) and widely spaced nipples. Cardiac problems include aortic dissection and, to a lesser extent, aortic stenosis.

TOP TIP!

Rheumatic fever is NOT a cardiac cause of clubbing.

Hands

Hand signs are often neglected and overlooked by doctors due to time constraints. However, it is important to note that the hands often reveal vital clues pointing towards underlying pathology.

- Observe for any evidence of tar staining indicating a smoker.
- Look at the colour of the nail beds; normal nail beds should be pink and flushed with colour, but blue nail beds represent peripheral cyanosis.
- Look at the nails for any evidence of splinter haemorrhages (brown-coloured thin vertical streaks found under the nail) which are associated with infective endocarditis.
- Check for signs of clubbing which could be due to infective endocarditis (IE), cyanotic congenital heart disease or atrial myxoma.

Next, ask the patient to turn their hands over to expose their palmar surfaces. Look for other features of infective endocarditis such as Osler's nodes and Janeway lesions. Osler's nodes are painful nodules found at the fingertips, whilst Janeway lesions are small painless erythematous macular or nodular lesions located on the palms of the hands or the soles of the feet.

Once you have inspected the hands check for temperature – the hands in a normal patient should be warm and well perfused, whereas cold peripheries may indicate inadequate peripheral circulation. Assess the capillary refill time by pressing down and blanching the nail bed for 5 seconds before releasing and watching for the blood to return – in healthy adults this should be less than 2 seconds.

Pulse

Move your attention to the patient's wrist. Palpate their radial pulse which can be found between the styloid process of the radius and the flexor carpi radialis tendon, just proximal to the wrist joint. Use three fingers to accurately locate and palpate it. You should note the rate, rhythm, volume and character of the pulse. However, be aware that the volume and character of the pulse is better assessed centrally, such as at the carotid artery, because the further you go away from the aorta the more the waveform is distorted.

Next palpate both radial pulses at the same time to assess for any asynchrony (radio-radial delay) which may be a sign of aortic dissection or co-arctation of

TOP TIP!

Co-arctation is a congenital narrowing of the descending aorta, usually just distal to the origin of the left subclavian artery, leading to higher blood pressure in the arms than legs. It is more common in boys. Most patients with this condition have usually been treated surgically and will be left with a left thoracotomy scar with no pulse in the left arm!

TOP TIP!

Avoid using the words *weak* or *strong* pulse in front of the patient as it may cause undue anxiety.

TOP TIP!

The aortic regurgitation pulse was coined 'water hammer' after a Victorian child's toy which consisted of a glass tube filled with either water or mercury within a vacuum. As the toy was turned upside down, the water or mercury would produce a characteristic knocking sound as it impacted against the glass.

TOP TIP!

Bisferiens orginates from Latin: *bis* – twice, and *ferio* – strike, describing the two peaks of the character.

TOP TIP!

Pulsus paradoxus (paradoxical pulse) is not really a paradox, but an exaggeration of the norm.

the aorta. Also check for a radio-femoral delay by simultaneously palpating the radial and ipsilateral femoral pulses. A delay between the two may be suggestive of co-arctation of the aorta.

Rate

Assess the rate of the radial pulse by counting the number of pulsations over 15 seconds, then multiply this value by 4 to get an approximation of the cardiac rate. The normal cardiac rate should be between 60 and 100 beats per minute. Tachycardia is when the rate is more than 100, whereas bradycardia is less than 60.

Rhythm

Feel the pulse for its rhythm and regularity:
- A normal regular pulse is said to be in sinus rhythm.
- A regularly irregular pulse is one whereby the irregularity of the pulse occurs at regular intervals. The most common cause of this is second degree heart block or sinus arrhythmia (when there is variation of the pulse with breathing – the pulse increases slightly on inspiration and slows on expiration).
- An irregularly irregular pulse, on the other hand, is when the irregularity of the pulse is unpredictable, such as in ectopic beats or atrial fibrillation.

Volume

As stated above, volume is best assessed at the carotids. The pulse volume may give some indication of the cardiac output. A weak or low volume pulse may be due to heart failure and aortic stenosis, whereas a strong or large volume pulse may be found in CO_2 retention, thyrotoxicosis or aortic regurgitation.

Character

A normal pulse has a firm upstroke with a slow paced downstroke. Diseases of the aortic valve affect how blood flows through the aorta which alters the character of the pulse (*Fig 2.2*). In aortic stenosis, with a narrowing of the aorta, blood flow is impeded, producing a slow rising pulse. In aortic regurgitation, the incompetent valve causes pooling of blood in the left ventricle, resulting in an increased stroke volume. This creates a tall initial upstroke with a collapsing downstroke, giving rise to a wide pulse pressure. This is known as collapsing or water hammer pulse and is best assessed by raising the patient's hand over their head and above the level of their heart whilst palpating their radial artery – an increased tapping sensation will be felt in the fingers held over the radial area.

In mixed aortic valve disease such as aortic stenosis with regurgitation, the pulse may have two upstrokes separated by a short mid-systolic downstroke. This is called the bisferiens pulse and may be felt as a double impulse with each beat of the heart over the radial pulse area.

If the pulse alternates from feeling strong to weak, this is known as pulsus alternans and is synonymous with severe left ventricular failure. Pulsus paradoxus is when there is an exaggeration of the normal physiological response with an increase in pulse volume during expiration – this sign is associated with cardiac tamponade or obstructive lung disease.

Blood pressure

After examining the pulse you should go on to measure the patient's blood pressure. In an exam setting, the examiner may give you a reading when you indicate that you wish to perform this task.

Face

Move your attention now to the patient's face, particularly focusing on the sclera, lips and the mouth. The face may give you clues to underlying heart valve problems, cardiovascular risk factors or genetic syndromes that can affect the heart, as follows:

- Take a look at the patient's sclera, warning them that you will be retracting their eyelid for a clearer view. Look for signs of a pale conjunctiva which may be suggestive of anaemia.
- Next look at the cornea, checking for an opaque grey ring around the iris, known as a corneal arcus. Although this may be a common sight in the elderly (where it is known as a senile arcus), in the younger patient it may signify lipid dysfunction.
- Look around the eyes for other signs of hyperlipidaemia, such as xanthelasma (yellow plaque-like deposits of fat around the peri-orbital area).
- Look at the patient's cheeks for a dusky pink discoloration known as malar flush that occurs in mitral stenosis.
- Check their lips and tongue for any blue discoloration which may be a sign of central cyanosis. It is often easier to visualize if the patient raises their tongue up against the roof of their palate. When looking in the mouth you should also check for a high arched palate which may be a sign that the patient has Marfan syndrome.
- Inspect the patient's dentition for poor dental hygiene as this can be associated with infective endocarditis in those with underlying valvular disease.

Neck

Carotid pulse

Look across to the patient's neck and check for any obvious pulsations which may be caused by a carotid pulse. Use your left thumb to assess the carotid pulse for volume and character. The pulse is usually located between the anterior border of the sternocleidomastoid muscle and the larynx around the level of the cricoid cartilage. Move on to examine the other carotid using your right thumb. Never compress both carotids simultaneously.

Jugular venous pressure

Whilst looking at the neck, try to elicit whether the patient has a raised jugular venous pressure (JVP). The JVP provides an indirect measurement of the central venous pressure and may help to distinguish between different types of heart or lung disease.

In order to do this the patient must remain reclined at a 45 degree angle with their head slightly turned to look to their left hand side (*Fig 2.3*); this should give you good visual access to the internal jugular vein which passes from behind the mastoid process vertically down between the sternal and clavicular heads of the sternocleidomastoid (SCM) muscle. In a healthy adult sitting upright, the JVP should not normally be visible. However, at a 45 degree angle, a faint pulsation may be seen at the level of the clavicle. The JVP may be seen from anywhere between the clavicle to just behind the ear lobe and, if visualized, its distance above the sternal angle should be measured in centimetres. A persistently raised JVP of more than 2 cm above the sternal angle is considered abnormal.

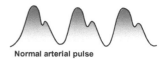
Normal arterial pulse

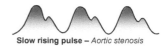
Slow rising pulse – *Aortic stenosis*

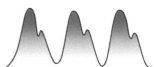
Collapsing pulse – *Aortic regurgitation, patent ductus arteriosus*

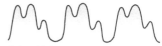
Pulsus alternans – *Left ventricular failure*

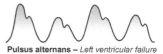
Pulsus bisferiens – *Aortic stenosis with aortic regurgitation*

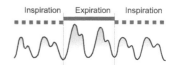
Pulsus paradoxus – *Cardiac tamponade, constrictive pericarditis*

Fig 2.2 Different pulse characters.

TOP TIP!

Suspect infective endocarditis in a patient presenting with a fever and an auscultable heart murmur.

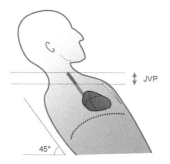
Fig 2.3 Measuring the JVP: the vertical height in centimetres between the sternal angle and the top of the venous column.

TOP TIP!

Always check behind the ear lobe if the JVP cannot be seen.

BOX 2.2 **Features to distinguish between the jugular and carotid impulses**

Jugular impulse	Carotid impulse
Pulse not palpable	Palpable pulse
Rapid inward movement	Rapid outward movement
Disappears when pressure applied to root of neck	Unaffected when pressure applied to root of neck
Two peaks per heartbeat (sinus rhythm)	One peak per heartbeat
Varies with position and respiration	Unaffected by position or respiration
Transient rise with abdominal pressure	No rise with abdominal pressure

If the JVP cannot be visualized you may wish to perform the hepatojugular reflux to confirm a normal right atrial pressure. Confirm that the patient does not have any pain in the abdomen and then apply firm pressure over the liver for around 10 seconds and observe the supraclavicular area. The pressure should cause a transient rise in the JVP such that it may be visualized above the level of the clavicle. This test may also be used to help distinguish between a carotid and jugular pulsation (see *Box 2.2*).

A raised pulsating JVP is a sign of right heart failure, whereas a raised non-pulsating JVP is a sign of superior vena cava obstruction, often due to bronchial carcinoma. A paradoxical rise in JVP during inspiration (normally venous return occurs with inspiration and brings the JVP down) indicates constrictive pericarditis and is known as Kussmaul's sign. See *Box 2.3* for further causes of raised JVP.

TOP TIP!

Do not confuse Kussmaul's sign (paradoxical rise of JVP during inspiration) with Kussmaul's breathing, which is deep, sighing respiration seen in severe metabolic acidosis, e.g. diabetic ketoacidosis or renal failure.

Waveform

When looking at the JVP you should try to discern its waveform. Although difficult at first, this skill often improves with experience. The normal waveform (see *Fig 2.4*) consists of two peaks (a and v) and two troughs (x and y) and a 'c' wave lying between the first peak and trough. The 'a' and 'v' waves can be distinguished by their timing against the carotid pulse: the 'a' wave occurs just prior to the pulse whereas the 'v' wave will be seen towards the tail end of the arterial pulsation.

The 'a' wave. This represents atrial contractions and is elevated if the pulmonary artery pressure is increased such as in pulmonary hypertension or right heart

BOX 2.3 **Causes of raised JVP**

Right heart failure

Fluid overload

Tricuspid regurgitation

Pulmonary stenosis, tricuspid stenosis

Pulmonary embolism, pericardial effusion

Constrictive pericarditis

Cardiac tamponade

failure (giant 'a' waves). It may be significantly prominent when the atrium contracts against closed tricuspid valves such as in atrial flutter or ventricular ectopics (cannon waves). If the 'a' waveform is not present, this may be the result of an absence of atrial contractions such as in atrial fibrillation.

The 'c' wave. This is not normally visible and represents the increased pressure caused by the tricuspid valve closing as well as pulsations from the carotid artery.

The 'v' wave. This represents passive atrial filling during ventricular systole whilst the tricuspid valve is closed. A large 'v' wave will be noted in tricuspid regurgitation as blood refluxes back into the right atrium from the right ventricle.

The 'x' and 'y' troughs. The 'x' descent denotes atrial relaxation whereas the 'y' trough signifies atrial emptying and ventricular filling.

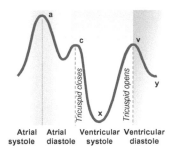

Fig 2.4 JVP waveform.

Precordium

Having inspected the patient's hands, face and neck, move down to inspect the precordial area. Look carefully for any obvious heaves or pulsations, including at the site of the apex beat. Also look out for any scars which may indicate previous cardiothoracic surgery. A median sternotomy scar that runs vertically along the sternum is suggestive of previous coronary artery bypass graft (CABG) or valve replacement. A left lateral thoracotomy scar found running diagonally from the left breast to the left axilla may indicate a mitral valvotomy or coarctation repair. Also look for an implanted pacemaker found usually on the left side below the level of the clavicle.

2.1.4 Palpation

You have now completed your inspection of the patient's cardiovascular system and so you can start to palpate the precordium. Confirm with the patient that they are not in any pain before commencing. Begin by palpating over any pacemaker scars for the presence of an implanted pacemaker.

Apex beat

Position the palm of your right hand over the patient's left precordial area. Feel for a pulsation over the 4th, 5th and 6th intercostal spaces along the mid-clavicular line. In a healthy adult a normal apex beat should be locatable in the left 5th intercostal space at the mid-clavicular line. Confirm its location by counting

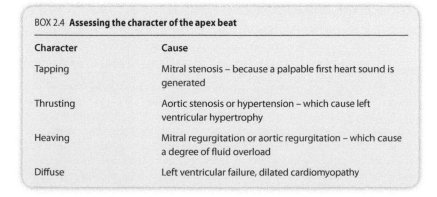

BOX 2.4 **Assessing the character of the apex beat**

Character	Cause
Tapping	Mitral stenosis – because a palpable first heart sound is generated
Thrusting	Aortic stenosis or hypertension – which cause left ventricular hypertrophy
Heaving	Mitral regurgitation or aortic regurgitation – which cause a degree of fluid overload
Diffuse	Left ventricular failure, dilated cardiomyopathy

down the intercostal spaces from the manubriosternal joint (2nd intercostal space).

Comment on whether or not the apex beat is displaced laterally. Cardiomegaly, large pleural effusions, pneumothorax and pneumonectomy can all displace the apex beat. If the apex beat is impalpable this may be due to obesity, pericardial effusions or dextrocardia (right-sided heart). Note the character of the apex beat, which is normally a brief outward early systolic pulsation (see *Box 2.4* for the cause of different characters).

Heaves and thrills

Whilst your hand is over the apex beat (hand position 1 in *Fig 2.5*) try to feel for a palpable thrill. Thrills are palpable murmurs and are always pathognomonic. They can be described as a feeling of a faint vibrating ripple underneath the hand. A thrill felt in the apex area is mostly likely due to mitral stenosis.

Next rotate your hand such that your fingers are now pointing to the patient's neck with the heel of the palm placed over the left sternal edge (hand position 2 in *Fig 2.5*). A palpable thrill here can be due to a ventricular septal defect. Whilst in this area check for a parasternal heave, which may be felt as a lifting sensation elevating your hand off the chest wall and is usually due to right ventricular hypertrophy (pulmonary hypertension).

Lastly, slide your hand vertically upwards to cover the sternal notch (hand position 3 in *Fig 2.5*). Aortic stenosis can often be felt as a palpable thrill at this location and over the neck.

Auscultation

This part of the examination is possibly the most critical in the entire cardio-vascular examination. You should use a good quality stethoscope that has both a diaphragm and dome-shaped bell. This will permit you to listen to the patient's heart sounds, looking out for any added sounds or murmurs.

Heart sounds

The heart sounds are the noises generated by the closure of the heart valves. In healthy adults, there are two normal heart sounds, the first heart sound (S_1) and second heart sound (S_2). This produces the classical *'lubb-dubb'* sound with the former (S_1) being louder than the latter (S_2).

First heart sound
The first heart sound is caused by the closure of the mitral and tricuspid valves and represents the beginning of systole – it is best heard at the apex. A loud S_1 is caused by a narrowing of the mitral valve (mitral stenosis) whilst a soft S_1 occurs in an incompetent mitral valve (mitral regurgitation).

Second heart sound
The S_2 heart sound is caused by the closure of the aortic and pulmonary valves and signifies the end of systole and the start of diastole. It is best heard in the left sternal edge at the second intercostal space. In a normal person it can be heard as a single heart sound with the aortic component being dominant, or as a split sound with two distinct noises in inspiration. The splitting of the heart sound can be physiological or due to a defect in the conduction pathway such as in right bundle branch block. A fixed splitting suggests an atrial septal defect.

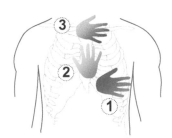

Numbers indicate the order in which the positions should be used.

Fig 2.5 Hand positions for palpating heaves and thrills.

TOP TIP!

Remember that the bell of the stethoscope is good for low pitched sounds (e.g. mitral stenosis) and should be applied gently. The diaphragm makes higher pitched murmurs easier to detect (e.g. aortic regurgitation). Pressing the bell too hard makes it act like the diaphragm.

Added sounds

Sounds heard in the heart other than the first and second heart sounds are usually abnormal.

Third heart sound

The third heart sound (S_3) represents ventricular filling and is best heard in the apex area. It is a low pitched sound that is best picked up by using the bell of the stethoscope. Although it may be present in normal individuals such as athletes or pregnant women, in the elderly it may signify heart failure.

Fourth heart sound

The S_4 heart sound can be heard just prior to S_1 and signifies atrial contraction. It is a low pitched sound heard in the apex area and is often due to left ventricular hypertrophy.

Opening snap

An opening snap is highly suggestive of mitral stenosis. It occurs shortly after S_2 and is described as a high pitched sound; it is best heard using the diaphragm of the stethoscope at the apex.

Midsystolic click

Midsystolic click, as the name suggests, occurs in systole. It is caused by mitral valve prolapse when one of the leaflets of the valve fails to close, often causing atypical chest pain. It can be associated with its own murmur occurring in late systole.

Mechanical heart valves

Mechanical heart valves are palpable and produce a distinctive metallic click – they are often heard without the need of a stethoscope. The timing of the sound depends on the valve that has been repaired. An aortic mechanical valve produces a metallic second heart sound click, whilst a mitral one produces a metallic first heart sound click. Patients should have a tell tale median sternotomy scar along with a lateral thoracotomy scar in the case of mitral valvotomy.

Pericardial frictional rub

A pericardial rub is synonymous with pericarditis. It is described as a low pitched scratching sound like the sound heard when walking on firm snow. It is due to the friction between the visceral and parietal pericardial layers.

> **TOP TIP!**
>
> Patients with mechanical heart valves will require life-long warfarin treatment. Look for a yellow warfarin INR booklet by the bedside to confirm this.

> **TOP TIP!**
>
> Try to listen to the heart sounds in as many patients (healthy and unwell) as you can because your ability to diagnose a murmur will only improve through experience.

Murmurs

Murmurs are audible sounds produced by turbulent blood flow through the heart valves. Not all murmurs signify valve disease. Some can be innocent and are caused by increased stroke volume in children, in pregnancy or during a fever. These murmurs are always systolic and soft in intensity.

If you hear a murmur on auscultation (see *Fig 2.6*) you should try to discern its location, timing (systolic or diastolic), character and pitch, radiation and intensity. To assess the murmur's timing in relation to the patient's heart beat, press your thumb over a carotid

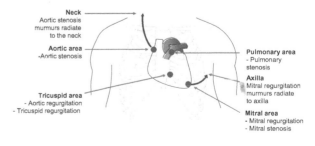

Fig 2.6 Best positions to hear heart murmurs.

TOP TIP!

As a rule, right-sided murmurs (pulmonary and tricuspid) are best heard in inspiration and left-sided murmurs (mitral and aortic) are best heard in expiration. This can be remembered by the acronym RILE: **R**ight **I**nspiration **L**eft **E**xpiration.

BOX 2.5 **Grading the intensity of a murmur**

Grade 1 (thrill absent)	Faint and hard to hear with stethoscope
Grade 2	Louder and heard easily with stethoscope
Grade 3	Very loud with stethoscope; no thrill present
Grade 4 (thrill present)	Heard with stethoscope on chest with thrill
Grade 5	Heard over wide area with stethoscope and thrill
Grade 6	Very loud; audible without stethoscope

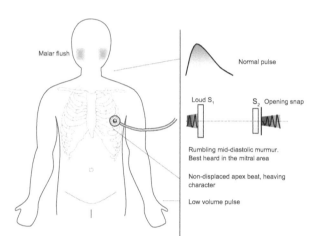

Fig 2.7 Mitral stenosis. This is typically asymptomatic but may present with angina, syncope or acute ventricular failure; ask the patient about past medical history of rheumatic fever.

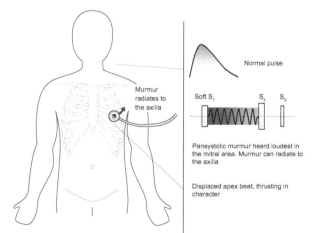

Fig 2.8 Mitral regurgitation. Has the same symptoms as congestive heart failure and may present acutely as left ventricular failure.

area to feel the carotid pulsation which represents systole. Note whether the murmur coincides with the pulse (systolic murmur) or not (diastolic murmur). Grade the murmur according to an agreed grading classification as described in *Box 2.5*.

When auscultating the precordium, begin with the bell of the stethoscope at the apex/mitral area and attempt to listen for mitral stenosis. Next use the diaphragm side of the stethoscope to listen for mitral regurgitation. Ensure that the patient holds their breath in expiration whilst leaning over to the left-hand side. If you do hear a murmur, check whether it radiates to the axilla. Move on to the tricuspid area, listening out for tricuspid regurgitation. Have the patient lean forward and hold their breath in expiration so that the aortic regurgitation murmur is accentuated. Next, move to the pulmonary area, looking out for pulmonary stenosis. Finally, listen in the aortic area for aortic stenosis; if heard, confirm whether it radiates to the carotids or not.

Mitral stenosis

Mitral stenosis (see *Fig 2.7*) is a disease of the valve characterized by a narrowing of the valve orifice which impedes blood flow from the left atrium to the left ventricle. It is commonly caused by rheumatic fever; however, rarer causes include SLE and bacterial endocarditis. The mitral stenotic murmur is a low pitched rumbling diastolic murmur for which the bell of the stethoscope should be used. On careful auscultation an opening snap can be heard shortly after S_2. The murmur is best heard in the mitral area and is accentuated by asking the patient to hold their breath in expiration whilst lying on their left side. You may wish to say to the patient: "*to help me listen better to this part of your heart can I ask you to lean over to the left and take a deep breath in, now breathe out and hold please.*"

Other features of mitral stenosis include malar flush on the cheeks, a non-displaced tapping apex beat, and a patient in AF. In severe mitral stenosis a Graham Steell murmur may be found. This is an early diastolic murmur due to pulmonary regurgitation heard loudest in the pulmonary area (second intercostal space, left sternal edge). This occurs because the chronically elevated pressure in the right atrium, which results from the stenosed mitral valve, leads to an increase in pulmonary capillary pressure and pulmonary hypertension, resulting in pulmonary regurgitation.

Mitral regurgitation

In mitral regurgitation (see *Fig 2.8*) there is an incompetence of the mitral valve leading to incomplete closure during systole. This allows blood to reflux back into the left atrium from the left ventricle. Common causes include mitral valve proplase, ischaemic heart disease, rheumatic fever and Marfan syndrome. Mitral regurgitation may also be a post-MI complication from rupture of the chordae tendinae or papillary muscles. It is best heard in the mitral area of the heart and presents with a soft S_1 and a blowing pansystolic murmur which radiates to the axilla. Additional features may include a displaced thrusting apex beat as well as an S_3.

Aortic stenosis

Aortic stenosis (*Fig 2.9*) is the narrowing of the aortic valve which obstructs blood flow from the left ventricle into the aorta. Causes include rheumatic heart disease, degeneration and calcification of a normal valve (presents in the elderly), or calcification of a congenital bicuspid valve (presents in the middle aged). Symptoms include angina, syncope or acute left ventricular failure. On auscultation, a high-pitched harsh crescendo–decrescendo ejection systolic murmur can be heard in the aortic area. Occasionally it can radiate to the carotids. Other signs may include a soft S_2, slow rising pulse, a thrusting apex beat and an aortic thrill.

Aortic regurgitation

Aortic regurgitation (*Fig 2.10*) describes a leaky aortic valve resulting in blood flowing back into the left ventricle from the aorta during diastole. Causes include rheumatic fever, infective endocarditis, Marfan syndrome, ankylosing spondylitis and syphilis. Since the murmur radiates from the aortic area downwards in the direction of blood flow, it can be auscultated in the tricuspid or aortic areas. Have the patient leaning forward with their breath held in end-expiration to hear it better. It is heard as an early blowing decrescendo diastolic murmur. It may also be accompanied by an Austin Flint murmur which is a mid-diastolic murmur caused by a reflux of blood partially shutting the mitral valve. Other features include:

- a collapsing arterial pulse
- de Musset's sign – head nodding with each pulse; classical sign of syphilitic aortitis
- Quincke's sign – capillary pulsations in nail beds
- Corrigan's sign – carotid pulsation
- Duroziez's sign – femoral diastolic murmur as blood flows backwards in diastole
- Traube's sign – 'pistol shot' sound over the femoral arteries.

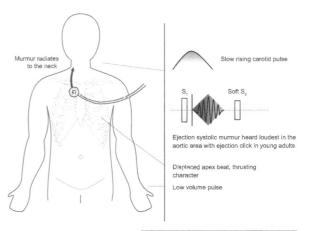

Murmur radiates to the neck

Slow rising carotid pulse

S_1 Soft S_2

Ejection systolic murmur heard loudest in the aortic area with ejection click in young adults

Displaced apex beat, thrusting character

Low volume pulse

Fig 2.9 Aortic stenosis. Typically asymptomatic, but may present with chest pain or syncope. Ask about a past medical history of rheumatic fever.

TOP TIP!

Mitral regurgitation is the most commonly found pathological murmur in the heart.

TOP TIP!

Do not confuse aortic stenosis with the more common aortic sclerosis, which is a senile degeneration of the valve. In aortic sclerosis there is also an ejection systolic murmur but no carotid radiation and a normal pulse.

TOP TIP!

Right-sided murmurs are much less common than left-sided murmurs and so are less likely to appear in your exams!

TOP TIP!

In an exam you are most likely to get a patient with aortic stenosis or mitral regurgitation because they are systolic and easily discernable.

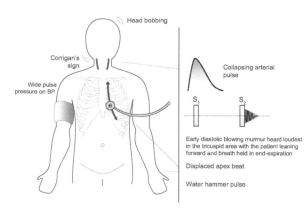

Head bobbing

Corrigan's sign

Wide pulse pressure on BP

Collapsing arterial pulse

S_1 S_2

Early diastolic blowing murmur heard loudest in the tricuspid area with the patient leaning forward and breath held in end-expiration

Displaced apex beat

Water hammer pulse

Fig 2.10 Aortic regurgitation. Asymptomatic or present with symptoms of ventricular or biventricular failure. Ask about past medical history of rheumatic fever, Marfan syndrome, and possibly syphilis or ankylosing spondylitis.

Pulmonary murmurs

Pulmonary stenosis and regurgitation are best heard in the pulmonary area which is around the second intercostal space, right sternal edge. The pulmonary stenosis murmur is similar to the aortic stenosis murmur in that it is ejection systolic in nature. Causes are usually congenital but it may also occur in rheumatic fever. Pulmonary regurgitation produces an early diastolic murmur similar to aortic regurgitation.

Tricuspid murmurs

Tricuspid murmurs are best heard in the tricuspid area which is located around the fifth intercostal space, left sternal edge. Tricuspid stenosis may be heard as an early diastolic murmur, whereas tricuspid regurgitation is a pansystolic murmur similar to mitral regurgitation. With tricuspid regurgitation there may also be a raised JVP and tender, pulsatile hepatomegaly associated with right heart failure. Ventricular septal defects (VSD) are also best heard at this point.

Carotids

Once you have auscultated the precordium, do not forget to listen over the carotids using the bell side of the stethoscope. Listen over each carotid artery for the radiation of an aortic stenosis murmur and for carotid bruits suggestive of atherosclerosis. A bruit is an audible vascular sound caused by turbulent blood flow through a narrowed vessel. Listen to one carotid at a time whilst asking the patient to take a deep breath in and hold. This will allow you to distinguish any noises heard from the patient's breath sounds.

Lung bases

With the patient leaning forwards, briefly listen to the lung bases to assess for the presence of crepitations or pleural effusions. These may be caused by pulmonary oedema secondary to left ventricular failure.

2.1.5 **Additional points**

Oedema

In the cardiovascular examination, oedema may signify the development of uncontrolled heart failure. In some situations the fluid overload may be so severe that it reaches the patient's sacrum, particularly if they are bed bound. Warn the patient that they may experience some discomfort when you check for this.

While the patient is leaning forward, examine for sacral oedema by applying firm pressure against the lower back and for pedal oedema by pressing down over the ankle. Observe for pitting oedema by looking for the indentation caused by your finger after applying pressure. It is useful while you are observing the legs to look out for any venous grafting scars – these are normally 10 cm long and located around the medial malleolus. Venous grafting scars together with a median sternotomy scar would suggest that the patient has had a CABG. Other signs to look for in the legs are pallor and ulcer suggestive of peripheral arterial disease.

TOP TIP!

Other causes of murmurs include congenital heart defects such as ventricular septal defect (VSD) which gives rise to a pansystolic murmur, atrial septal defect (ASD) which causes an ejection systolic murmur, and a patent ductus arteriosus (PDA) which results in a continuous machinery murmur throughout systole and diastole, radiating through to the back.

TOP TIP!

Remember that grafts can also be taken from the radial artery or internal mammary arteries for CABG, so do not forget to inspect for scars in these areas.

Peripheral vascular examination

Your examination of the cardiovascular system will not be complete if you do not examine the rest of the vascular system. Arterial disease in the heart is more than likely to be replicated elsewhere in the body and so you should ask to perform a full peripheral vascular examination (see *Chapter 2.14*) including the femoral, popliteal, posterior tibial and dorsalis pedis pulses.

2.1.6   Summing up

If you have found a cardiac murmur you should consider referring the patient for an echo cardiogram which will provide detailed structural information about the heart. If you have not already done so, indicate that you would like to measure the blood pressure. If the patient is found to have raised blood pressure you should ask to perform a urine dipstick to look for protein and carry out a fundoscopy to look for evidence of retinopathy.

Also, as with any examination, it is useful to request some bedside tests that may help in the diagnosis, such as an ECG and a chest X-ray of the patient. Indicate that you would also like to have a look at the patient's oxygen saturations, respiration and temperature chart.

Thank the patient for their co-operation and offer to cover them with a blanket to protect their dignity. Keep the curtain around them drawn and give them appropriate time to dress themselves. Whilst waiting you may wish to collect your thoughts about what information you have gained from the examination before conveying it back to the patient.

2.1.7   Common clinical scenarios

The following are a list of common cardiology cases which you may encounter. For each one, consider:
- what the likely diagnosis is
- what key features you would look for
- what questions you would ask or further investigations you would order to refine or confirm your diagnosis

You could use role play with a friend, using the histories in the cases below as a framework.

CASE 1

A 45 year old lady presents with shortness of breath with exercise, which has been getting progressively worse over the last 4 months. Her past medical history is only significant for rheumatic fever at the age of 10. On examination, she is in AF and the apex beat is tapping but not displaced. On auscultation there is a rumbling low-pitched mid-diastolic murmur best heard at the apex, which does not radiate – it is of 3/6 intensity. The lung bases are clear and there is no peripheral oedema.

CASE 2

A 60 year old gentleman, who is 3 days post MI, has presented with sudden onset of shortness of breath and a cough productive of frothy pink sputum. He is sitting up and finding it very difficult to breathe. On examination, he is in sinus tachycardia with a rate of 115. Auscultation reveals a pansystolic murmur loudest at the apex, which radiates to the axilla. The lung bases show evidence of crepitations and he has pitting oedema in the legs to the level of the knees.

CASE 3

A 70 year old gentleman presents to the GP with episodes of chest pain and fainting while running for the bus. These problems never happened while he was resting. He was given a spray to put underneath his tongue by his GP which helps the pain but the fainting is now becoming more frequent and he is worried. On examination the pulse is 75 beats per minute and regular but is slow rising in nature at the carotids. On auscultation a harsh ejection systolic murmur is heard following an ejection click. The murmur is noted to radiate to the carotids. Otherwise the heart sounds were normal. He did not appear to be in heart failure.

CASE 4

A 47 year old patient with a congenital bicuspid aortic valve was admitted from A&E as he had been feeling unwell for the last 6 weeks. He describes feeling fatigued, sweating at night and sometimes notices blood in his urine. He has unintentionally lost about 5 kg in the last 6 weeks. The only recent history of note is that he had a tooth extraction at the dentist. On examination, he has a temperature of 38.5°C and his nails are boggy with 1 mm red lines in the nail beds. He complains of pain when capillary refill time is assessed and there are a few red nodules present on the palms and finger tips. He was noticed to have a collapsing pulse and the apex beat was thrusting in nature and displaced to the anterior axillary line. Auscultation reveals a loud early diastolic murmur all over the precordium but loudest in the tricuspid region with the patient sitting forward.

CASE 5

A 65 year gentleman attends a new registration check at the GP surgery. He brings along a warfarin diary with INRs currently controlled at 3.5. On examination he is found to have a median sternotomy scar and an audible click coinciding with a second heart sound.

Chapter 2.2
Respiratory examination

What to do . . .

- Introduce yourself to the patient – establish rapport and seek consent
- Appropriately position and expose the patient
- Inspection: look at the hands, face, neck and chest
- Palpation: feel the trachea and apex beat, assess for chest expansion and feel for tactile vocal fremitus, and check for cervical lymph nodes
- Percussion: percuss over the anterior, lateral and posterior areas comparing the left with the right side
- Auscultation: listen over the same areas comparing the left with the right side – if vocal resonance is assessed then tactile vocal fremitus is not required
- Examine for oedema at the sacrum and in the legs
- Thank the patient and conclude the examination

Respiratory disease includes diseases of the lung, pleural cavity, bronchial tubes, trachea and upper respiratory tract. They may range from being mild and self-limiting such as the common cold, to life-threatening such as pulmonary embolism. Disorders of the respiratory system manifest in only a handful of principal symptoms, including dyspnoea, cough, sputum, haemoptysis, wheeze and pleuritic chest pain. Although a good history may point you in the right direction, the respiratory examination is vital in distinguishing the actual cause from a whole host of other possibilities.

The respiratory examination is a comprehensive assessment of the entire respiratory system, with the aim of ascertaining the presence of any pathology, rather than just listening to a patient's chest with a stethoscope.

Anatomy of the chest

The respiratory tract runs from the oro-nasal pharynx to the alveoli of the lungs. It plays a primary role in oxygenating the blood as well as removing harmful by-products of respiration such as carbon dioxide. It also has a secondary role in thermoregulation and maintaining the acid–base balance of the body.

Air enters the respiratory system through the nasal passages as well as the oro-pharynx. It passes down into the larynx before entering the lower respiratory tract. As food and air can both enter the oro-pharynx, a thin fibrocartilage, known as the epiglottis, acts to guide each to their appropriate orifice.

The trachea is the first part of the lower respiratory tract. It is a cartilaginous tube that lies in front of the oesophagus. At its end it bifurcates into the right and left bronchi within the lungs. The right bronchus is wider and more vertical than the left and is a common site of inhaled foreign bodies such as peanuts. The bronchi further divide and subdivide into lobar bronchi, segmental bronchi and then bronchioles, before branching out into individual alveoli.

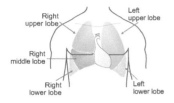

Fig 2.11 Anatomy of the lungs.

There are two lungs within the thoracic cavity (see *Fig 2.11*) which contains millions of alveoli that aid respiration. The right lung consists of three lobes, the upper, middle and lower, whilst the left lung has two lobes, the upper and lower. The lingula is a division of the left upper lobe that corresponds anatomically to the middle lobe of the right lung. The left lung is smaller in volume than the right because of the presence of the heart within the thoracic cavity. Each lung is encapsulated by a pleural sac which is a double-layered membrane with the inner layer (visceral pleura) covering the lungs and the outer layer (parietal pleura) attached to the chest wall. In between the two layers is a cavity known as the pleural space which is filled with pleural fluid. The pleura's primary function is to facilitate respiration by helping the lung remain attached to the chest wall.

2.2.1 **Beginning the examination**

Introduce yourself to the patient stating your name and job title. Ask the patient's name and age and check to see if they are in any discomfort. Explain to the patient what you intend to do and gain consent to proceed.

Female patients may have to disrobe to their bra and may feel uncomfortable – always check to see if they would like a chaperone to be present.

2.2.2 **Patient exposure and position**

Before requesting the patient to undress, ensure that adequate privacy is maintained. Lay the patient at a 45 degree angle on the couch as this should help in the examination of their JVP later on. Expose their chest and ensure that you have a clear view of their lower limbs so that you can assess for any evidence of pedal oedema or relevant skin changes such as erythema nodosum (seen in tuberculosis) or sarcoidosis.

Give the patient a sheet or blanket to maintain their modesty when they are not being examined. Make sure that you wash your hands thoroughly before commencing your examination.

2.2.3 **Inspection**

Observe the patient from the end of the bed and look to see if they are comfortable at rest.
- Check if they are in respiratory distress, looking for the use of accessory muscles, intercostal recession, nasal flaring or tachypnoea.
- See if the patient purses their lips to breathe as this is suggestive of COPD.
- Comment on whether the patient is obviously cyanosed.
- Note if the patient is suffering with an obvious cough, wheeze or stridor (stridor is a high-pitched inspiratory sound originating from upper airways and suggests possible airway obstruction).
- Look around the bed for nebulizers, inhalers, chest drains, sputum pots, peak flow meters or oxygen masks.

Nails and hands

Begin the examination by inspecting the patient's hands. Look closely at the nails for a dusky blue discoloration which may be a sign of peripheral cyanosis. Note for tar staining, particularly on the nails and fingers – smoking is an important risk factor for bronchial carcinoma and COPD. Inspect the fingers from the sides for loss of the nail bed angle which occurs in clubbing. Respiratory causes of clubbing include bronchial carcinoma, pleural and mediastinal tumours, chronic suppurative lung disease (CF, bronchiectasis, abscesses) and lung fibrosis.

Assuming the patient is not in pain, gently take hold of their hands and feel the palmar surfaces for sweat and warmth. Patients with chronic respiratory disease may have warm red palms as a result of dilatation of the vessels from CO_2 retention. Ask the patient to hold their hands out with their fingers splayed and look for a fine tremor in the fingers – this can be caused by overuse of β-agonist drugs such as salbutamol inhalers. Now ask the patient to stretch their arms out in front of them and cock their wrist back – ask them to close their eyes and hold the pose for up to 30 seconds. Observe for a flapping tremor (asterixis) which is a late sign of CO_2 retention; note that this feature is also seen in liver disease and cannot be distinguished by simple observation.

Pulse and respiratory rate

Once you have finished with the hands, inform the patient that you wish to feel for their pulse. Palpate the radial pulse for 15 seconds and multiply the number of pulsations by 4 to determine their heart rate in beats per minute. In addition to the rate, you should assess the rhythm and character of the pulse, particularly feeling for a bounding pulse caused by CO_2 retention (also present in sepsis).

Move on to assess the patient's respiratory rate. Count the number of breaths the patient takes in 15 seconds and multiply this number by 4 to obtain an estimate of the patient's respiratory rate. Determine if this is tachypnoeic (> 20 breaths per minute), bradynoeic (< 12 breaths per minute) or normal (12–20 breaths per minute). Next, assess the pattern of breathing, paying particular attention to the inspiratory and expiratory phases. A prolonged expiratory phase suggests a degree of airflow obstruction such as in asthma or COPD. The presence of alternating phases of hyperapnoea and apnoea is known as Cheyne–Stokes respiration. This occurs in severe left ventricular failure and in brain stem ischaemia. If the patient has a normal respiratory rate but is taking excessively deep breaths, this could suggest they have Kussmaul respiration which is seen in severe metabolic acidosis and renal failure.

> **TOP TIP!**
>
> The length of inspiration should be two-thirds of the total respiratory cycle.

Look at the chest wall for any asymmetry during respiration. In the absence of structural deformity or phrenic nerve involvement, a reduced chest wall movement may be due to underlying pathology preventing air from entering the lung on the unilateral side.

Face

Move your attention now to the face. Look at the conjunctivae for evidence of anaemia. Ask the patient to look up and gently pull down the lower eyelids. Normal conjunctivae are healthy red in colour but anaemic individuals will have a pale conjunctiva. Look at the pupil, noting any pupillary constriction as well as ptosis of the eyelid which can occur in Horner's syndrome, secondary to a Pancoast tumour (an apical lung tumour causing sympathetic palsy).

> **TOP TIP!**
>
> Assess the respiratory rate whilst you are at the wrist (checking the pulse), otherwise the patient may feel uncomfortable and anxious if you seem to be staring at their chest.

Look inside the mouth for evidence of central cyanosis. Ask the patient to open their mouth as wide as possible and stick their tongue up against the roof of their mouth. Look at the under-surface of the tongue for any bluish tinge, which signals central cyanosis.

Observe the neck for any evidence of a raised JVP (see *Section 2.1*). Raised JVP can be seen in congestive heart failure, cor pulmonale (right heart failure caused by chronic lung disease) and also in superior vena cava obstruction, secondary to bronchial carcinoma.

Chest

Move your attention on to the patient's chest wall. Inspect for any obvious thoracic cage deformities such as:

- pectus excavatum – this is a congenital deformity of the chest wall whereby there is dysplasia of the sternum and ribs, giving rise to a sunken and depressed appearance to the sternum
- pectus carinatum – also known as 'pigeon chest', this is an abnormal protrusion of the sternum, which can occur in adults with a history of severe asthma in childhood.

Look for any spinal-shaped deformities such as scoliosis or kyphosis which may give rise to chest wall abnormalities. Kyphosis is the abnormal outward curvature of the upper spine forming a 'hump' whereas in scoliosis there is increased lateral curvature of the spine.

Inspect for any operative scars found on the chest wall (*Fig 2.12*).

- A midline sternotomy scar may be seen and is suggestive of a previous CABG or valve replacement.
- A thoracoplasty scar refers to a scar that is caused by removal of a number of ribs from the chest wall to induce lung collapse.
- A lobectomy scar denotes surgical removal of a lobe of the lung.
- A phrenicotomy (phrenic nerve crush) scar suggests the use of an old surgery technique employed to treat tuberculosis. It involves surgically resecting the phrenic nerve to reduce unilateral diaphragmatic movements and decreased lung volume. The scar is often found above the clavicle.

Look at the antero-posterior diameter of the chest wall for signs of hyperinflation, also known as barrel chest. The size of the chest diameter is often proportional to the severity of the airflow obstruction.

2.2.4 Palpation

The purpose of palpation of the chest is to determine the mediastinum position by locating the position of the trachea and apex beat, the degree of chest expansion to note for any lung pathology, and finally vocal fremitus to distinguish between types of lung disorders. You should also complete your palpation by checking for any lymph nodes.

Gentle chest wall palpation is indicated if the patient has chest pain; local tenderness can be identified, the causes of which include bone, muscle and cartilage disease.

Position of the trachea and apex beat

The trachea and the apex beat are both good markers of mediastinal position. Because the trachea is located in the upper part of the thoracic cage, lung lesions causing upper mediastinal shifts are more likely to affect it. On the other hand, the apex beat is in the lower end of the thoracic cage and so it is a good indicator of lower mediastinal shift. For example, a moderately sized pleural effusion will cause a displacement of the apex beat, whereas a larger effusion will also cause tracheal deviation.

TOP TIP!

Kyphosis is where the spine is shaped like a letter 'K' whereas in scoliosis it is shaped like an 'S'.

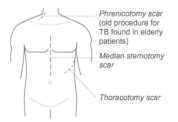

Phrenicotomy scar (old procedure for TB found in elderly patients)

Median sternotomy scar

Thoracotomy scar

Fig 2.12 Common surgical scars seen on the chest.

TOP TIP!

Do not forget to inspect the back of the chest in addition to the front so that you do not miss a thoracotomy scar. Consider doing this when examining the back so that you do not move the patient too often.

Feel for the trachea at the sternal angle (see *Fig 2.13*). This can be done by placing your index finger and ring finger on either side of the trachea and noting whether the distances are equal from the adjacent sternomastoid tendons. Confirm this by resting your middle finger on the trachea itself and feeling for the cricoid cartilage. Warn the patient prior to commencing this test as it can be uncomfortable for them.

The trachea is the central airway column in the chest and so is a good indicator of the position of the mediastinum. The trachea can be displaced by localized neck masses such as goitre and, more importantly, lung lesions causing mediastinal shift can also displace it. Tracheal deviation to one side can be caused by a lesion either pushing it away from the midline or by pulling it towards itself. Conditions such as pneumothorax or a very large pleural effusion can shift the trachea away as air or fluid, respectively, collect within the pleural space. On the other hand, conditions such as a collapsed lung or lung fibrosis may reduce the volume of the affected lung and may pull the trachea towards it.

Palpate the apex beat starting at the 5th intercostal space mid-clavicular line. In the absence of cardiomegaly, any lateral shift in the apex beat may indicate mediastinal displacement.

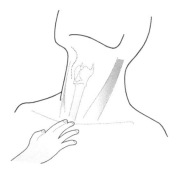

Fig 2.13 Method to palpate the trachea.

TOP TIP!

Complete your examination on the anterior chest wall before asking the patient to lean forwards and repeating the steps on the back – this will reduce the number of times they are moving and so will help to minimize any discomfort they experience.

Chest expansion

Chest expansion should be assessed to establish the depth and quality of movement on each side of the chest. Both sides of the chest wall should be assessed for symmetry. If there is a unilateral loss of chest expansion this may indicate pathology on that side, for example due to an underlying pneumothorax, pleural effusion, or a collapsed lung. If the chest expansion is bilaterally reduced then this could be caused by hyperinflation of the chest as seen in asthma and COPD.

Rest the palms of your hands on either side of the upper part of the patient's chest (see *Fig 2.14*). Ask the patient to take a deep breath in and then look for any obvious asymmetry in the movements of your hands as the chest expands. Next move your hands down to the lower ribcage around the 10th ribs. Gently wrap the fingers of both your hands around the patient's chest with your thumbs meeting at the midline [note that they don't meet on the figure]. Ensure that your thumbs are free from the patient's skin to avoid impeding chest expansion. Ask the patient to take another deep breath and note the degree to which the chest expands by measuring the distance the thumbs oppose one another – normal chest expansion should be at least 5 cm. Complete the assessment of chest expansion by repeating the procedure on the patient's back.

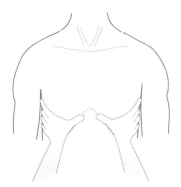

Placement of hands to measure chest expansion

Tactile vocal fremitus

Tactile vocal fremitus refers to the vibrations that can be felt on the chest wall which are transmitted through the lung when the patient speaks. These vibrations can be assessed by placing the ulnar border of each hand horizontally at two comparable positions on the patient's chest and asking the patient to say 'ninety nine' when doing so. Compare the vibrations felt between the two sides to note if there are any abnormalities.

In normal lungs, the vibrations felt on the two sides of the chest should be similar, except over the heart. The mechanism and alterations of vibrations in disease are the same as for vocal resonance, with increased vibrations more on one side possibly indicating the presence of lung consolidation. In lung consolidation there is inflammation of the parenchyma as the alveoli fill with fluid and this

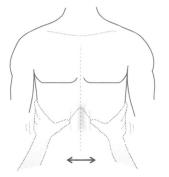

Ask the patient to take a deep breath in. Measure distance created between your thumbs

Fig 2.14 Measurement of chest expansion.

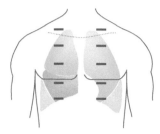

Anterior chest wall

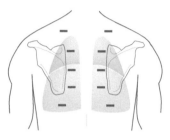

Posterior chest wall

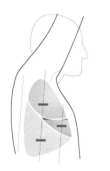

Lateral chest wall

Fig 2.15 Areas to percuss on anterior, posterior and lateral chest wall.

results in sound being transmitted faster than in a normal aerated lung – because the sound waves travel quicker through a solid than through a gas. If the vocal fremitus vibrations are reduced, it may suggest the presence of a pneumothorax or an effusion. This is because the sound has to be transmitted through an extra cavity (i.e. pleura) between the lung and the chest wall that is filled with air, fluid or blood (haemothorax).

2.2.5 **Percussion**

The purpose of percussing the chest (see *Fig 2.15*) is to determine the resonance of the structures that lie within the chest wall. Place your non-dominant hand on the patient's chest, ensuring that your fingers are spread out and your middle finger rests within an intercostal space. Tap the interphalangeal bone using the tip of your middle finger of the dominant hand. Make sure that the strike is short and sharp with the action arising from the wrist. Hit the finger at right angles to obtain the optimal sound. Ensure that you withdraw your finger immediately after the tap has ceased to prevent damping out the vibrations and percussion note. Tap over the same area two to three times before moving on to another area.

Divide the anterior chest into three zones: upper, middle and lower. When tapping, compare the left and right sides of each zone before moving downwards. Complete your examination of the anterior chest wall by percussing the apices of the lung by tapping directly over the clavicles and finish off by examining the axillary areas. Move on to examine the back in a similar fashion.

When percussing the chest it is important to be aware of the underlying anatomical structures. The anterior chest wall largely corresponds to the upper lobes of the lung, whereas the posterior wall reflects the location of the lower lobes. The examination of the lateral chest wall gives a good cross-section of all the lobes in the chest and permits you to examine the upper, middle and lower lobes.

The percussion note changes depending on whether the underlying structures contain air, fluid or solid mass. The percussion note of the normal air-filled lung should be resonant. An increased or hyper-resonant note suggests the presence of large volumes of air, possibly due to a pneumothorax, large bullae, or air trapping as seen in obstructive airway disease. A dull note is heard in any lung tissue that is solid such as in consolidation or fibrosis. If the percussion note is particularly dull or stony dull this may indicate pleural effusion because fluid fills the pleural cavity and prevents vibration from transmitting into the lung from the chest wall. In obese patients the percussion note may be uniformly reduced due to the extra fat overlying the chest wall.

2.2.6 **Auscultation**

Auscultation of the chest is perhaps the most important part of the examination and allows you to hear the breath sounds that the patient makes as well as any added sounds that may arise from underlying pathology.

When auscultating, you should largely listen over the same areas employed during percussion. Begin with the bell side of the stethoscope to examine the apices of the lung before using the diaphragm for the rest of the chest. Alternate between the left and right sides, comparing the two for any differences. Instruct the patient to breathe through their open mouth to allow for good air entry into the lungs.

TOP TIP!

Demonstrate to the patient how you would like them to breathe when auscultating the chest.

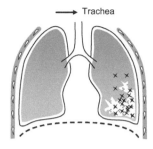

Trachea →

Lung fibrosis
Chest expansion   Decreased bilaterally
Trachea position   Shifted to affected side
Vocal fremitus   Increased
Percussion note   Dull
Breath sounds   Bronchial
Added sounds   Coarse crepitations

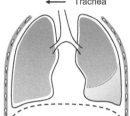

← **Trachea**

Pleural effusion
Chest expansion   Decreased on affected side
Trachea position   Shifted to opposite side
Vocal fremitus   Absent
Percussion note   Stony dull
Breath sounds   Absent (bronchial above fluid)
Added sounds   Absent (may be pleural rub above fluid)

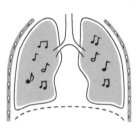

Wheeze
Chest expansion   Decreased bilaterally
Trachea position   Central
Vocal fremitus   Normal or decreased
Percussion note   Increased
Breath sounds   Decreased
Added sounds   Polyphonic wheeze

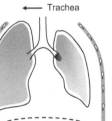

← **Trachea**

Lung collapse
Chest expansion   Decreased on affected side
Trachea position   Shifted to affected side
Vocal fremitus   Absent
Percussion note   Dull
Breath sounds   Decreased
Added sounds   Absent or decreased

← **Trachea**

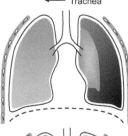

Pneumothorax
Chest expansion   Decreased on affected side
Trachea position   Shifted to opposite side
Vocal fremitus   Decreased
Percussion note   Increased (hyper-resonant)
Breath sounds   Decreased
Added sounds   Absent or decreased

Consolidation
Chest expansion   Decreased on affected side
Trachea position   Central
Vocal fremitus   Increased
Percussion note   Dull
Breath sounds   Bronchial breathing
Added sounds   Crepitations

Fig 2.16 Diagnostic findings
on auscultation with common
lung abnormalities.

Breath sounds

Breath sounds are generated by the turbulent air flow passing through the upper airways. Because they are conducted through the lower respiratory tract and then into the lung parenchyma, the sound becomes attenuated. The sounds heard on the chest wall are usually vesicular in nature and are generally soft pitched and with a rustling character. The sounds are heard steadily throughout inspiration and tail off at the beginning of expiration.

Bronchial breath sounds are sounds heard over the trachea and main bronchi. They are described as a loud, harsh sound with almost equal inspiratory and expiratory phases. They are characterized by a short pause between the two phases which distinguishes them from vesicular breathing. If bronchial sounds are heard in other parts of the lung rather than just in these areas, this is considered abnormal and is known as bronchial breathing. The most common cause of this is consolidation whereby the solid lung facilitates conduction of the bronchial sounds directly to the chest wall.

Breath sounds can be decreased or absent which suggests lung abnormalities (see *Fig 2.16*). Causes include pleural effusions, lung collapse, pneumothorax or emphysema. In pleural effusion, breath sounds may be absent or reduced beneath the level of the effusion but have bronchial breathing just above. This is because the lung volume is compressed by the effect of the effusion beneath it, giving rise to sounds similar to those heard in consolidation. In emphysema the reduced breath sounds are heard bilaterally because there is significant lung damage and air trapping that restricts the patient's ability to take in large tidal volumes. Hence, little air is inhaled to generate a sound.

Added sounds

Added sounds are sounds that are not normally heard in the healthy adult. Their presence is always suggestive of underlying pathology that should be investigated further. The most commonly heard sounds include wheezes, crackles and a pleural rub.

Wheeze

Wheezes tend to be high-pitched musical sounds that are caused by air passing through narrowed airways. In fact, the narrower the airways the higher the pitch heard. Wheezes are normally heard in expiration, are polyphonic in nature and can be heard throughout the chest wall, such as in COPD and asthma. A localized low-pitched monophonic wheeze may indicate single airway obstruction, possibly due to an enlarged lymph lobe, bronchial carcinoma or foreign body.

Crackles

Crackles are also known as crepitations and are caused by the snapping open of the airways that have been collapsed by fluid or exudate. They produce a unique, instantly recognizable crackling sound in the lung that is heard during inspiration. Crackles that are heard earlier on in inspiration suggest larger airway disease such as bronchiectasis or bronchitis, whereas those heard at the end of inspiration point towards small airways involvement, such as in pulmonary fibrosis and congestive heart failure. Crackles are often divided into two categories depending on the sound generated. Fine crackles are heard in pulmonary fibrosis and congestive heart failure whereas coarse crackles are more common in bronchiectasis and pneumonia. When eliciting crackles you should indicate whether they are unilateral and localized or bibasal or widespread. Localized crackles are often due to pneumonia, whereas bibasal crackles are due to fibrosis or mild pulmonary oedema. Widespread crackles can be heard in severe pulmonary oedema.

Pleural rubs

Pleural rubs describes a leathery sound created when the two pleural layers rub against one another. This can occur if the pleura is inflamed or thickened such as in pneumonia or in pulmonary infarction. The sound occurs on chest movements and hence is heard both in inspiration and in expiration.

Vocal resonance

The stethoscope is used to assess the degree of vibration conducted through the lung. Place the diaphragm of the stethoscope over the lung areas and ask the patient to make a resonating sound by saying 'ninety nine'. Compare the quality of vibration between right and left sides to determine if there is any disease pathology. The changes to the sound and their causes are similar to that seen in tactile vocal fremitus.

> **TOP TIP!**
>
> You should perform either tactile vocal fremitus or vocal resonance during your examination but not both, because they give similar information.

Posterior chest wall

It is important to complete your examination by repeating inspection, chest expansion, percussion and auscultation on the posterior chest wall, if you have not already done so. This is particularly important because the posterior chest wall houses the right and left lower lung lobes. Ask the patient to sit forward so that you can get good access to their back.

You should consider palpating for lymphadenopathy, feeling for the sub mental, sub-mandibular, anterior cervical, supra-clavicular, posterior cervical, pre-auricular and occipital nodes of the head and neck. These areas are commonly affected in upper respiratory tract infections, tuberculosis and in cancers.

2.2.7 **Additional points**

Oedema

In the respiratory system shortness of breath may be due to congestive cardiac failure. This is commonly associated with oedema affecting the legs and in severe cases the sacral areas. As part of your routine respiratory examination you should therefore examine both the legs and sacrum for evidence of oedema. Press the pulp of your finger against the patient's ankles and sacrum looking for any indentation marks left behind. Warn the patient that this may be uncomfortable before checking for this. Note the level to which the oedema rises and describe it against local anatomical structures such as the mid-shin, knee and thighs. This may act as a useful reference to denote response to treatment.

2.2.8 **Summing up**

After you have completed your examination it may be necessary to undertake some investigatory tests to form a working diagnosis. Ask to see the patient's observation chart and look particularly at their temperature, pulse, blood pressure and oxygen saturations. It may be necessary to perform an ABG if the patient is in respiratory distress. If the patient has a wheeze or is known to be asthmatic, a peak flow measurement may be useful.

Request an ECG (looking for signs of pulmonary embolism or P pulmonale) in addition to a chest X-ray as an initial investigatory work-up. Chest X-rays are helpful in diagnosing pneumonias, pleural effusions, pneumothorax, collapsed lung and occasionally bronchial carcinomas.

If the patient has a productive cough, ask for a sputum sample that can be sent to microbiology for acid-fast bacilli testing, microscopy, culture and sensitivity (M, C & S) and cytology if clinically indicated. If a sputum sample is forthcoming inspect it for colour and consistency:

- typical green–yellow coloured sputum is found in both viral and bacterial pneumonias. Bronchiectasis and lung abscess produce a green–yellow coloured sputum that is also foul smelling
- rusty coloured sputum may suggest that the patient is suffering from pneumococcal pneumonia
- frothy pink sputum associated with shortness of breath points towards pulmonary oedema
- red streaks in the sputum may simply be caused by violent coughing; however, a significant amount of blood may be due to pulmonary embolism, bronchial carcinoma and tuberculosis. A greyish-white phlegm is typically seen in a smoker or a patient suffering from COPD.

Thank the patient for their co-operation and offer to cover them with a blanket to maintain their dignity. Draw the curtain around them and give them appropriate time to dress themselves. Whilst waiting you may wish to collect your thoughts about what information you have gained from the examination before conveying it back to the patient.

2.2.9 Common clinical scenarios

The following are a list of common respiratory cases which you may encounter. For each one, consider:

- what the likely diagnosis is
- what key features you would look for
- what questions you would ask or further investigations you would order to refine or confirm your diagnosis

You could use role play with a friend, using the histories in the cases below as a framework.

CASE 1
A 23 year old man who plays professional basketball presents with sudden onset of shortness of breath and pleuritic chest pain. On examination he is found to have a respiratory rate of 32, reduced chest expansion on the left side with increased percussion and decreased breath sounds.

CASE 2
An 85 year old woman presents and complains of a four day history of shortness of breath, fever and productive cough. On examination she is noted to be pyrexic and tachycardic in addition to having a raised respiratory rate. She has increased vocal fremitus over the right lower base with bronchial breathing and crepitations. Percussion note is dull.

CASE 3

A 28 year old lady presents with a five day history of increasing shortness of breath, wheeze and nocturnal cough. On examination her peak flow was 50% of her normal expected value. Her chest revealed a polyphonic wheeze throughout.

CASE 4

A 58 year old heavy smoker presents with shortness of breath and haemoptysis. On examination he is cachexic, with tar stains on his fingers and with finger clubbing. Chest signs include absent breath sounds on the right side, absent vocal fremitus and a stony dull percussion note.

CASE 5

An 8 year old boy attended a party and is brought to A&E with acute shortness of breath. On examination he is noted to have absent breath sounds on the right side, slight tracheal deviation to the right as well as reduced expansion on the right side.

Chapter 2.3
Abdomen examination

What to do . . .

- Introduce yourself to the patient – establish rapport and seek consent
- Appropriately position and expose the patient
- Inspection: look around the bedside and then at the abdomen, face, hands and body
- Palpation: feel for Virchow's node, palpate all the abdominal quadrants with light and then deep palpation; palpate the liver, spleen, kidney and aorta
- Percussion: percuss the liver, spleen ascites and bladder
- Auscultation: listen to the abdomen for bowel sounds, the aorta for aortic bruits and the renal arteries for renal bruits (renal artery stenosis)
- Examine for inguinal hernias – check for a positive cough impulse
- Consider performing a full inguino-scrotal examination and PR examination
- Thank the patient and conclude the examination

Patients presenting with abdominal symptoms such as pain, nausea, vomiting and constipation are commonly seen in all specialities; from the neonate presenting with colicky abdominal pain to the elderly patient presenting with bowel obstruction, performing the abdomen examination is a fundamental skill. To excel at the abdominal examination a systematic approach is needed so that the maximum amount of information can be established about the patient and their presenting problems.

A common misconception held by medical students is that the abdominal examination is simply an exercise to locate the source of the patient's pain. It is important to remember that the examination should not just focus on the abdomen, but a more holistic approach is required, with the examination also covering the hands, face, and lower groin.

Signs and symptoms of abdominal disease are often closely correlated to the major organs of the abdominal cavity, and a good knowledge and awareness of anatomical landmarks and the locations of vital organs is therefore essential in determining the pathology of the presenting complaint.

Abdominal cavity

The abdominal cavity spans the length of the abdomen and is defined superiorly by the lower limits of the costal margins of the ribs, and inferiorly by the inguinal ligaments which run from the anterior superior iliac crest to the pubic tubercle. The cavity encases a number of organs, including the lower segment of the oesophagus, stomach, gallbladder, liver, spleen, pancreas, kidneys, abdominal aorta, small and large bowel, bladder and ovaries. Both the liver and spleen can be found tucked up underneath the domes of the diaphragm behind the ribs, with only their edges exposed in the abdomen.

Quadrants

It is useful, for descriptive purposes, to divide the abdomen into quadrants or areas which will help focus the examination and help in developing a working diagnosis (*Fig 2.17*).

One approach is to divide the abdomen into four quadrants consisting of right and left, upper and lower areas. In this method, the abdomen is delineated using an imaginary vertical line running down from the xiphisternum to the symphysis pubis bisected by a horizontal line passing through the umbilicus. Whilst this approach may not be very exact, it does provide a snapshot of the general area where the organs may lie.

An alternative approach is to use a more comprehensive nine region method. This subdivides the abdomen into nine segments, allowing for a more precise description and delineation of any pathology. The areas are formed using hypothetical lines running down vertically from both mid-clavicular points, trisected by two imaginary lines, the first of which runs horizontally across the subcostal plane and the second of which runs across the anterior superior iliac spines.

2.3.1 **Beginning the examination**

Start by introducing yourself to the patient by stating your name and job title. It is also courteous to ask the patient for their name, ask how they are feeling and establish whether they are in any pain or discomfort.

It is important to explain clearly to the patient what you intend to do when examining the abdomen. For female patients it may be necessary to seek the assistance of a chaperone if you feel this is appropriate. For example, you may say to the patient, '*In view of the problem you have been complaining about, I wish to perform an abdomen examination. This will involve me examining and pressing on your tummy as well as looking at your hands and eyes. Before I proceed may I ask if you are in any pain or discomfort?*'

Once the patient has understood what you have said, seek consent to proceed with the examination.

2.3.2 **Patient exposure and position**

Before beginning the examination and asking the patient to undress, ensure that adequate privacy is maintained. You may wish to draw curtains around the cubicle or close any doors. Ask the patient to lie comfortably flat on the couch and expose them from nipple to knee – offer the patient a sheet or blanket to maintain their modesty.

Ensure that there is good lighting to observe the patient as some signs may be missed with poor lighting. Try to make the patient feel comfortable and at ease because an anxious patient may tense their abdominal muscles which makes palpation difficult. You may offer the patient a soft pillow to rest their head on but ensure that the neck is not overly flexed as this can also affect palpation. You should always make a habit of washing your hands thoroughly before commencing your examination.

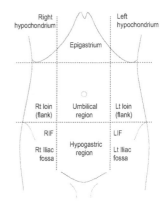

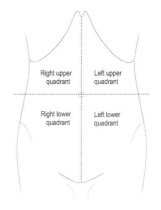

Fig 2.17 The nine area and four quadrant approach to examining the abdomen.

TOP TIP!

In an exam situation it is very important to read the vignette clearly because you may be asked to perform a focused abdominal examination and some medical schools may also expect you to take a brief history.

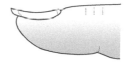

Fig 2.18 Koilonychia.

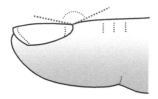

Normal finger
Less than 160 degrees

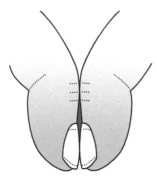

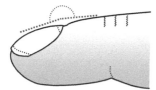

Clubbed finger
Greater than 180 degrees

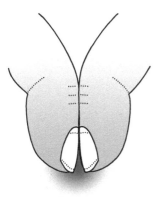

Fig 2.19 Finger clubbing with loss of the diamond sign.

2.3.3 Inspection

Start by observing the patient from the end of the bed to see if they are grimacing with pain or lying comfortably. Look around the bed for any IV cannula drips, PEG or nasogastric feeds, urinary catheters or stoma bags. Move closer to the patient and proceed in a systematic way, inspecting the hands, face and abdomen in more detail.

Hands

Hand signs are often overlooked, but it is important to note that the hands often reveal vital clues with regard to underlying pathology, particularly in the abdominal examination.

Begin your inspection of the hands by looking at the nails. A whitening of the nails is known as leukonychia and is found in liver cirrhosis and low albumin states (hypoalbuminaemia). Disfigurement of the nails resembling a spoon shape is known as koilonychia (*Fig 2.18*), and is commonly found in iron deficiency anaemia.

Another significant sign found in the nails is clubbing (see *Fig 2.19*), which has a variety of causes including liver cirrhosis, inflammatory bowel disease and coeliac disease. A simple way of testing for clubbing is to look for a loss in the angle between the nail bed and the nail – ask the patient to bring together the nail beds of the right and left middle fingers to form an 'M' shape. Normally a small gap, known as the 'diamond sign', is visible at the base of the adjacent nail beds, and the disappearance of this sign indicates the presence of clubbing.

Next ask the patient to turn their hands over to expose their palmar surfaces. Look for redness of the palms, known as palmar erythema, which often

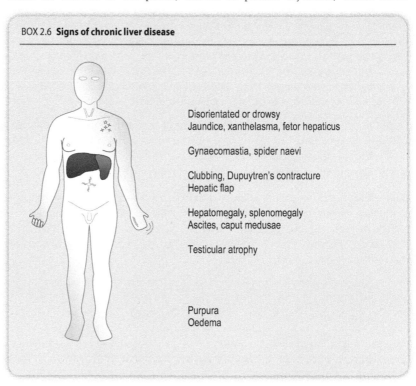

BOX 2.6 **Signs of chronic liver disease**

Disorientated or drowsy
Jaundice, xanthelasma, fetor hepaticus

Gynaecomastia, spider naevi

Clubbing, Dupuytren's contracture
Hepatic flap

Hepatomegaly, splenomegaly
Ascites, caput medusae

Testicular atrophy

Purpura
Oedema

indicates chronic liver disease, and look for a flexion deformity of the small and ring fingers, known as a Dupuytren's contracture. This may be a sign of liver cirrhosis, but can also be due to injury (commonly in manual labourers or carpenters).

Ask the patient to stretch out their arms in front of them with their fingers splayed out and then get them to cock back their wrists – observe for a flapping tremor. If present this is known as asterixis and may be due to liver failure (see *Box 2.6* for signs of chronic liver disease); note that the sign is not diagnostic and may also be found in respiratory, renal or cardiac failure.

Face

Move your attention now to the patient's face, focusing particularly on the sclera, lips and mouth. Before looking at the sclera warn the patient that you will be retracting their lower eye lids for a better view. Look for signs of jaundice, which is a yellow discoloration of the sclera occurring when the serum bilirubin rises above 35 µmol/l. Also look for signs of a pale conjunctiva which may be suggestive of anaemia. Remember to look out for greenish-brown rings occurring in the periphery of the cornea which are known as Kayser–Fleischer rings and are suggestive of Wilson's disease.

Look around the eyes for xanthelasma which are deposits of lipids and appear as yellow flat plaques around the periorbital area. This sign may be seen in primary biliary cirrhosis or raised serum cholesterol (hypercholesterolaemia).

Look down to the mouth and check the lips for brownish freckles which may be associated with Peutz–Jeghers syndrome. Ask the patient to open their mouth and stick their tongue out. Observe the oral cavity for ulcers and poor dentition which may be found in Crohn's disease and coeliac disease. Look more closely at the tongue for:
- enlargement (macroglossia) – occurs in acromegaly and hypothyroidism
- atrophy – occurs in iron, folate and B_{12} deficiency
- dryness – a sign of dehydration.

Do not forget to check for any abnormal breath odour for ketosis, ethanol or fetor hepaticus. Fetor hepaticus is a sweet smelling odour occurring in portal hypertension whilst a ketotic breath is more characteristically a fruity smell laden with ketones found in diabetic ketoacidosis.

Abdomen

Move down to the abdomen noting any:
- gynaecomastia – enlargement of the male breast with palpable granular tissue
- spider naevi – spider-shaped vessels originating from a central arteriole; applying a simple pressure to the central arteriole causes blanching; five or more spider naevi is indicative of concurrent liver disease. Campbell de Morgan spots, on the other hand, are non-blanching small red or violet lesions on the chest and are a common incidental finding.
- caput medusa – engorged dilated abdominal veins found around the umbilicus. They are suggestive of portal hypertension whereby blood is shunted from the portal venous system to the umbilical veins
- petechiae – pinhead-sized bruises found on the skin or occur in low platelet counts.

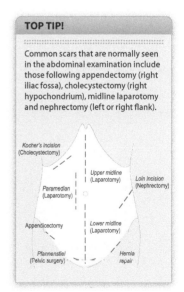

TOP TIP!

Common scars that are normally seen in the abdominal examination include those following appendectomy (right iliac fossa), cholecystectomy (right hypochondrium), midline laparotomy and nephrectomy (left or right flank).

Kocher's incision (Cholecystectomy)

Upper midline (Laparotomy)

Loin incision (Nephrectomy)

Paramedian (Laparotomy)

Appendicectomy

Lower midline (Laparotomy)

Pfannenstiel (Pelvic surgery)

Hernia repair

These are all common findings in chronic liver disease (*Box 2.6*).

Spend some more time inspecting the abdomen. Look at its overall size and shape as well as noting any obvious distension, scars (see figure in Top Tips box), masses or hernias. Causes of distension can easily be remembered using the 'five Fs' mnemonic:, **F**at (obesity), **F**luid (ascites), **F**latus (gaseous distension), **F**aeces and **F**etus (in females).

Also look out for stoma bags and any indwelling catheters. A stoma bag is a bag attached to the abdominal wall which collects faeces. It may be temporary or permanent and is usually inserted into the colon or the ileus depending on the type of operation. Colostomy bags are often located in the left iliac fossa and collect faecal material from the large intestine. Ileostomy bags are found in the right iliac fossa and collect unformed faecal matter from the small bowel.

When describing the abdominal shape, state whether the contour is flat, scaphoid (sunken) or protuberant. Note any gastric peristalsis or pulsations:
- pulsations may be a normal finding in thin adults; however, in the elderly one must always rule out an abdominal aortic aneurysm
- gastric peristalsis is normally seen as a wave-like movement passing over the upper abdomen; when seen, signs of small bowel obstruction should be excluded.

Finally, look for special signs such as Grey Turner's and Cullen's sign which are ecchymoses appearing as bruises located in the flanks and umbilical areas, respectively. They are usually found in patients suffering with pancreatic trauma or acute pancreatitis.

2.3.4 Palpation

Now that you have gained sufficient information about the patient from inspection, you can move on to palpation. Before you begin palpating it is important to reconfirm that the patient is not in any pain and also ensure that your hands are clean and warm.

Initially palpate the patient's left supraclavicular fossa by placing the pulp of your fingers over the area and feeling for a Virchow's node (an enlarged lymph node associated with gastric carcinoma).

Kneel down besides the patient such that their abdomen is at your eye level. If the patient stated that they were suffering with some discomfort, ask them to point towards it so that you may avoid examining this area until the end. Begin by palpating the abdomen with your hand, applying a light pressure systematically in all quadrants. Only palpate for a few seconds using the tips of your fingers. Whilst palpating, focus your attention on the patient's face looking for signs of grimacing, a sure sign that the patient is experiencing some discomfort at the point of palpation.

Light palpation

Superficial palpation is helpful to elicit signs of widespread tenderness, guarding and rigidity as seen in generalized peritonitis. Grossly enlarged abdominal masses may also be felt during light palpation.

Peritonitis is inflammation of the abdominal lining known as the peritoneum. It presents with severe pain and generalized tenderness over the whole abdomen and is associated with fevers and a sensation of nausea and vomiting. On

> **TOP TIP!**
>
> When palpating, look at the patient's face not the stomach – it is the face that grimaces with pain and not the abdomen.

examination the patient is acutely unwell, has a hard rigid abdomen with signs of guarding. Peritonitis may be caused by a perforation of one of the abdominal viscera such as a burst ulcer or appendix or, in women, by an ectopic pregnancy or a ruptured cyst. Guarding is the reflex contraction of the patient's abdominal muscles caused by palpation, whereas rigidity is the constant involuntary contraction of these muscles, whether palpated or not.

Deep palpation

Having superficially examined the abdomen, now proceed to examine more closely using deep palpation. Deep palpation is useful to establish organomegaly, to localize pain and to locate and describe any abdominal masses.

Begin by deeply palpating the nine areas of the abdomen (see *Fig 2.17*), using either one or two hands, depending on your preference. When palpating you should apply firmer pressure and for a longer period compared to when you were lightly palpating.

Start, for example, in the right upper quadrant and work your way around the abdomen in a clockwise motion, finishing up in the umbilicus. Whilst you are examining, ensure that you take into consideration the underlying structures of each area. In the right hypochondrium, you are likely to encounter the liver and gallbladder. Pain in this area is usually caused by either of these two organs. The epigastric area contains the stomach, lower part of the oesophagus, pancreas and the aorta. Common causes of epigastric pain are reflux, ulcers and pancreatitis. In the left hypochondrium the border of the stomach, spleen and the descending flexure of the large colon can all be found.

The right iliac fossa consists of the appendix, bowel, the right ovary and Fallopian tube. If you elicit pain in this area, it is essential that you exclude an acute appendix. In acute appendicitis you will normally find localized pain over McBurney's point, rebound tenderness and guarding along with a positive Rovsing's sign (the reproduction of pain in the right iliac fossa when gentle but firm pressure is applied over the left iliac fossa). Rebound tenderness can be elicited either by the patient complaining of pain on percussion of the area or upon the releasing of pressure applied by your hand on the abdomen.

Palpation of the organs

It is important to palpate the large organs of the abdomen including the liver, spleen, kidneys and abdominal aorta to look for signs of pathology such as chronic liver disease, polycystic kidneys or an aortic aneurysm.

Liver
Although the liver is located in the right hypochondrium, you should begin your assessment of it starting from the right iliac fossa. This is because when the liver enlarges due to pathology, it expands downwards towards the right iliac fossa. The liver is usually located between the 5th intercostal space anteriorly down to the 10th rib and is not normally palpable in a healthy adult. However, in a normal thin individual it may be possible to feel the liver edge in deep expiration.

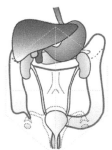

Epigastric pain
Stomach: Gastritis, peptic ulcer
Oesophagus: GORD, malignancy
Pancreas: pancreatitis

RUQ pain
Liver: Hepatitis, cancer, right ventricular failure
Gallbladder: Biliary colic, cholecystitis
Kidney: Pyelonephritis

LUQ pain
Liver: Hepatitis, cancer, right ventricular failure
Gallbladder: Biliary colic, cholecystitis
Kidney: Pyelonephritis

RLQ pain
Bowel: Appendicitis, IBD, Meckel's diverticulum, diverticulitis, malignancy
Fallopian tubes: Salpingitis, ectopic pregnancy, PID
Kidney: Ureteric stone

LLQ pain
Bowel: Diverticulitis, Ulcerative colitis, malignancy
Fallopian tubes: Salpingitis, ectopic pregnancy, PID
Kidney: Ureteric stone

Suprapubic pain
Bladder: Urinary tract infection
Uterus: Pelvic inflammatory disease

Fig 2.20 Causes of abdominal pain.

TOP TIP!

McBurney's point is found one-third of the distance from the anterior superior iliac spine to the umbilicus.

TOP TIP!

When examining for appendicitis you may wish to perform the psoas test by raising the patient's right leg up whilst keeping their knees extended. A positive psoas sign would be eliciting abdominal pain when doing so and may indicate appendicitis.

TOP TIP!

Always warn the patient that they may experience pain before examining for rebound tenderness.

Place your hand in the right iliac fossa parallel to the border of the costal margin and ask the patient to take in deep breaths. Using the radial aspect of your right index finger, advance 2 cm upwards towards the liver edge in a dipping motion during the expiratory phase of respiration. With each breath the patient takes, work your way up until you reach the lower costal margin.

Using this technique, attempt to locate the liver edge. If found, you should describe it in finger breadths below the costal margin. Note whether the liver edge is smooth or irregular in shape, tender or non-tender, hard or soft or pulsatile in nature. A normal liver should have a smooth and regular shape and be non-tender; in early cirrhosis the liver can be extremely large, smooth and non-tender, whereas in late cirrhosis the liver is often shrunken and not always palpable. In right heart failure a smooth pulsatile and often tender liver edge may be felt, whilst in liver carcinomas an enlarged hard craggy edge is usually palpable.

Gallbladder

Complete your palpation of the liver by attempting to palpate for an enlarged gallbladder. The gallbladder is not normally palpable, unless it is obstructed. The gallbladder is located approximately in the junction between the right mid-clavicular line and the right costal margin. An enlarged gallbladder may be tender in acute cholecystitis and Murphy's sign may be useful in establishing this. Murphy's sign is performed by asking the patient to breathe out fully whilst resting two of your fingers on their right hypochondrium. Next, instruct the patient to take a deep breath in. If the patient is overwhelmed with pain and abruptly stops breathing then this may indicate a tender and inflamed gallbladder. Repeat the exercise in the left hypochondrium. In the absence of pain on the left hand side Murphy's sign is considered to be positive.

Spleen

Normally the spleen is impalpable and can only be felt once it has doubled or trebled in size. It is located between the 9th and 11th ribs extending to the anterior axillary line on the left-hand side. When the spleen enlarges in size it expands diagonally downwards towards the right iliac fossa.

When palpating the spleen (see *Fig 2.21*) employ a similar technique to examining the liver. Start in the right iliac fossa and palpate towards the left hypochondrium, co-ordinating your actions with the patient's respiration. Work your way up to the left costal margin, feeling for a splenic notch.

An enlarged spleen is commonly the result of infective causes such as glandular fever, malaria and tuberculosis, and cancers such as leukaemia and Hodgkin's lymphoma. A massive spleen felt over the umbilicus is suggestive of chronic myeloid leukaemia or myelofibrosis.

When both the spleen and liver are enlarged this is known as hepatosplenomegaly. Common causes include portal hypertension, lymphoproliferative disorders and chronic malaria.

Kidneys

The kidneys are usually impalpable in a healthy adult. However, in a thin individual, the right kidney is more likely to be palpated than the left. This is because the right kidney is located two centimetres lower than the left behind the 12th rib, whereas the left kidney is located behind the 11th and 12th thoracic ribs.

Start by examining the right kidney by sliding your left hand underneath the patient's back, resting your hand under their right loin area (see *Fig 2.22*). Place

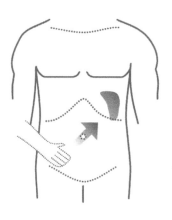

Fig 2.21 Technique for palpating the spleen.

TOP TIP!

Examining the kidney is a difficult skill to master and it will be obvious to an examiner if you have not practised it.

the pulp of the fingers of your right hand over their right flank. Attempt to ballot the kidney by caressing the kidney between the two hands.

For the left kidney use the same technique: place your left hand underneath the kidney and your right hand on top. Similarly, attempt to ballot the kidney between the two surfaces of your hands.

If the kidney is tender possible causes to be considered are infection (pyelonephritis) or obstruction (hydronephrosis). Infection can be confirmed by eliciting renal angle tenderness: ask the patient to sit up and place the palmar surface of your hand over the renal angle, then form a clenched fist with your other hand and gently knock the dorsal surface of your resting hand – a positive sign is noted if the patient complains of increased pain over the kidney.

A unilateral enlarged kidney is usually due to renal carcinoma whilst bilaterally enlarged kidneys are caused by polycystic kidneys or bilateral hydronephrosis.

Due to the proximity of the left kidney to the spleen, you may find if difficult to distinguish one from the other. It is important to remember that there are a number of subtle signs in your examination that will help differentiate between the two. The kidney is ballotable, smooth in shape with no palpable notch and moving late in inspiration, whereas the spleen has a palpable notch, enlarges towards the right iliac fossa, moves with inspiration and is dull to percussion over Traube's space. Do not forget that you cannot palpate above the spleen, whereas in the kidney you can.

Aorta

Do not forget to palpate for an abdominal aortic aneurysm in the abdominal examination as its presence is a grave sign.

The abdominal aorta may be located in the lower epigastrium or umbilical area. It can normally be palpated (see *Fig 2.23*) in thin individuals but may be impalpable in muscular or obese patients. Use the edge of your fingers to locate the border of the palpating mass. Establish its size and whether it is expansile or not – this can be done by placing your two index fingers either side of the mass and observing if they are being pushed apart in an upwards and outwards direction. An expansile mass could indicate an aortic aneurysm. If the mass is greater than 5 cm in size, surgical intervention may be required. A pulsatile mass suggests a non-aneurysmal abdominal aorta. In this case your fingers will be pushed only in an upwards direction.

Aortic aneurysms are expansile masses that push the palpating fingers upwards and outwards.

2.3.5 **Percussion**

Having completed your palpation the abdomen should now be percussed; percussion is a very useful tool to confirm the presence of organomegaly. It can also be used to help establish the characteristics of masses found on deep palpation. It is also helpful to determine if abdominal distension is due to gas or fluid. You should begin your percussion with the major organs.

Liver

To determine the size of the liver, its upper and lower borders need to be percussed (see *Fig 2.24*). To detect the upper border begin percussing from the clavicle down the chest along the mid-clavicular line. The lower border can be found by percussing upwards from the right iliac fossa in the mid-clavicular line. The liver edge is noted when the percussion note changes from resonant to dull.

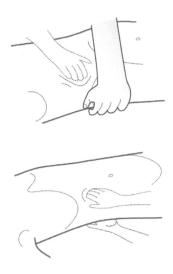

Fig 2.22 Technique for palpating the kidneys.

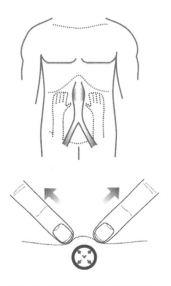

Fig 2.23 Palpation of the aorta to look for an aortic aneurysm.

TOP TIP!

A ruptured aortic aneurysm is a surgical emergency. If an elderly patient complains of abdominal pain with associated back pain and is found to have low blood pressure, tachycardia and epigastic tenderness with an expansile mass, you should suspect a ruptured aortic aneurysm. Immediately fluid resusitate the patient and inform the on-call vascular surgeon.

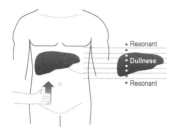

Fig 2.24 Percussion and palpation of the liver.

The normal liver is located between the 5th intercostal space down to the lower costal margin. It is important to percuss for the upper border of the liver because on occasions the whole liver may be shifted downwards. In such circumstances you may find a liver edge despite the fact that the liver is not physically enlarged.

Spleen

As for the liver, you should percuss to check for an enlarged spleen. You should start from the right iliac fossa and work your way up diagonally towards the left hypochondrium. A change in percussion note from resonant to dull may signify the lower border of the spleen. Detection of a lower edge of the spleen confirms splenomegaly as the spleen is always impalpable in the adult.

Bladder

The bladder is not normally percussable unless it is distended or obstructed. Start percussing from the umbilicus down towards the symphysis pubis – in normal adults the percussion note should remain tympanic all the way down. If you detect any dullness this could represent an enlarged bladder or an enlarged uterus in women. Further examination may be warranted if this is the case.

Ascites

Ascites is the accumulation of fluid in the abdominal cavity. In the majority of cases it is caused by cirrhosis. However, there is a significant minority which is associated with malignancy, cardiac failure, tuberculosis and pancreatitis.

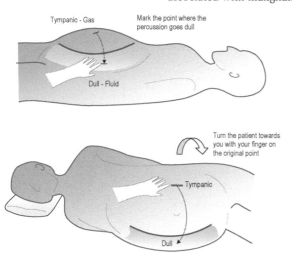

Fig 2.25 Percussing for shifting dullness in ascites.

In the supine patient gas moves upwards and gathers centrally in the abdomen, whereas fluid, which is denser, collects in the flanks. Hence when percussing for ascites begin centrally over the umbilicus and work your way horizontally down towards the flanks (see *Fig 2.25*). Your initial percussion note will be tympanic over the central gas, but as you percuss down towards the flank this will change to a dull note if ascites is present. Note the point where the percussion note changes by keeping your finger at this location. Next, ask the patient to roll towards you and maintain this position for around 30 seconds, allowing the fluid to shift away from the flank. Repercuss over this point and observe whether the percussion note has transformed from a dull to a tympanic sound. This technique is known as demonstrating shifting dullness.

If you suspect that the patient is suffering from massive ascites, a useful way to check for this is by demonstrating a fluid thrill (*Fig 2.26*). Seek the assistance of a colleague or the patient, and ask them to place the ulnar border of their hand over the patient's umbilicus. Ask them to exert mild pressure over this area. Position your hands on either side of the patient's abdomen. With one hand flick the flank area of the abdomen gently whilst feeling for a vibration or thrill on the other side with the other hand. Presence of a fluid thrill suggests severe ascites.

2.3.6 **Auscultation**

Listening for bowel sounds

Bowel sounds are generated from the rhythmic contractions of loops of bowel, moving gas and fluid in a unilateral direction. In order to check for bowel sounds, place the diaphragm of the stethoscope over the umbilical area for 30 seconds; if bowel sounds are present, they should be assessed for pitch and frequency.

Normal bowel sounds are soft, sporadic and are gurgling in nature, occurring every 5–15 seconds. Hyperactive bowel sounds can be caused by diarrhoea or inflammatory bowel disease. In bowel obstruction, bowel sounds tend to be high pitched, more frequent and are described as 'tinkling' because the fluid is held under higher pressure due to the peristaltic activity of the bowel. Absence of, or hypoactive bowel sounds usually suggest paralytic ileus or generalized peritonitis.

Listening for bruits

Move the stethoscope over the abdominal aorta and listen for bruits. Bruits are sounds created by turbulent blood flow passing through altered vasculature, suggesting the presence of an aortic aneurysm or arteriosclerosis.

Place the diaphragm of the stethoscope over the approximate position of the renal arteries, roughly 2–3 centimetres above and lateral to the umbilicus to check for renal artery stenosis. Renal artery stenosis is the narrowing of the renal artery, most often due to atherosclerosis. The narrowing restricts blood flow to the kidney and may lead to raised blood pressure and in the long term chronic kidney disease and failure.

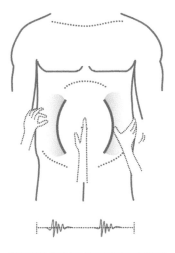

Fig 2.26 Checking for fluid thrill.

While you have your stethoscope to hand, you may wish to perform the liver scratch test. This is performed by placing the diaphragm over the liver, usually in the xiphersternal area. Next, using your index finger, gently scratch over the surface of the skin just below where you suspect the liver edge to lie. Methodically lightly scratch upwards until the sounds are amplified in the stethoscope, signifying the lower edge of the liver. This will help confirm whether the liver is enlarged or not.

2.3.7 Additional points

An examination of the abdomen is not complete without a check for hernias – a patient presenting with acute bowel obstruction could be suffering with a strangulated inguinal hernia.

In the abdominal examination it is appropriate to simply observe and feel for the presence of any hernias over the inguinal canal, requesting that the patient cough whilst doing so. If the cough impulse is positive then this is suggestive of a hernia and you should then proceed to complete a full inguinal scrotal examination of the patient (see *Chapter 2.4* for full details).

Conclude the examination by informing the patient that you would like to perform a per rectum (PR) examination. The PR examination (see *Chapter 2.5* for details) is an important assessment tool and should be carried out on every patient on whom you undertake an abdomen examination. This is because it may give important clues towards underlying pathology such as piles, Crohn's disease, acute appendicitis and rectal carcinoma, and it allows you to check for melaena in a suspected upper GI bleed.

2.3.8 Summing up

Thank the patient for their cooperation and offer to cover them with a blanket to protect their dignity. Draw the curtain around them and allow for sufficent time for them to dress themselves. Whilst waiting you may wish to collect your thoughts about what information you have gained from the examination before conveying it back to the patient.

2.3.9 **Common clinical scenarios**

The following are a list of common cases which you may encounter when examining an abdomen. For each one, consider:

- what the likely diagnosis is
- what key features you would look for
- what questions you would ask or further investigations you would order to refine or confirm your diagnosis

You could use role play with a friend, using the histories in the cases below as a framework.

CASE 1

A 30 year old man smelling of alcohol presents with chronic right upper quadrant pain. On examination he is found to have clubbing, palmar erythema and a liver flap. He also has eight spider naevi and gynaecomastia on his chest with caput medusa around his umbilical area. On palpation, there is a tender smooth liver edge 3 cm below the costal margin.

CASE 2

A 48 year old cachectic man is found to have yellowish discoloration of the sclera, scratch marks over his abdomen and distension. On examination, he is noted to have a 3 cm craggy hard liver edge with associated ascites demonstrated by shifting dullness.

CASE 3

A 25 year old athletic man presents complaining of pain in his right iliac fossa. On examination, he is found to have tenderness over McBurney's point. The pain increases on the release of the palpating hand. There is also localized guarding over the right iliac fossa and the patient complains of pain in this area when an adjacent point in the left iliac fossa is palpated. The pain is increased when passively extending the patient's right thigh with their knee extended (psoas sign). On PR examination, there is significant tenderness over the right side.

CASE 4

A 66 year old cachectic man presents with abdominal distension and a dull ache in the left upper quadrant. On examination, he looks pale and wasted with pallor of the conjunctiva noted. He has a large mass in the left hypochondrium extending to the umbilicus. It is smooth with a notched edge and dull to percussion. Palpation is not possible above the mass.

CASE 5

A 65 year old man, on routine examination, is found to have an abdominal swelling in the gastric region. On palpation, he has an expansile pulsatile mass which measures 5 cm. On auscultation a bruit is heard over the same area.

CASE 6

A 58 year old man is found to have a right iliac fossa mass. The patient has a yellow tinge to his skin and a right nephrectomy scar. He has an arteriovenous fistula in his left arm. A 10 cm smooth mass can be felt in the right iliac fossa – it is firm, non-tender and dull to percussion.

Chapter 2.4
Inguinal scrotal examination

What to do . . .
- Introduce yourself to the patient – establish rapport and seek consent
- Appropriately position and expose the patient

External genitalia
- Inspection: inspect the penis, scrotum and groin on both sides
- Palpation: feel the scrotum for the presence of both testes and for any lumps; proceed to examine the epididymis and spermatic cord
- Describe lumps in terms of site, size, shape, consistency, and transillumination

Hernias
- Inspection: inspect for obvious hernias and scars
- Palpation: palpate the hernia noting its position with regard to the inguinal ligament
- Ask the patient to reduce the hernia whilst placing two fingers over the deep ring, then ask the patient to cough; repeat the test over the superficial ring
- Percussion and auscultation: check the lump for presence of bowel
- Ask to perform a full abdominal examination, examining inguinal lymph nodes and femoral pulses
- Thank the patient and conclude the examination

Lumps in the inguinoscrotal area may cause stress and anxiety in the male patient. Despite heightened awareness of the seriousness of lumps in the testes, male patients are still quite embarrassed to attend their doctor for assessment and examination and so it is important that you deal with the patient in an empathetic way before examining them.

A scrotal lump does not automatically mean testicular cancer, nor does it necessarily have to originate from the scrotum. When considering scrotal lumps it is important to decide first where the lump arises from and whether it is solely confined to the testes – this will help distinguish between a simple hernia or a scrotal mass. An understanding of the embryonic development and anatomical structures of the male genitalia will help you distinguish between common pathologies.

Embryology of the testicular descent

During pregnancy in the male fetus, the testes descend from the lumbar area into the scrotal sac led by the gubernaculum. As it descends, it drags with it an evagination of the peritoneal wall known as the processus vaginalis. This helps direct the testes through the inguinal canal to their final resting destination.

Normally shortly after birth, the processus vaginalis obliterates leaving the distal remnant, a small serous sac surrounding the testes, known as the tunica vaginalis. Occasionally, failure of the processus vaginalis to obliterate will leave a patent communication between the abdominal wall and the scrotal sac. In later life, this may allow fluid and abdominal contents to pass through, giving rise to a hydrocele or an indirect inguinal hernia.

Anatomy of the inguinal scrotal region

The inguinal scrotal region is defined superiorly by the inguinal canal. The canal is a passage that runs obliquely across the inferior part of the lower abdominal wall and parallel with the inguinal ligament. It is approximately 4 cm long and originates from the deep inguinal ring ending at the superficial ring. It contains blood and lymphatic vessels as well as the ilio-inguinal nerve. In males, it carries the spermatic cord whereas in females it holds the round ligament of the uterus.

Hernias

A hernia is a protrusion of an organ or fascia through its containing cavity. With respect to the inguinal scrotal region the most commonly found hernias include the inguinal (direct or indirect), femoral and incisional (viscus protruding through a previous scar).

Inguinal hernias are broadly divided into two categories depending on where they protrude from:
- Indirect inguinal hernias are the most commonly seen and account for 80% of inguinal hernias. They arise from the deep (internal) ring passing through the inguinal canal before exiting through the superficial ring.
- Direct hernias represent the remaining 20% of inguinal hernias and herniate through a weakness or defect in the posterior wall of the inguinal canal. Occasionally they may also emerge out of the superficial ring but rarely descend into the scrotum.

Femoral hernias are the protrusion of bowel content through the femoral canal found medial to the femoral vessels. The femoral ring, in contrast to the superficial ring, is found below the level of the inguinal ligament. Hence femoral hernias are noted to be below and lateral to the pubic tubercle as opposed to inguinal hernias that are found above and medial to the pubic tubercle.

When examining for hernias you should note whether or not the swelling can be pushed back into the abdomen. A hernia that can be returned is known as a reducible hernia. Irreducible hernias containing a loop of bowel that cannot be reduced are more likely to become obstructed. They may present with colicky abdominal pain, vomiting, abdominal distension and an inability to pass flatus or stool. Obstructed bowel may lead to localized swelling particularly at the neck of the hernia. This can interrupt the blood supply to the bowel resulting in strangulation and infarction (strangulated hernia). Bowel viability may become impaired, leading to pain and redness at the site of the hernia. This is a surgical emergency as it may result in gangrene of the affected bowel.

As indirect inguinal hernias have to travel through the narrow inguinal canal, they are more likely to strangulate than a direct inguinal hernia. Similarly, because femoral hernias pass through the femoral canal, which is inflexible and has tough firm borders, strangulation is more likely.

2.4.1 **Beginning the examination**

Introduce yourself to the patient, stating your name and job title. Establish the patient's name and age and ask if they are in any pain. Explain to the patient the nature of the examination you wish to perform and gain their consent before commencing.

Before you begin examining the patient it may be useful to ask them a few questions pertaining to their inguinal scrotal complaint. If the patient presented with a lump you should ask where it is located and when it was first noticed. If the lump is noted to be outside the scrotal area, ask if it has ever become tender or painful (possible strangulation), and then check for the four cardinal signs of obstruction: abdominal pain, swelling, vomiting and absolute constipation. Briefly check for predisposing causes for hernias, which includes anything that increases intra-abdominal pressure, such as a chronic cough, heavy lifting and straining when opening bowels.

If the lump is noted to be within the scrotum, ask the patient when they first noticed it and if it is painful. Enquire about other associated symptoms including fever, dysuria, urgency and frequency. A painless testicular lump that is gradually increasing in size in a young adult must be taken seriously and diagnosis of testicular cancer must be considered. Torsion of the testis presents with acute onset of unilateral pain within the scrotum, often in teenage boys, which is severe enough for them to seek medical assistance. Epididymo-orchitis often occurs as a result of a urinary tract infection or from a sexually transmitted infection in a sexually active adult; patients often complain of localized pain within the scrotum that has being ongoing for a few days and which can be associated with swelling, fevers and urinary symptoms.

2.4.2 **Patient exposure and position**

When examining the patient's inguinoscrotal area you must bear in mind that the patient may be acutely embarrassed at being examined. It is important to relax the patient by employing a sensitive approach as well as fully explaining the examination that you wish to perform. As the inguinoscrotal examination is an intimate examination it is recommended that you have a chaperone present. This is particularly pertinent if you are a female doctor examining a male patient.

Before you start it is extremely important to maintain strict privacy by closing any doors or drawing curtains around the cubicle. Ensure that you wash your hands before commencing. Initiate the examination by asking the patient to undress to expose the area between the umbilicus and their knees. Have the patient standing so that you can inspect the inguinoscrotal area clearly. Although the inguinoscrotal examination comes under one heading, it is best to approach this task by separating out the two systems. Begin your examination with the external genitalia before completing it by examining for a hernia.

External genitalia

Inspection
Inspect the patient's inguinal scrotal area by kneeling down on one knee at a slight angle to the patient. Inspect the anterior genitalia generally for hair distribution, and the size of the penis and scrotal sac for sexual maturity. Move down to observe the scrotum, looking at the colour of the skin, skin lesions such as ulcers, swellings and presence of scars (previous orchidectomy or orchidopexy). The

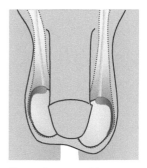

Normal testes: Two testicles around 4cm in size with right held slightly higher than the left

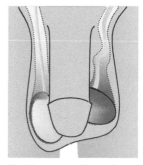

Testicular torsion: Acutely tender, enlarged and firm testis. Testis can be held transversely and at a higher position in the scrotal sac compared to the other side.

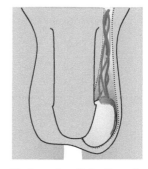

Varicocele: Collection of dilated veins in the pampiniform plexus often found on the left side

Fig 2.27 Common findings on examination of the scrotum.

normal scrotal sac is slightly more pigmented than the rest of the body skin. It contains two ovoid-shaped testes that are approximately 3–4 cm in size with the right testis lying slightly more superiorly to the left (see *Fig 2.27*).

Once you have carefully inspected the front, warn the patient that you are going to gently draw forwards their scrotal skin so that you can inspect the posterior aspect of the scrotum. Make sure you have also inspected the penis for any ulcers, discharge or abnormalities of the foreskin. Examine the glans of the penis, looking at the position of the urethra. A low-set urethra is known as hypospadias and is a developmental abnormality that results in the urethra opening on the lower surface of the penis.

2.4.3 Palpation

Ask if the patient has any pain in their groin and if so, to point towards where they feel the pain. Make sure you observe the patient's face at frequent intervals when palpating in case they grimace with pain. Warm your hands before commencing as cold hands may induce the cremasteric reflex causing the testis to retract upwards.

Testes

Palpate the testes by rolling them gently between your thumb and index and middle fingers from behind. Check that both testicles are palpable. In cases where only one testicle is present it may be due to an orchidectomy following torsion or testicular cancer or a congenital undescended testis. If two testicles are present examine each testicle in turn. Note any difference in size, shape or tenderness between the testicles and whether any lumps are present. If you notice a lump you must describe it like any other swelling in terms of site, size, shape, colour (of skin overlying it), consistency and whether it transilluminates. To transilluminate a lump you should use a small pen torch to shine a light from one side of the swelling and watch it become bright from the other side.

A painless firm lump that arises from the testis may be suggestive of testicular cancer (*Fig 2.28*). The lump often has poorly defined margins that make it difficult to distinguish from the testis itself. A hot severely tender testicle in a young adult may be caused by testicular torsion (*Fig 2.28*). It may also be associated with lower abdominal pain and nausea and vomiting. The testis is held transversely and at a higher position in the scrotal sac compared to the other side. In orchitis, there is diffuse swelling and inflammation of the testis, usually secondary to infection.

If the testis feels diffusely swollen and difficult to palpate, it may be because of a hydrocele (*Fig 2.28*). This is caused by fluid collecting within the tunica

TOP TIP!

When inspecting the posterior aspect of the scrotum, gently draw the scrotal skin NOT the testis.

TOP TIP!

An acutely tender, enlarged and firm testis is suggestive of torsion (*Fig 2.27*) and is a surgical emergency! There is no pain relief on elevating the testis (a negative Prehn's sign), and the cremasteric reflex may be absent.

TOP TIP!

Make sure you know what a normal testis feels like – they are usually of equal size, have a firm consistency and are oval in shape with a smooth surface.

TOP TIP!

Indirect inguinal hernias often pass into the scrotum whereas direct inguinal hernias rarely do. This is because of the embryological origins of the inguinal canal described above.

Indirect inguinal hernia. The most common type of inguinal hernia. It arises from the deep ring and passes through the inguinal canal and exits via the superficial ring. Presents as a lump in the scrotum that you cannot get above.

Testicular cancer. Firm non-tender swelling that is continuous with the surface of the testis. May be concealed within a hydrocele.

Hydrocele. Collection of fluid in the scrotum. Transilluminates well. Most causes are unknown but may be due to trauma, infection or tumours.

Testicular torsion. Usually present in the young male as an acute onset of severe pain in one testicle. Patients usually present with a hot red exquisitely tender testicle.

Fig 2.28 Possible findings on a testicular examination.

vaginalis and feels fluctuant on palpation. When a light is applied over the swelling it transilluminates well, with a visible red glow occurring throughout the scrotal sac. This will easily distinguish it from swellings or tumours arising from the testis which do not illuminate well.

Epididymis

After palpating the testes, now locate the epididymis which lies in the posterior lateral surface of each testicle. It is normally soft and palpable just behind the testicles. Feel the epididymis for any obvious lumps or tenderness. A palpable non-tender cystic mass in the epididymis may represent an epididymal cyst (*Fig 2.29*). This can be confirmed on transillumination whereby a well-defined red glow is noted around the cyst, compared to the red glow throughout the whole scrotum as seen when transilluminating a hydrocele. If the cyst contains spermatozoa (i.e. spermatocele), a less pronounced greyish glow would be noted.

If the patient complains of tenderness whilst palpating the epididymis this could be caused by epididymitis (*Fig 2.29*). The pain may be relieved by slightly elevating the ipsilateral testicle (Prehn's sign).

TOP TIP!

Do not forget to examine both sides of the groin.

TOP TIP!

Make sure you note if there is a scar close to the hernia. It does not necessarily have to be on top of the hernia to be an incisional one.

Epididymal cyst. These are smooth cysts over the epididymis that are palpated separate to the testis. They may present bilaterally and are well defined.

Epididymitis. Infection of the epididymis usually caused by an STI in the young and *E. coli* in the older age group. Usually presents with localized pain and tenderness during ejaculation.

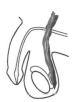

Varicocele. Collection of dilated veins in the pampiniform plexus; the vast majority are found on the left side. Felt as a 'bag of worms' behind and above the testicles. A sudden onset of varicocele in the elderly has been associated with kidney tumour.

Fig 2.29 Possible findings on examination of the epididymis.

Spermatic cord

Feel along the spermatic cord found above the epididymis, tracking back into the lower abdomen. Examine for any swellings (hydrocele of the cord, epididymal cyst) and a varicocele (*Fig 2.29*) which may feel like a 'bag of worms' which disappears when the patient lies flat.

Lymph nodes

Examine the inguinal and para-aortic lymph nodes as part of the examination of the male genitalia. Inguinal lymph nodes are normally not in the groin and so their presence may represent a localized infection in the groin area. It is important to examine para-aortic lymph nodes because testicular carcinomas may metastasize to this area.

DIFFERENTIAL DIAGNOSIS

for scrotal lumps

Site and transillumination	Diagnosis
Separate to testis and transilluminates	Epididymal cyst
Separate to testis and no transillumination	Varicocele
Part of the testis and transilluminates	Hydrocele
Part of the testis and no transillumination	Tumour, orchitis

2.4.4 **Examining for hernias**

Inspection

Ask the patient to lie down on the couch before you begin examining for the presence of any hernias. Observe the patient from the end of the bed, looking to see if their abdomen is distended and for any obvious swellings or scars (hernia repair).

Ask the patient to raise their head off the couch and then cough to make any hernias become more apparent. This may help reveal the presence of an umbilical or incisional hernia that may have been missed at first glance. If you do see a lump, describe its site in relation to any nearby anatomical landmarks, its size, its shape, and whether there are any overlying skin changes; redness of skin over a hernia may suggest the presence of a strangulated hernia.

Now ask the patient to stand with their feet apart for the remainder of the examination; this should help increase the patient's intra-abdominal pressure, making any swelling become more prominent. Inspect the groin area again, looking for any obvious lumps. Describe its location in relation to the pubic tubercle and whether it is above and medial (inguinal hernia) to it, or below and lateral to it (femoral hernia). Ask the patient to cough again and look for a visible cough impulse.

Palpation

Check with the patient that they are not in any pain before proceeding. Use your examining hand to feel for any obvious lumps in the groin (*Fig 2.30*). Feel over the lump, describing its site, size, shape (circular or irregular) and consistency (firm, hard, soft). Determine if the lump is hot as this may be caused by a strangulated hernia.

Whilst keeping two fingers over the lump ask the patient to turn their face away from you and cough. A positive cough impulse would be felt if the swelling bulged forward and touched the tip of your fingers.

Direct and indirect hernias

If a lump is noted in the inguinal area that is thought to be an inguinal hernia, you should try to determine whether it is a direct or indirect (see *Fig 2.31*). To do this you should start by locating the inguinal ligament which lies between the anterior superior iliac spine (ASIS) and pubic tubercle. Next locate the superficial ring, one centimetre superior and medial to the pubic tubercle, and the deep ring, found at the mid-point of the inguinal ligament.

Ask the patient to reduce the hernia. It is better that the patient performs this instead of attempting it yourself as they will have a better insight in how to do this causing minimal discomfort. Once the lump has been fully reduced, place two fingers over the deep ring and ask the patient to cough, feeling for a cough impulse at this point

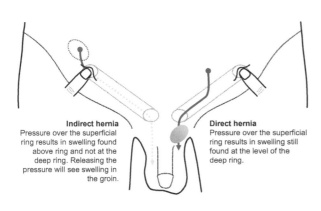

Indirect hernia
Pressure over the superficial ring results in swelling found above ring and not at the deep ring. Releasing the pressure will see swelling in the groin.

Direct hernia
Pressure over the superficial ring results in swelling still found at the level of the deep ring.

Fig 2.30 Position of hands when examining for hernias.

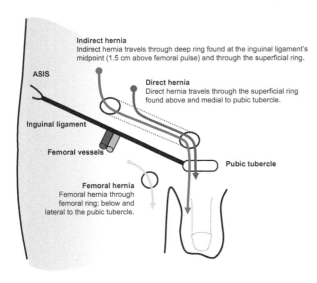

Indirect hernia
Indirect hernia travels through deep ring found at the inguinal ligament's midpoint (1.5 cm above femoral pulse) and through the superficial ring.

ASIS

Direct hernia
Direct hernia travels through the superficial ring found above and medial to pubic tubercle.

Inguinal ligament

Femoral vessels

Pubic tubercle

Femoral hernia
Femoral hernia through femoral ring: below and lateral to the pubic tubercle.

Fig 2.31 Difference between the hernias in the groin.

whilst observing for an appearance of a lump in the groin. If a cough impulse is felt over the deep ring with no lump emerging from the superficial ring, then the hernia is contained by your fingers and therefore is likely to be an indirect hernia. If, however, there is no cough impulse at the deep ring and a hernia is visualized over the superficial ring, it is likely that the hernia is directly protruding through a weakness in the inguinal canal and exiting out of the superficial ring.

Perform the tests on both sides to rule out the presence of a hernia on the contralateral side.

2.4.5 **Percussion and auscultation**

Percuss gently over the lump to elicit for a resonant percussion note if there is bowel involvement. Confirm this by listening for bowel sounds over the swelling with your stethoscope.

2.4.6 **Summing up**

The inguinal scrotal examination is not complete without examining the regional lymph nodes. If you have not already done so, feel along the inguinal ligament for the horizontal chain and over the medial thigh for the vertical chain. You should also ask to palpate the femoral arteries (mid-inguinal points) and auscultate them for bruits in case of a femoral aneurysm. As hernias involve bowel, it may be a good idea to also suggest performing a full abdominal examination for completeness, including a PR if you suspect obstruction.

Thank the patient for their cooperation and offer to cover them with a blanket to protect their dignity. Draw the curtain around them and give them appropriate time to dress themselves. Whilst waiting you should collect your thoughts about the information you have gained from the examination before conveying it back to the patient. Do not forget to wash your hands at the end of the examination.

2.4.7 **Common clinical scenarios**

The following are a list of common cases which you may encounter when checking for an inguinoscrotal hernia. For each one, consider:
- what the likely diagnosis is
- what key features you would look for
- what questions you would ask or further investigations you would order to refine or confirm your diagnosis

You could use role play with a friend, using the histories in the cases below as a framework.

> **TOP TIP!**
>
> Do not confuse the mid-point of the inguinal ligament (half way between the ASIS and pubic tubercle) and the mid-inguinal point (half way between the ASIS and pubic symphysis, the landmark of the femoral pulse).

> **TOP TIP!**
>
> It is impossible to truly differentiate between an indirect and a direct inguinal hernia from examination alone, except if the hernia migrates down into the scrotum (i.e. indirect hernia).

CASE 1	A 63 year old lady presents with severe colicky abdominal pain in the left iliac fossa. She has also noticed mild abdominal swelling and has not passed any stool or wind over the past day. On examination, she has a distended abdomen with a red, hot and tender swelling lateral and inferior to the pubic tubercle in the left groin. The swelling has a positive cough impulse and is irreducible.

CASE 2

A 53 year old man presents with a 4 year history of a lump in his right groin. He is worried that he can now feel it move into his scrotum. There are no changes to his abdominal pain or change in bowel habit. On examination there is a 2 x 3 cm non-tender lump lying superior and medial to the pubic tubercle in the right iliac region. It is reducible and contained with pressure over the deep ring.

CASE 3

A 49 year old gentleman has presented because he noticed a swelling in the centre of his abdomen. He had an urgent laparotomy for bowel obstruction a number of years ago. On examination there is a large 4 x 6 cm swelling with a positive cough impulse adjacent to the umbilicus with an accompanying laparotomy scar. Percussion is resonant and auscultation is positive for bowel sounds.

CASE 4

A 17 year old keen rugby player presents to the GP with a large tense swelling over the left scrotum. He mentions that he sustained a blow to the groin area during training the day before. On examination, the testis is not palpable on the left side due to the swelling. The swelling is fluctuant, dull to percussion, has a fluid thrill and transilluminates brilliantly.

CASE 5

A 37 year old retired footballer presents to his GP as his wife noticed a lump on his right testicle. He does not know how long it has been present and he denies any pain. On examination, there is a 1 x 2 cm firm non-tender swelling in the body of the right testis. The lump feels irregular and nodular. On further examination, lymphadenopathy is found in the para-aortic region.

CASE 6

A 65 year old man presents with a 3 week history of a swelling in his left testicle. On examination his left scrotum appears like a bag of worms. The swelling has a bluish tinge and does not transilluminate. When the patient was lying down, the swelling disappeared.

Chapter 2.5
Rectal examination

What to do . . .
- Introduce yourself to the patient – establish rapport and seek consent
- Appropriately position and expose the patient
- Wash hands, wear gloves and apply lubricant gel to index finger
- Inspection: part the buttocks and inspect for blood, skin tags, prolapsed haemorrhoids, ulcers, abscesses, fissures and fistulas
- Warn patient prior to palpation and then feel in a clockwise and anticlockwise direction in the rectum
- Palpate the prostate anteriorly in males, looking for tenderness, enlargement, lumps and the presence of the central sulcus
- Palpate anteriorly in females for uterus and ovarian masses
- Examine anal tone and comment on faecal impaction
- Withdraw finger and inspect for faeces (colour), blood and mucus
- Dispose of gloves and rubbish in clinical waste bin
- Consider performing a full abdominal examination, proctoscopy or sigmoidoscopy
- Thank the patient and conclude the examination

The digital rectal examination, although relatively quick and simple to perform, is often embarrassing for both the doctor and the patient. For this reason it is commonly overlooked or avoided, resulting in an incomplete assessment of the patient's presenting complaint.

The rectal examination is usually a component or extension of the abdominal and genito-urinary examinations and is rarely performed in isolation. It provides useful information for the diagnosis of rectal tumours, benign prostatic hypertrophy or prostatic tumours in males. It is also employed in the assessment of anal sphincter tone in neurologic cases, gynaecological palpation of internal organs in females, assessment of faecal impaction and in the evaluation of haemorrhoids. Symptoms such as PR bleeding, melaena, pelvic pain and urinary or faecal incontinence should warrant a digital rectal examination in the patient.

Signs and symptoms of rectal disease and dysfunction are often closely related to the major organs that lie within and adjacent to the rectal canal. General awareness and knowledge of the anatomy within the rectum will help allow you to rationalize what you are palpating and allow you to localize possible pathology.

The rectum

The rectum is the terminal end of the large bowel connecting the sigmoid colon to the anus. It measures around 12 cm and is located in the concavity of the sacrum. The upper anterior part of the rectum is covered by peritoneum. In males the anterior rectal peritoneum shares a border with the base of the bladder, whereas in females it reflects to form the pouch of Douglas. The lower part of the anterior segment of the rectum in men lies adjacent to the prostate, membranous urethra and bladder base, whereas in women it lies next to the vagina. The lower part of the rectum ends in the anus which is an opening into the perineum. Within the area where the anus and rectum join, around 3 cm from the surface, is an important anatomical landmark known as the pectinate line. Above this line there is an absence of somatic nerve fibres and hence lesions located above this point tend not to cause pain. Below the pectinate line, somatic nerves innervate the area and thus localized pathology can induce pain here.

The anus and rectum are supported by a number of complex ligaments and muscles that work together to form two main sphincters that maintain continence and allow for voluntary defecation. The internal sphincter involuntarily relaxes to permit faecal matter to be loaded into the rectum from the sigmoid colon. Once the rectum is loaded a reflex contraction of the external sphincter occurs to prevent any incontinence. Faecal matter is then released through the anus through voluntary control of the external sphincter.

2.5.1 Beginning the examination

Before beginning your examination you should introduce yourself to the patients stating your name and job title. Ask the patient their full name and age and also ask how they are currently feeling.

The rectal examination is an extremely intimate procedure and at times can be quite discomforting for the patient. Informing them of what you intend to do and what they should expect to experience may, to a small degree, lessen the impact of such a procedure. You may wish to say: *'In view of your symptoms I would like to perform an examination of your back passage. This is a quick procedure that will involve me inserting my gloved finger into your back passage to feel if there are any problems there. Although it may feel slightly uncomfortable it should not be too painful. However, if you find that it causes you undue discomfort, do not hesitate to tell me and I will immediately terminate the procedure.'*

It may also be pertinent to warn the patient that during the procedure they may experience rectal fullness and the desire to defecate. If they do feel this inform them that it is a completely normal sensation to have.

Inform the patient that you would like to request a chaperone to be present, particularly if you are examining an individual from the opposite gender. Gain consent before proceeding with the examination.

2.5.2 Patient exposure and position

Before beginning the examination and asking the patient to undress, ensure that adequate privacy is maintained. You should draw curtains around the cubicle or close any doors. Ask the patient if they can remove all clothing below the waist, including their undergarments, and then ask them to lie on their left hand side with their knees drawn up to their chest. Ensure that their buttocks are at the edge of the bed to facilitate inspection and palpation.

Offer the patient a sheet or blanket to maintain their modesty. Wash your hands thoroughly before commencing your examination and then put on a pair of gloves. Ensure that you have a pack of tissues by your side so that you can clean the patient after the examination.

> **TOP TIP!**
>
> Remember that some people may have religious and cultural sensitivities about having a rectal examination. In such situations you should explain clearly how and why you wish to do the examination. If they would prefer a doctor of the same gender to undertake the procedure, try your best to facilitate this if possible.

> **TOP TIP!**
>
> Due to the intimate nature of this examination, ensure that you maintain the patient's dignity at all times. Tell them that if they feel uncomfortable at any point to let you know so you can stop the examination.

2.5.3 **Inspection**

With the patient lying on their side gently part their buttocks to allow for good visualization of the natal cleft and anus. Thoroughly inspect the anus as well as the surrounding skin for evidence of skin changes such as excoriations, scars, skin tags, genital warts (human papilloma virus) and ulcers. Observe the anal perimeter more closely, looking for any sinuses, anal fissures or fistulas, polyps and external haemorrhoids. Ask the patient to bear down as if they were passing a motion to reveal any rectal prolapse or prolapsing haemorrhoids.

Anal fissures are cracks or tears of the superficial skin of the anus. They are most commonly found posteriorly, i.e. in the 6 o'clock position; however, they may be found anteriorly, in the 12 o'clock position, after child birth. They present with a sharp pain on defecation with occasional streaks of fresh blood noted on the toilet tissue. Fissures may present with a sentinel pile which is a skin tag found on the anal verge as the fissure extends downwards.

Haemorrhoids, more commonly known as piles, are pads of tissue engorged with blood located at the anorectal junction. They are part of the normal anatomical structure of the anus and aid the passage of stool motion through the rectum. They become pathological when they swell up and exhibit symptoms such as bleeding, prolapse and occasionally pain. They can usually be seen at the 3, 7 and 11 o'clock positions when the patient is in the lithotomy position. They are graded according to the degree of prolapse experienced (see *Box 2.7* and *Fig 2.32*).

> **TOP TIP!**
>
> Sinuses, anal fissures and abscesses can be a sign of perianal Crohn's disease.

> **TOP TIP!**
>
> Many anal skin conditions are described in terms of the patient in the lithotomy position, so try to align yourself with this to be able to recognize the findings on examination: 12 o'clock describes anterior and 6 o'clock describes posterior.

> BOX 2.7 **Grading the degree of haemorrhoid prolapse**
>
> Grade I: Internal haemorrhoid with no prolapse
> Grade II: Prolapse during defecation but which spontaneously reduces
> Grade III: Prolapse during defecation but which can be manually reduced
> Grade IV: Prolapsed haemorrhoid that cannot be reduced

Palpation

Once you have finished inspecting the anorectal area you should inform the patient that you would now like to proceed in palpating the rectum. Do not forget to lubricate your gloved examining finger. Request that the patient takes some deep breaths in and out in order to relax them. Advise them to strain down as if they are trying to open their bowel as this will help relax the external sphincter and ease the entry of the examining finger. If the patient is in extreme pain and discomfort, this could be caused by an anal fissure. Consider applying some local anaesthetic gel before repeating your attempt.

Place the fingertip of your examining finger on the posterior anal margin (at the 6 o'clock position). Gently insert your finger into the anus following the sacral curve. Continue to insert the finger a further few centimetres to examine the rectum and note any pain, masses or tenderness whilst doing so.

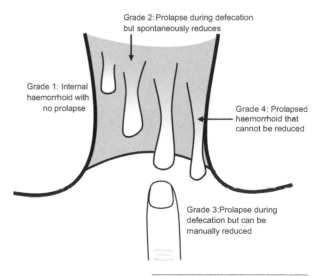

Grade 2: Prolapse during defecation but spontaneously reduces

Grade 1: Internal haemorrhoid with no prolapse

Grade 4: Prolapsed haemorrhoid that cannot be reduced

Grade 3: Prolapse during defecation but can be manually reduced

Fig 2.32 Grading of haemorrhoids.

Palpate the rectum by moving the finger through 180 degrees whilst feeling the walls of the rectum. Swivel both in a clockwise and anticlockwise motion trying to detect for any masses, such as a polyp or tumour, which may be attached to these walls. Note whether the rectum is loaded with stool and whether it is impacted or not.

Rotate your finger to the anterior position and feel for the prostate in men. In women a retroverted uterus may occasionally be palpable.

Prostate

The normal size of the prostate is approximately 3cm in diameter and it will slightly protrude into the lumen of the rectum. It consists of an anterior, posterior, medial and two lateral lobes (right and left) with a palpable midline sulcus. It has a rubbery and firm texture with a smooth surface and is usually painless to touch.

When examining the prostate during the rectal examination, note its size, consistency, and texture, as well as for the presence of the midline sulcus. You should try to run your index finger across the lobes of the prostate and rest it on the sulcus and try to elicit whether the prostate is enlarged and if so whether it is smooth (BPH) or craggy (cancer).

The normal anatomical description of the prostate does not accurately represent the cell types or the potential risk of pathology, i.e. prostate cancer. The concept of zones was therefore postulated by McNeal and this approach divides the prostate into four areas including the peripheral, central, transitional, and anterior fibromuscular zones. The peripheral zone represents up to 70% of the prostate gland. It is also the most common site (80%) for prostate cancers to develop (see *Fig 2.33*).

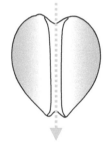

Normal prostate
Smooth prostate, central sulcus
and normal urine flow

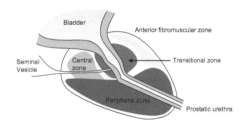

Fig 2.33 Zones of the prostate.

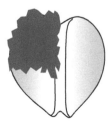

Benign prostate hypertrophy
Enlarged smooth prostate with
restricted urine flow

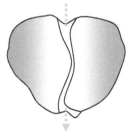

Prostate adenocarcinoma
Enlarged, asymmetrical, hard with
an irregular border

Fig 2.34 Normal and altered prostate.

Benign prostatic hypertrophy (BPH; see *Fig 2.34*) is a common condition in elderly men whereby the prostate is enlarged which puts pressure on the urethra, causing symptoms such as frequency, hesitation and poor stream. The prostate is found to be enlarged, smooth, rubbery and with an intact midline groove.

Prostatic adenocarcinoma (see *Fig 2.34*) usually arises from the posterior lobe in the peripheral zone of the prostate. On examination the gland is usually found to be large, asymmetrical and hard, with an irregular border. The midline sulcus can be obliterated. As the cancer grows and infiltrates the surrounding areas, the rectal mucosa may become tethered to the underlying gland and therefore may no longer be mobile. Patients may present with haematuria as well as symptoms similar to BPH.

Tenderness or pain when examining the prostate may suggest prostatitis (inflammation of the prostate), whereas pain felt over the rectovesical pouch may represent irritation of the peritoneum caused by appendicitis. In women, pelvic inflammatory disease and ovarian cysts, as well as ectopic pregnancy may cause pain on deep palpation.

Anal tone

Before you withdraw your examining finger you should not forget to assess the patient's anal tone. This is particularly important if you suspect spinal injury or cord compression. With your finger still remaining in the anus, request the patient to squeeze your finger. Reduced anal muscle tone may indicate cord compression, cauda equina syndrome or multiple sclerosis causing paraplegia.

Once you have finished examining all the relevant areas you may withdraw the index finger. Observe the tip of the glove for the presence of stool and note its colour. Black stools may suggest melaena, iron tablet or bismuth ingestion. Red stools may be due to acute bleeding from the lower GI tract. Pale stools and dark urine can occur in obstructive hepatobiliary disease.

2.5.4 Summing up

To finish up, wipe off any lubricant that remains on the patient's anus and remove any faeces from the anal margin using gauze or tissue. The patient may feel more comfortable doing it themselves and so you should ask them if they would prefer to do so. Ensure that you remove and dispose of any gloves and waste into the clinical waste bin.

Thank the patient for their cooperation and offer to cover them with a blanket to protect their dignity. Draw the curtain around them and give them appropriate time to gather themselves and get dressed. Remember to wash your hands again at the end of the examination.

2.5.5 Additional points

Depending upon your examination findings you may wish to pursue further lines of investigation, the most common of which includes a proctoscopy or sigmoidoscopy. A proctoscope is useful to examine the anal cavity and rectum and helps visualize internal haemorrhoids or rectal polyps. A sigmoidoscope allows deeper visualization of the upper rectum as well as the sigmoid colon. It is helpful in the diagnosis of inflammatory bowel disease as well as localized tumours.

In cases where an enlarged prostate is palpable, you may wish to consider performing a serum Prostate Specific Antigen (PSA) measurement. This may help differentiate between BPH and prostatic carcinoma. PSA increases yearly in men over the age of 40 and the range depends on the age (see *Medical Guidelines*

Medical Guidelines
Interpretation of the PSA value

Age (years)	PSA cut-off (ng/ml)
50–59	≥3.0
60–69	≥4.0
70 and over	>5.0

Prostate Cancer Risk Management Programme: Age-related referral values for total PSA levels (2009)

TOP TIP!

It is important to measure prostate specific antigen (PSA) prior to rectal examination, as PR can cause false elevation of this marker.

BOX 2.8 **Causes of elevated PSA levels**

Prostatitis
Benign prostatic hyperplasia (BPH)
Prostate carcinoma
Transurethral resection of the prostate (TURP)
Acute urinary retention
Recent sexual activity (ejaculation)
Urinary catheterization or cystoscopy
Urinary tract infection (UTI) or prostatitis
Medication: cyclophosphamide (Cytoxan, Neosar), diethylstilbestrol, methotrexate

box for details). Keep in mind that there is considerable overlap in raised PSA levels in men with BPH and prostate cancer (see also *Box 2.8*). The patient will require appropriate counselling before arranging this test.

2.5.6 **Common clinical scenarios**

The following are a list of common cases which you may encounter when undertaking a rectal examination. For each one, consider:

- what the likely diagnosis is
- what key features you would look for
- what questions you would ask or further investigations you would order to refine or confirm your diagnosis

You could use role play with a friend, using the histories in the cases below as a framework.

CASE 1

A 53 year old man presents to his GP with a 3 month history of difficulty passing urine. He notices a weak stream, dribbling, frequency and nocturia. There is no weight loss or appetite change and he is otherwise well. Rectal examination reveals a smooth prostate with a midline sulcus. His PSA is mildly elevated.

CASE 2

A 72 year old man presents with lower back pain for the last 3 weeks which is noticeably worse at night. Further history reveals unintentional weight loss and loss of appetite. Recently he has been suffering with nocturia and haematuria. On examination of his back, there is tenderness over the lumbar spine on palpation, but no warmth or swelling. PR reveals a hard irregular prostate with a firm nodule on the right lobe causing obliteration of the midline sulcus. PSA is 102.

CASE 3

A 32 year old man presents to A&E after passing 1 cupful of fresh bright red blood via his rectum. He reports no pain during the episode and this is the first time anything like this has happened. The bleeding occurred just after he had opened his bowels. He has a long history of constipation and always has to strain to pass stool. On examination he is haemodynamically stable, abdomen is soft and non-tender and PR examination reveals red bulging areas at the 3 and 11 o'clock positions which are irreducible.

CASE 4

A 24 year old woman presents to her GP because of painful defecation. She describes the pain like passing glass from her back passage. This happens on and off every few weeks when she opens her bowels, especially when she passes a large, hard stool. She has noticed some bright red blood on the toilet paper but denies abdominal pain. On rectal examination there is a skin tag and what looks like a small paper cut at the 6 o'clock position.

CASE 5

A 22 year old student presents with a bout of bloody diarrhoea and mucus for the last 2 weeks. There is minor weight loss and night sweats. He has not recently travelled abroad. On examination, he has painful nodular rash on the skin. Rectal examination reveals numerous skin tags, as well as abscess and anal ulceration. Mucus and blood is noted on the glove.

Chapter 2.6
Cranial nerves examination

What to do . . .

- Introduce yourself to the patient – establish rapport and seek consent
- Appropriately position and expose the patient
- Enquire about the patient's sense of smell and taste
- Assess the patient's visual acuity (oculomotor nerve), fields and pupillary reflexes; offer to perform fundoscopy
- Inspect the eyes for ptosis and examine the external ocular muscles' movements by asking the patient to follow your finger as you move it in an 'H' sign, checking if they have any double vision or pain whilst doing so
- Test light touch over the face using cotton wool
- Test the muscles of mastication by asking the patient to clench their teeth and move their jaw from side to side; assess the corneal reflex using cotton wool; check for the presence of a brisk jaw jerk
- Enquire about change in taste sensation and offer to test formally using tasting objects
- Inspect the face for asymmetry – ask the patient to raise their eyebrows to look for forehead sparing; examine the muscles of facial expression by asking the patient to screw their eyes tight shut, show their teeth and blow out their cheeks
- Test the VIII nerve by assessing gross hearing in each ear using the whisper test; then use a tuning fork to carry out Rinne and Weber tests before examining the ear drums using an otoscope
- Ask the patient to open their mouth and say 'Aaah'; inspect the uvula for any signs of deviation and offer to check the gag reflex using an orange stick
- Inspect the patient's tongue for fasciculation and wasting and ask them to move it from side to side
- Inspect the sternocleidomastoid muscle for wasting and check power by asking them to turn their head against resistance, then ask them to shrug their shoulders
- Thank the patient and conclude the examination

Examining the neurological systems is not easy and can cause much anxiety and frustration in doctors and medical students alike. Notwithstanding the complex nature of the examination itself but also the complex signs that may be elicited, the neurological examinations can be a real challenge to master. Having a good foundation and knowledge of neurological physiology and basic anatomy should prepare you to interpret all the common cases you can expect to encounter.

When undertaking any neurological examination you should be systematic and methodical in your approach so that signs and symptoms elicited are taken in the context of the overall neurological function. This will help you localize any lesion and reveal any potential underlying pathology.

TOP TIP!

Due to time constraints in an exam, it is very unlikely that you would be expected to perform a full examination on all 12 cranial nerves. It is more likely that you would be expected to carry out a detailed assessment of a selected range of nerves. It is also unlikely that you would be required to take a full patient history in addition to examining the cranial nerves. However, it is good practice to elicit a focused history regarding any physical signs that you may find.

TOP TIP!

You should familiarize yourself with all equipment required for the exam to ensure that you are confident and comfortable when using them.

TOP TIP!

If tropicamide is used be aware that it may take up to 10 minutes for its effects to take place. In the examination, the patient may have already had eye drops applied.

TOP TIP!

Most people will not volunteer the fact that they cannot smell, and so it is always sensible to explicitly enquire about their sense of smell.

The anatomy

The cranial nerves are the twelve pairs of nerves that emanate directly from the brain innervating structures mainly located in the head and neck. The first two nerves are located between the mid-brain and medulla, whereas the remainder emerge from the brain stem. They play an important role in the body by controlling taste, smell, auditory and visual senses, as well as motor and sensory function of the face. The motor nuclei of the cranial nerves are mainly located in the brainstem, though for nerves I and II they are in the cerebrum. Sensory ganglia, equivalent to the dorsal root ganglia in the spinal cord, are located outside the brain and are the origin of the sensory components of cranial nerves.

2.6.1 Beginning the examination

Start by introducing yourself to the patient by stating your name and job title. Ask the patient for their full name and age and then ask them how they are currently feeling. Explain to the patient the nature of the examination you wish to perform and gain their consent before commencing.

The examination of the cranial nerves does not conform to the rigid inspection, palpation, percussion and auscultation model as seen in other systems. Instead it requires a different but still very structured format to elicit the relevant signs in each cranial nerve. This requires much practice to master and make your examination efficient.

Patient exposure and position

Have the patient sitting upright in a chair and ensure that you have all your equipment to hand, including a pin, piece of cotton wool, tuning fork, tendon hammer, aromatic smells and pen torch.

2.6.2 Olfactory nerve (I)

The olfactory nerve is the first cranial nerve and derives its name from its main function which is to transmit information pertaining to smell. Sensory impulses (sense of smell) from the olfactory filaments located in the cribiform plate of the ethmoid pass via the olfactory tract to the medial temporal lobe. Any disruption to this tract may lead to anosmia, the loss of sense of smell. This can occur after severe head injury, local compression or a space-occupying lesion. However, the most common cause of loss or reduction of smell (hyposmia) is nasal congestion or upper respiratory tract infection.

When examining the olfactory nerve you should ask the patient if they have noticed any change in their sense of smell. If they have and a detailed examination is required, you should begin by inspecting the patient's nasal passages to ensure that they are unoccluded and offer to use a range of aromatic bottles for formal testing. These may include peppermint, camphor, coffee or orange peel. Make sure that you test each nostril individually in turn by occluding the other with your thumb or finger.

2.6.3 Optic (II), oculomotor (III), trochlear (IV) and abducens (VI) nerves

These nerves are primarily involved in controlling vision, pupillary reflexes, in addition to extraocular movement. Please refer to *Chapter 2.12* on the eye examination for a comprehensive assessment of these cranial nerves.

2.6.4 **Trigeminal nerve (V)**

The trigeminal nerve carries both motor and sensory information from the facial region. The sensory limb is usually divided into three branches:

- ophthalmic (V1) – the ophthalmic branch supplies sensation to the cornea (corneal reflex), forehead, scalp, upper eyelid and nose
- maxillary (V2) – the maxillary division supplies sensation to the upper mouth, teeth and gums
- mandibular (V3) – the mandibular division supplies the lower mouth, anterior two-thirds (not taste) of the tongue, and cutaneous lower lips and jaw.

The trigeminal nerve also supplies the motor innervation to the muscles of mastication (chewing) which include the masseters, temporalis, and the medial and lateral pterygoids.

When examining the trigeminal nerve you should test both its sensory function and motor function as well as eliciting the two reflexes (jaw jerk and corneal reflex).

Sensory function

Before examining, ask the patient if they have any numbness or altered sensation in the face. Begin by testing the response to light touch by using a wisp of cotton wool. Initially place this over the sternum as a point of reference for the type of sensation they would be expected to feel. Next, gently place the cotton wool over the ophthalmic, maxillary and mandibular regions (see *Fig 2.35*), comparing like for like on the left and right sides. Ask the patient if they are able to feel the cotton wool and whether it is the same for both sides. If there are any abnormalities, consider testing for pain and temperature over the same areas.

Pain can be tested by using the sharp and blunt end of a neurological pin and asking the patient to differentiate between the two. Although rarely performed, temperature sensation can be tested by using two glass tubes that contain hot and cold water; again, ask the patient to describe correctly what they felt from each tube in turn.

Motor function

Inspect for wasting of the muscles of mastication, particularly around the temples (temporalis) and the temporo-mandibular joint (masseters). Ask the patient to clench their teeth and then subsequently relax. Palpate the temporalis and masseter muscles whilst their jaw is clenched, feeling for its muscle bulk and asymmetry.

Test the power by feeling the belly of the temporalis and masseters whilst the jaw is clenched. Also test the medial and lateral pterygoids and masseters by asking the patient to move their jaw from side to side. Next ask the patient to open their jaw and keep it open against the resistance of your hand: a weakness of the pterygoids will result in a deviation of the jaw to the side of the lesion. This is because the left and right pterygoids both exert an inward pressure upon the jaw towards the midline and, as a result, a unilateral weakness will result in the jaw being pushed towards that side.

Isolated lesions to the trigeminal nerve, causing loss of sensation to one side of the face, could be caused by facial fractures or local tumour invasion. Cavernous sinus lesions (nasopharyngeal, meningiomas, aneurysms, pituitary tumours) cause an interruption to the corneal reflex and ophthalmic regional sensation often associated with III, IV and VI involvement.

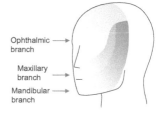

Ophthalmic branch

Maxillary branch

Mandibular branch

Fig 2.35 Regions to test for the three branches of the trigeminal nerve.

TOP TIP!

Always give the patient a reference point when testing light touch, by using the sternum.

Reflexes

Having assessed the motor and sensory components of the trigeminal nerve, offer to test its reflexes. The corneal reflex is rarely performed due to the discomfort it may cause the patient. However, it can play a useful role in assessing the functionality of the trigeminal and facial nerves. Ask the patient to look up and away from you, whilst retracting the lower eyelid softly. Touch the outer edge of the cornea with a wisp of cotton wool. Observe the ipsilateral eye (direct) as well as the contralateral (consensual) for blink responses.

The blink reflex is made up of both a sensory (trigeminal) input and motor (facial) output to the orbicularis oculi. In patients without any lesions both eyes should blink simultaneously. In patients with a unilateral trigeminal nerve lesion, a blink reflex will be lost in the ipsilateral eye as well as a loss of the consensual reflex in the other eye. However, in patients with a lesion affecting the seventh nerve, such as in Bell's palsy, the blink reflex is lost only on the affected side and the consensual reflex remains intact.

The jaw jerk can be elicited by asking the patient to relax their jaw and open their mouth loosely. Place two of your fingers on their chin and slowly tap against your fingers with a tendon hammer. You should be able to observe a brief sharp reflex contraction. Brisk jaw jerks are a sign of upper motor lesions and can help distinguish between pseudobulbar palsy (present) and bulbar palsy (absent).

2.6.5 **Facial nerve (VII)**

The facial nerve originates in the pons, emerging at the pontomedullary junction, along with the auditory (VIII) nerve. Both nerves pass into the internal acoustic meatus, with the facial nerve continuing via the facial canal and eventually passing through the parotid gland before subdividing into five separate branches.

The seventh nerve provides sensory innervation to the anterior two-thirds of the tongue in the form of taste via the chorda tympani division. The seventh nerve also supplies parasympathetic innervation to the lacrimal, submandibular and sublingual glands. The nerve's motor fibres innervate the muscles of facial expression, as well as giving off a motor division to the stapedius muscle in the ear. This muscle acts to dampen sounds and therefore a nerve lesion here may cause hyperacusis (sounds are louder than normal).

Sensation

Assess the sensory component of the facial nerve by checking the patient's sense of taste. Ask the patient if they have noticed a change in their taste in the anterior two-thirds of the tongue. Offer to objectively assess this by presenting varying tasting objects to the tongue, such as sugar and salt. Ask the patient what they can taste, and whether it has changed in any way.

Motor

The primary function of the facial nerve is to innervate the muscles of facial expression and so any lesion affecting the facial nerve will lead to facial asymmetry. Begin your examination of this nerve by closely inspecting the patient's face. Particularly focus on the nasolabial fold and the corner of the mouth, because they are good indicators for asymmetry. Look for any asynchronies in blinking as this may be a subtle indicator of weakness to the orbicularis oculi muscle.

Other signs to look for include drooling or dribbling from the corner of the mouth or an asymmetrical smile. Check for forehead sparing if there is any indication of asymmetry. Also, offer to inspect and examine the ipsilateral ear, looking for vesicular eruptions within the external auditory meatus (Ramsay Hunt syndrome).

Test the different muscle groups in the face by asking the patient to make a number of facial expressions:
- ask them to wrinkle their forehead by raising their eyebrows (frontalis muscle), screw their eyes up tight and then try and gently prise them open (orbicularis oculi)
- ask them to show you their teeth (orbicularis oris)
- ask them to blow out their cheeks.

Observe for any asymmetry or weakness when testing.

Facial nerve palsies may occur due to an upper or lower motor neuron lesion, but it can often be difficult to distinguish between the two clinically; however, there may be some subtle signs that help:
- upper motor neuron (UMN) lesions (stroke, space-occupying lesion, MS) will often have forehead sparing whereby there is no weakness to the muscles of the forehead; this is because there is bilateral cortical innervation of the upper facial muscles
- lower motor neuron (LMN) lesions (Bell's palsy, see *Box 2.9* and *Fig 2.36*) will present with loss of forehead wrinkling as well as facial symmetry; look for Bell's phenomenon, where the eye rolls up due to an inability to wrinkle the forehead and close the eyes.

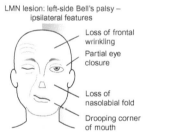

LMN lesion: left-side Bell's palsy – ipsilateral features

Loss of frontal wrinkling

Partial eye closure

Loss of nasolabial fold

Drooping corner of mouth

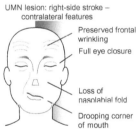

UMN lesion: right-side stroke – contralateral features

Preserved frontal wrinkling

Full eye closure

Loss of nasolabial fold

Drooping corner of mouth

Fig 2.36 Difference between upper and lower motor neuron presentation of a facial nerve palsy.

2.6.6 **Vestibulo-cochlear nerve (VIII)**

The vestibulo-cochlear nerve (also known as the acoustic or auditory nerve) carries sensory information from the inner ear to the brain. The nerve has vestibular and cochlear branches which are responsible for equilibrium, balance and the transmission of sound. It emerges from the medulla and enters the skull via the internal auditory meatus in the temporal bone, along with the facial nerve.

BOX 2.9 **Bell's palsy**

Bell's palsy is an LMN lesion of the facial nerve. It is caused by inflammation of nerve VII within the facial canal. However, its underlying pathology is unclear and it is therefore a diagnosis of exclusion. Its symptoms resolve spontaneously in over 85% of cases in 6 months, but corticosteroids have been shown to be helpful to reduce symptom duration. A LMN VII nerve lesion associated with vesicles within the ear is the Ramsay Hunt syndrome, caused by herpes zoster infection.

> BOX 2.10 **Causes of deafness**
>
> ---
>
> *Conductive hearing loss:*
> Wax, otitis media or glue ear, head injury, perforated ear drum, otosclerosis
> *Sensorineural hearing loss:*
> Presbycusis, Ménière's disease, congenital infection (mumps, rubella), meningitis, noise
> pollution, acoustic neuroma, drugs (gentamicin)

When assessing the auditory nerve try to establish whether the patient has any loss of hearing and determine whether it is conductive or sensorineural in nature (see *Box 2.10*). Carry out a simple whisper test by positioning yourself behind the patient and whispering a short sequence of numbers and letters in one ear whilst gently rubbing the tragus of the other. Perform this test in both ears and consider repeating up to three times if a mistake is made.

Complete your examination by using a 512 Hz tuning fork to conduct the Rinne and Weber tests before finally using the otoscope to examine the outer ear. Please refer to *Chapter 2.13* on the ear examination for a more detailed account.

2.6.7 Glossopharyngeal (IX) and vagus nerve (X)

Both the glossopharyngeal and vagus nerves arise at the lateral medulla and exit the skull via the jugular foramen, passing as they do so in between the internal carotid artery and internal jugular vein. The glossopharyngeal nerve mainly carries sensory information, supplying sensation for both the pharynx and tonsils. The nerve also carries taste and sensation from the posterior third of the tongue as well as supplying parasympathetic fibres to the parotid gland.

The vagus nerve runs down in the carotid sheath before entering the thorax where it sends off motor branches as the pharyngeal and recurrent laryngeal branches; these go on to innervate the soft palate, pharyngeal and laryngeal muscles. The uvula is also innervated by the vagus nerve, and a vagus nerve lesion will cause deviation of the uvula to the contralateral side (*Fig 2.37*).

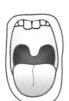 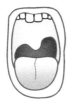

Normal   Right palatal
                      palsy

Fig 2.37 A vagus nerve palsy; a right-sided palatal palsy causes the uvula to deviate to the left side.

From the thorax, the vagus continues its course down into the abdomen, providing visceral innervation. All the organs of the thorax and abdomen lying from the neck down towards the transverse colon are supplied via the motor parasympathetic fibres of the vagus nerve, except for the adrenal glands. Subsequently, the vagus nerve is responsible for controlling a variety of important bodily functions ranging from gastrointestinal peristalsis, heart rate and sweating to speech (via the recurrent laryngeal nerve), and is also responsible for maintaining laryngeal patency for breathing.

Begin the examination by asking the patient an open question. Listen carefully to the patient's response, particularly noting any signs of dysarthria or dysphonia that may be caused by a vagus nerve lesion. Ask the patient to open their mouth and using a pen torch inspect the uvula and palate. Ask the patient to say 'Aaah' and observe the movement of the uvula for any signs of deviation. Move on to test pharyngeal sensation by using an orange stick (note that this test is rarely performed in an exam situation). Press the tip of an orange stick on one side of the pharynx and repeat on the other side; ask if they felt the sensation and whether there was a difference in sensation between the two sides.

Finally, attempt to elicit the gag reflex as this will assess both the IX (afferent) and X (efferent) nerves. With a tongue depressor gently touch the posterior pharyngeal wall to help induce the gag reflex.

Unilateral lesions of IX and X can be caused by basal skull tumours or a fracture, and also by lateral medullary syndrome. Recurrent laryngeal nerve lesions can be caused by mediastinal tumours, thyroid surgery and lung cancer and will result in a 'bovine cough' and dysphonia.

2.6.8 Hypoglossal nerve (XII)

The hypoglossal nerve (XII) nucleus lies in the dorsal medulla just beneath the floor of the fourth ventricle. The nerve travels through the hypoglossal canal, and then passes behind the vagus nerve lying between the internal carotid artery and internal jugular vein. It then passes through the digastric muscle into the submandibular region before entering the tongue to supply most of its motor fibres.

Ask the patient to stick out their tongue and inspect it for signs of wasting, fasciculation or deviation. Next, get the patient to wiggle their tongue from side to side before getting them to close their mouth and push out each cheek with it. You can further check the strength of the tongue muscle by applying resistance on the patient's cheek as they push it out. Finally, assess the patient's ability to articulate by asking them to repeat the phrases 'British Constitution' (labial sounds) and 'yellow lorry' (lingual sounds).

An LMN lesion of the hypoglossal nerve will cause wasting and fasciculation of the tongue with deviation to the side of the lesion (see *Box 2.11*). UMN lesions are more often than not bilateral, and therefore lead to a uniformly spastic tongue, with a rutted appearance.

2.6.9 Accessory nerve (XI)

The accessory nerve is the only one of the 12 cranial nerves to originate from outside the skull. It is located in the lateral horns of the upper spinal cord (C1–5). The nerve fibres ascend through the foramen magnum, and exit via the jugular foramen together with nerves IX and X. The lateral horns of C1–5 are continuous with the nucleus ambiguus from the medulla, from which the cranial component of the nerve is derived. The spinal accessory nerve is therefore the only cranial nerve to both enter and leave the skull. The spinal accessory nerve

> **TOP TIP!**
>
> Eliciting the gag reflex is usually quite uncomfortable for the patient and so you must warn them first. In an exam, you are more likely to be asked to talk through how you would do it, rather than actually perform it.

BOX 2.11 Bulbar and pseudobulbar palsy

When an LMN lesion in the hypoglossal nerve (wasted tongue) is involved with deficits in nerves IX, X and XI it is referred to as bulbar palsy. This occurs due to LMN lesions of the lower cranial nerves outside the brainstem. Bulbar palsy is the term given to the collective symptoms that this produces and is not in itself a disease process. Causes include motor neurone disease, Guillain–Barré syndrome, space-occupying lesion and syringobulbia.
Pseudobulbar palsy results from an UMN lesion to the corticobulbar pathways in the pyramidal tract within the internal capsule. Patients have difficulty chewing and swallowing and demonstrate slow, forced and indistinct speech, often described as 'Donald Duck speech'. Causes include motor neurone disease, vascular bilateral hemisphere infarction, progressive supranuclear palsy, MS, brainstem space-occupying lesion, trauma and amyotrophic lateral sclerosis.

> **TOP TIP!**
>
> Bulbar and pseudobulbar palsy can often be distinguished by the presence of wasting of the tongue (bulbar palsy) as well as brisk reflex (pseudobulbar palsy).

> **TOP TIP!**
>
> Although the cranial nerves are labelled I to XII, it is often easier to examine nerves IX, X and XII together as they supply similar anatomical areas. In addition it reduces the need to move the patient unnecessarily.

runs posterior and inferiorly after exiting the cranium, and provides motor innervation to the sternocleidomastoid and trapezius muscles.

Before beginning to inspect, ensure that the patient removes any items of clothing that prevent access to the supraclavicular area. Inspect closely for wasting of the trapezius and sternocleidomastoid muscles; the bellies of these muscles can also be palpated to assess their bulk. Go on to test the power in the left sternocleidomastoid by asking the patient to turn their head to the right side. Gently apply pressure using your examining hand by trying to push the patient's cheek back to the mid-line. Repeat this on the other side. Place your hands on the trapezius muscle, between the base of the patient's neck and their shoulders. Ask the patient to shrug their shoulders as you push down.

Isolated accessory nerve lesions can be caused by a mass within the posterior triangle of the neck, by trauma or by surgery within this region.

2.6.10 **Summing up**

Once you have completed your examination of the cranial nerves, ask the patient to get dressed if necessary and gather your thoughts before presenting your findings back to them. Thank the patient and acknowledge any concerns they may have.

2.6.11 **Common clinical scenarios**

The following are a list of common cases which you may encounter when undertaking a cranial nerve examination. For each one, consider:
- what the likely diagnosis is
- what key features you would look for
- what questions you would ask or further investigations you would order to refine or confirm your diagnosis

You could use role play with a friend, using the histories in the cases below as a framework.

CASE 1

A 22 year old actor wakes up with dribbling from the corner of his mouth and difficulty completely closing his right eye. On examination he is found to have right-sided facial asymmetry which is more pronounced when he attempts to smile. There is a loss of wrinkles of the right side of his forehead.

CASE 2

A 67 year old smoker complains of an increasingly husky voice for the last 3 months and this has been associated with weight loss and general lassitude. On examination you find him cachectic with drooped right-sided eyelid and a unilateral small pupil that does not change with light.

CASE 3

A 70 year old widower complains of tinnitus and reduced hearing to the right side as well as feeling that the room is spinning around. On examination, the Rinne test is positive bilaterally, whereas the Weber test localizes to the left side. When touching different areas of the face there was a diminished light touch response to the right side.

CASE 4

A 25 year old Afro-Caribbean lady presents with a recurrent history of episodal weakness and unsteadiness in the legs. More recently she has noted pain in the eye with loss of red colour vision. She also has difficulty swallowing and has slurred speech. On examination of the cranial nerves she is found to have a brisk jaw jerk, slow slurred speech, but with no wasting and fasciculation of the tongue.

CASE 5

A 36 year old man complains of severe pain in his left ear with a red rash over his ear and right side of his forehead. On examination he has a painful blistering rash with vesicles in his right ear. You also note right-sided facial asymmetry and loss of nasolabial folds.

Chapter 2.7
Upper limb motor examination

What to do . . .

- Introduce yourself to the patient – establish rapport and seek consent
- Appropriately position and expose the patient
- Inspection: look around the bedside, check for abnormal posturing or tremor; look at the skin and muscles
- Pronator drift: ask the patient to hold their arms straight out with their eyes closed and look for pronation of a supinated arm
- Tone: assess for tone in the arms, looking for increased tone or hypotonia
- Power: assess the power in the different muscle groups and grade according to the MRC scale; compare both sides
- Reflexes: assess the biceps, triceps and supinator reflexes and grade them
- Co-ordination: perform the finger-to-nose test and assess for dysdiadochokinesis
- Ask to perform an upper limb sensory examination in addition to a full lower limb neurological examination
- Thank the patient and conclude the examination

A commonly held misconception is that the neurological examination of the motor system is simply an assessment of muscle function and provides little other detail. Whilst the assessment of motor function and power plays an important role in this examination, other information such as muscle tone, reflexes and co-ordination helps to provide insight into the possible underlying causes of dysfunction.

The motor system comprises the motor cortex, basal ganglia and corticospinal tracts as well as spinal nerve roots, peripheral nerves, neuromuscular junctions, muscle fibres and cerebellum. It can be broadly divided into two systems:
- pyramidal – this plays an important role in the initiation of movements
- extra-pyramidal – this system focuses on modifying and refining any motion.

The pyramidal system consists of an upper motor neuron originating from the primary motor cortex, passing down through the lateral and corticospinal tracts within the spinal cord, before terminating at the anterior horn cells. The motor cortex is located in the precentral gyrus of the frontal lobe. This region maps out motor function in a stereotypical topographical way. Movements of the face, hands and mouth are over-represented compared to the legs and lower limbs due to the number of neuron connections arising from these areas. This is often depicted as a homunculus with a large distorted image of a human body mapped over the motor cortex (*Fig 2.38*).

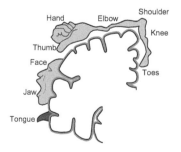

Fig 2.38 Homunculus showing the location of motor functions in the motor cortex.

Axons pass from the motor cortex through the corona radiata and internal capsule before extending down to the medulla. They congregate in a dense orderly fashion, forming a pyramid-like structure; hence the name. Axons representing information from the face are located medially and go on to form the corticobulbar tract synapsing with lower motor neurons of the cranial nerves. The remaining axons of the body go on to form the corticospinal tract. At the level of the pyramids, 80% decussate, i.e. cross over, to form the lateral corticospinal tract (see *Fig 2.39*). The remaining axons continue on the ipsilateral side and enter the anterior corticospinal tract. These axons pass down the spinal cord and synapse in the anterior horn with the lower motor neurons. The lower motor neuron exits the spinal cord and travels to the muscle end-plate via peripheral nerves.

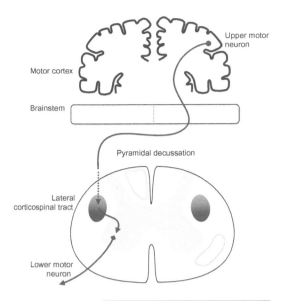

Fig 2.39 Lateral corticospinal tract.

Lesions of the upper and lower motor neurons

Disorders of the motor system often manifest themselves as abnormalities in muscle strength and tone. They have a variety of characteristic signs, as described in *Table 2.1*. Muscle weakness can be due to a lesion at:

- the level of the motor cortex and corticospinal tracts – such a lesion will present with upper motor neuron (UMN) signs
- the anterior horn cells, spinal nerve roots, peripheral nerves, the neuromuscular junction or muscle fibres – such a lesion will present itself with lower motor neuron (LMN) signs.

Upper motor neuron lesions

Motor lesions of the corticospinal tract usually present with contralateral signs. An internal capsule infarct (as seen in most strokes) presents with contralateral hemiparesis, i.e. weakness of the opposite arm, trunk and leg. However, not all UMN lesions present in the same way.

- A unilateral spinal cord lesion that occurs below the level of decussation will result in ipsilateral signs, i.e. Brown-Séquard syndrome.
- Bilateral injury to the corticospinal tract within the cervical spinal cord will result in tetraparesis, i.e. weakness of all four limbs. This is most commonly caused by trauma to the neck area.
- A similar injury to the spinal cord below T1 will result in paraparesis, with weakness only limited to the legs. Other causes include spina bifida or a spinal tumour.

TOP TIP!

Not all patients who have had a stroke present with contralateral symptoms. Brainstem infarction, also known as the lateral medullary syndrome, may present with cranial nerve palsies and generalized ataxia.

Table 2.1 Characteristic signs of upper and lower motor neuron disorders	
UMN Signs	**LMN Signs**
Signs on opposite side to lesion	Signs on same side as lesion
Spasticity ± clonus	Hypotonia
Brisk reflexes	Depressed or absent reflexes
No fasciculation	Fasciculation
Usually no wasting (may be disuse atrophy)	Wasting
Muscle weakness	Muscle weakness
Extensor plantar response	Down-going plantar response

Lower motor neuron lesions

Lesions in the LMN always present with ipsilateral signs and often display features of weakness associated with flaccid paralysis, fasciculation and absent reflexes. It is best to divide up the causes depending on the location of the lesion along the LMN pathway.

- Diseases that affect the anterior horn cell include poliomyelitis and motor neurone disease.
- At the level of the spinal root, dysfunction such as disc prolapse, spinal trauma, tumour or spinal artery infarction can also give rise to LMN signs.
- The peripheral nerve from the spinal root up to the motor end-plate can be affected by trauma, injury or disease processes such as polyneuropathy (Guillain–Barré, diabetic amyotrophy).
- Dysfunction at the motor end-plate, as seen in myasthenia gravis, may produce weakness of the muscles, characteristically after exertion, without any muscle wasting.

TOP TIP!

Be aware that motor neurone disease can present with both upper and lower motor neuron signs.

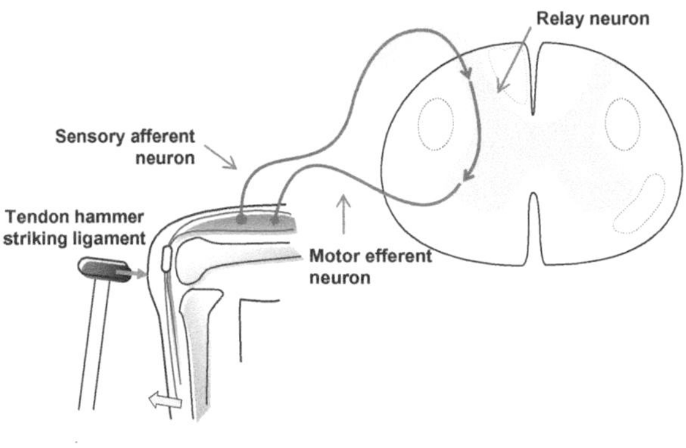

Fig 2.40 The reflex arc.

TOP TIP!

After an acute UMN lesion, such as following a stroke, an initial period of hypo-reflexia may be observed (instead of the more brisk response expected) – this is due to spinal shock. However, after a short period of time hyper-reflexia will manifest and persist.

TOP TIP!

Disease processes that affect the muscle directly, such as myopathies, may result in pronounced muscle weakness and stiffness but invariably do not affect the reflex arc.

TOP TIP!

A wide variety of neurological equipment is usually available in an examination room so familiarize yourself with what you need so you do not appear to be confused.

Reflex arc

There are other pathways that invoke a motor response but without direct connection or involvement of the cerebrum. These responses are subconscious and usually involuntary in nature and are known as the reflex arc (*Fig 2.40*). They are particularly helpful in the neurological examination because they provide an unambiguous objective response that cannot be altered and they require little cooperation or input from the patient.

Most reflex arcs require a sensory (afferent) input synapsing within the spinal cord to a motor output (efferent) directly enervating muscle fibres. Because the arc does not directly pass to the brain its responses are virtually instantaneous. Absence of response, or a brisk response, may therefore point to the location of the lesion: UMN lesions often present with a more brisk reflex response (hyper-reflexia) because although the reflex arc does not directly communicate with the brain, a number of descending inhibitory pathways exist that originate from the brain stem, cerebellum, spinal cord, basal ganglia or the cerebral cortex, and these act as a damper to the reflex response. In a UMN lesion some, if not all, of these pathways are affected, reducing their inhibitory effect on the motor neurons, leading to a more pronounced and excitatory reflex. In contrast, an LMN lesion may affect either the afferent or efferent limbs of the reflex arc, resulting in a reduced or absent response.

2.7.1 Beginning the examination

Before beginning the examination ensure that you have washed your hands thoroughly and collected any necessary equipment such as a tendon hammer. Introduce yourself to the patient, stating your name and job title. Establish the name and age of the patient before proceeding with the examination itself.

As the motor examination will involve you actively moving parts of the patient's upper limbs you should regularly check that they are comfortable and not in any pain. Briefly explain to the patient the steps that you wish to carry out and obtain consent to proceed. You may wish to say: *'In view of the problem you have presented with, I would like to perform a neurological examination of your upper limbs today. This will involve moving your arms and testing their strength. Before I proceed, are you in any pain or discomfort?'*

You may wish to ask the patient some questions before you begin the examination. Useful neurological questions include establishing whether the patient is right- or left-handed, asking if they have noticed any weakness or stiffness in hands or arms, and asking whether the patient's limbs become fatigued easily, especially after carrying out repetitive movements.

Patient exposure and position

Before beginning the examination and asking the patient to undress, ensure that adequate privacy is maintained. Lay the patient comfortably on a couch or have them sit upright in a chair. Expose their arms fully by requesting them to remove their upper garments. Female patients may keep their undergarments on to maintain their modesty.

2.7.2 Inspection

Observe the patient from the end of the bed, noting any signs or symptoms of neurological dysfunction. Look around the room for any obvious walking aids such as a stick, Zimmer frame or wheelchair. Look for an abnormal posture such as a flexed upper limb that may be apparent in hemiplegia. Note for any tics, obvious tremors (resting as seen in Parkinson's disease, or intentional as seen in cerebellum disease) or choreiform movements. Then move closer to the patient and proceed in a systematic way, inspecting the arms in more detail.

Skin

Look closely at the skin for neurofibromas or café au lait (milky coffee-coloured) spots consistent with neurofibromatosis.

Muscle

Observe the patient's general muscle bulk for evidence of any asymmetry. Move closer and inspect for signs of wasting, paying particular attention to the muscles of the hand, i.e. thenar and hypothenar eminence. Note any hand deformities such as a claw hand (ulnar nerve palsy), Klumpke's paralysis (inferior brachial plexus lesion), or Erb's palsy (superior brachial plexus lesion) which is otherwise known as waiter's tip. Do not forget to look for fasciculation which is a sign of an LMN lesion.

> **TOP TIP!**
>
> In Erb's palsy the arm is held in an adducted and pronated position with wrist flexion and fingers fully extended. Klumpke's paralysis, on the other hand, results in a flexed and supinated elbow with an extended wrist and fingers fully flexed.

Pronator drift

Before testing the muscle tone of the upper limb, first assess for the presence of pronator drift. This is a useful screening test because it can help reveal signs of mild spasticity due to a UMN lesion. Ask the patient to stretch out their arms in front of them with the palms of their hands facing upwards in the supinated position. Ask them to briefly close their eyes and observe for an intentional pronation and downward drift of any of the upper limbs.

> **TOP TIP!**
>
> In cerebellar disease there is also a pronator drift; however, unlike in UMN lesions, the drift is upwards.

Tone

Next move on to formally assess the patient's muscle tone. Ask the patient to relax their limbs so that their arms go floppy. Ensure that the patient is not in any pain before beginning your assessment. Hold the patient's hand and passively flex and extend the wrist whilst securing the elbow. Next pronate and supinate the forearm before flexing and extending at the elbow joint.

When assessing the patient's tone, try to establish whether there is an increased (hypertonia) or reduced (hypotonia) level of muscle tone. In UMN lesions a supinator catch and a clasp knife phenomenon may be found; a supinator catch as well as a clasp knife can be felt at the wrist joint when passive supination is met with initial high resistance which later releases as movement is continued. A clasp knife phenomenon may be noted in a patient with a cerebral vascular accident and is commonly seen in the upper limbs. Similar to the mechanism of opening or closing a 'flick knife', tone is increased initially before rapidly subsiding. In contrast to this, lead-pipe rigidity is when there is an increased level of tone experienced throughout the whole range of movement. This is classically seen in Parkinson's disease and affects both flexors and extensors equally. If the patient has an associated resting tremor than the rigidity becomes interspersed in a cogwheel motion, otherwise known as cogwheel rigidity.

Whilst it may be difficult to elicit, hypotonia may be seen in LMN lesions, cerebellar disorders and in the initial stages of an acute UMN lesion. It usually presents as flaccid floppy limbs that lie in a slump-like posture.

Power

Test the strength of the different muscle groups in the arms by having the patient perform manoeuvres against resistance. Always compare one side to the other and start with the normal side first. Each joint should be tested in isolation and the strength should be graded on a scale from zero to five against the MRC scale.

When testing the power of a muscle group you should consider whether the strength of the muscle is typical for the patient's physique, whether there are notable differences between the same group of muscles on either side, and if the weakness is present all the time or improves when the patient is rested (myasthenia gravis).

When testing different muscle groups you should try to explain clearly to the patient what posture they should hold. It may be a good idea to demonstrate this first. Begin examining muscle power by assessing the proximal muscles first, i.e. shoulder, before moving distally to the elbow and then the hand.

Shoulder

Start proximally at the patient's shoulder joint by testing for abduction. This will assess the power of the deltoid muscle supplied by C5/axillary nerve. Ask the patient to: *'put both arms out by your sides with the elbows slightly bent like chicken wings'.* Place your hands just superior to the patient's elbow joint and push down whilst asking the patient to resist your efforts.

Elbow

Test power at the patient's elbow by assessing elbow flexion. This is largely controlled by the biceps muscle which has C5/C6 supply (musculo-cutaneous nerve). Ask the patient to bring their arms up to form a boxing stance. Stabilize their elbow with your non-dominant hand before placing your dominant hand on their forearm. Ask the patient to pull you towards them to isolate their biceps muscle. Keeping the patient in this position, ask the patient to push you away. This will test for elbow extension influenced by the triceps muscle which is innervated by the radial nerve (C7, C8).

Wrist

Move your attention to the hand and particularly to the wrist joint. Examine the wrist extensors that are innervated by the radial nerve (C6, C7, C8). Get the patient

---

Medical Guidelines
MRC scale for muscle power

0 No visible muscle contraction

1 Flicker of muscle contraction visible but no movement of joint

2 Movement of muscle at joint when gravity is eliminated

3 Movement of muscle at joint sufficient against effect of gravity

4 Movement overcomes effect of gravity and mild resistance

5 Normal power

Medical Research Council: Aids to examination of the peripheral nervous system (1976)

TOP TIP!

It is important to differentiate true weakness from tiredness or slowness, such as in myasthenia gravis or Parkinson's disease. Weakness will usually be confined to a specific distribution such as a whole limb or a muscle group, whereas tiredness and slowness will lead to generalized changes of different muscle groups.

to make a fist and cock their wrist back at the wrist joint. Attempt to push their fist downwards whilst asking the patient to prevent you from doing so.

Thumb and fingers

Test finger extension by asking the patient to straighten out their fingers whilst resisting your attempts to flex them down using the ulnar border of your hand. Make sure that you support their wrist when performing this action. Finger extension is largely governed by the extensor digitorum muscle which takes its supply from the posterior interosseous nerve (C7/C8).

Rest your index and your middle fingers in the palm of the patient's hands and ask them to grip them as hard as possible. Try to dislodge your fingers out of their grasp to test for finger flexion. Finger flexion is performed by a number of different muscle groups that are supplied by branch nerves of the median and ulnar nerve (C7, C8, T1).

Ask the patient to splay out their fingers in a fan-like distribution and, using your index finger and thumb, attempt to adduct their index and small fingers. Perform this manoeuvre whilst stabilizing their hand by holding onto the MCP joints. Finger adduction is governed by the dorsal interossi muscle that is supplied by the ulnar nerve (T1).

With the palmar surface facing upwards, ask the patient to point their thumbs vertically up towards the ceiling. Attempt to force the thumb back down into the palm whilst asking the patient to resist this motion. Thumb abduction utilizes the adductor pollicis brevis muscle that is innervated by the median nerve (T1).

Both upper and lower motor neuron lesions can cause reduced muscle power. It is important to correlate this sign with other findings that will help differentiate between the two. Generally speaking, UMN lesions tend to affect one side of the body including the arm, leg (hemiplegia on the contralateral side of the lesion) and often the face. LMN lesions tend to affect either an arm in isolation or specific muscle groups, e.g. the small muscles of the hand in a T1 root lesion.

> **TOP TIP!**
>
> You should try to oppose 'like with like' whenever possible in order for your assessment of power to be more accurate; so try to push down the patient's thumb with your own thumb.

> **TOP TIP!**
>
> Myotonia can be assessed by asking the patient to clench their fists for a length of time and then asking them to release the clench whilst immediately extending their fingers. A significant delay will be observed in myotonia because there is an impairment of muscle relaxation directly after contraction.

Reflexes

When testing for the deep tendon reflexes, otherwise known as muscle stretch reflexes, you should avoid improvised tools such as the edge of a stethoscope and stick to specifically designed tendon hammers (the 'Queens square tendon hammer' is preferred by most neurologists).

To test their reflexes the patient must be relaxed and positioned properly before starting. In the upper limb exam ensure that the patient is sitting upright and facing you with their arms relaxed and held slightly flexed. The force of your stimulus will determine the reflex response and you should use no more force than you need to provoke a response. Prior to testing the reflexes, it is important to show the tendon hammer to the patient and explain that you are going to be tapping lightly on their arm in different places and that it should not cause significant discomfort. During your examination try to elicit the three reflexes in the upper limb: the biceps, triceps and supinator reflexes. Test each reflex individually and compare with the other side. If you are finding it a struggle to elicit a reflex, you should use a reinforcement technique such as asking the patient to clench their teeth to help exaggerate the response.

Biceps

The biceps reflex is innervated by spinal root C5, C6. It is best tested with the patient's arms resting in their lap with palms supinated. The elbow should be slightly flexed such that the biceps tendon is relaxed. Place two fingers over the

> BOX 2.12 **Grading reflexes**
>
> | | |
> |---|---|
> | **0** | Completely absent |
> | **+/−** | Present only with reinforcement |
> | **1 or +** | A hypoactive slight jerk |
> | **2 or ++** | A normal average response |
> | **3 or +++** | A hyperactive reflex not associated with clonus |
> | **4 or ++++** | An extremely hyperactive reflex associated with clonus |

tendon in the anterior cubital fossa and gently strike your digits with the tendon hammer. Look for an involuntary contraction of the biceps tendon.

Supinator
Next locate the supinator tendon on the radial margin of the forearm, place three fingers over it and strike it lightly. Observe for flexion and supination of the forearm which represents a supinator reflex (C5, C6).

Triceps
Finally, test the triceps reflex (C7) by having the elbow flexed to 90 degrees and the arm resting across the patient's chest. Strike the triceps tendon gently just proximal to the elbow.

TOP TIP!

If you notice both UMN and LMN signs in a patient over the age of 40, think of motor neurone disease.

Exaggerated reflexes are seen in UMN lesions, whereas LMN lesions usually produce a diminished or absent response. Isolated loss of a reflex may point towards a localized radiculopathy affecting that level. For example, in a C5–C6 disc prolapse you may find a loss of the biceps reflex. All reflexes should be graded on a scale of 0–4 or 'plus' scale (see *Box 2.12*).

Co-ordination

Co-ordination is evaluated by testing the patient's ability to perform point-to-point and rapidly alternating movements correctly.

Finger-to-nose test
Perform the finger-to-nose test by asking the patient to touch their nose and then your finger as fast as possible with their eyes open. Look for intention tremor and past pointing (dysmetria), suggestive of cerebellar disease. Repeat this test on both sides.

Rapid alternating movement
The next test is to assess rapidly alternating movement. The patient should have one palm facing upwards. With their other hand they should tap the palmar surface of the resting hand, alternating between the palmar and dorsal surfaces. Ask the patient to perform this manoeuvre a number of times and as quickly as possible. Repeat for the other side. Note that they must lift the second hand between each movement and touch the same point on the other palm without stroking the hand. Look for dysdiadochokinesis which is poor co-ordination, or an inability to perform this test; this can be due to a disorder of the ipsilateral cerebellar hemisphere.

2.7.3 **Additional points**

In order to wrap up your examination, ask to perform a full sensory exam of the upper limbs and examine the sensory and motor system of the lower limbs.

2.7.4 **Summing up**

Thank the patient for their co-operation. Draw the curtain around them and give them appropriate time to get dressed. Make sure to wash your hands again once you have completed the examination. Whilst waiting you may wish to collect your thoughts about what information you have gained from the examination before conveying it back to the patient.

2.7.5 **Common clinical scenarios**

The following are a list of common cases which you may encounter when undertaking an upper motor limb examination. For each one, consider:
- what the likely diagnosis is
- what key features you would look for
- what questions you would ask or further investigations you would order to refine or confirm your diagnosis

You could use role play with a friend, using the histories in the cases below as a framework.

CASE 1

A 69 year old man with hypertension presents with a 2 day history of weakness and heaviness of his left arm. On inspection there is no wasting or fasciculation of the muscles or any skin changes, but there is some increased tone with a supinator catch in the left arm. He has power of 2/5 in the left arm; however, the right side was all 5/5. His reflexes were brisk. His sensation and lower limbs were all normal.

CASE 2

A 45 year old woman presents with a 3 month history of morning headaches and vomiting. The headaches get better towards the end of the day. She complains that recently she has tended to walk into things and her friends have told her that they have noticed some personality changes, such as losing her inhibitions over the last few months. The power in her right arm is reduced to 3/5, with increased tone and reflexes. She also has a right-sided pronator drift.

CASE 3

A 32 year old obese woman presents with a 4 week history of numbness and tingling in the left lateral 3½ digits of her hand. This sensation wakes her up in the middle of the night and is relieved by shaking her hand. On inspection she has wasting and fasciculation of the thenar eminence and difficulty in abducting her thumb.

CASE 4

A 35 year old woman presents with a 3 week history of drooping eyelids and double vision. She has noticed that her voice deteriorates when she talks for a long time and she has difficulty chewing food for long periods of time. On testing power it becomes evident that she cannot keep her arms outstretched for more than a few minutes as they start to become weak. Once she has rested the power becomes normal again. Her reflexes are normal.

CASE 5

A 19 year old male medical student is found by A&E confused and smelling of alcohol. He complains of inability to extend his wrist and numbness at the back of the hand. On examination, you find a weakened wrist extension.

Chapter 2.8
Lower limb motor examination

What to do . . .

- Introduce yourself to the patient – establish rapport and seek consent
- Appropriately position and expose the patient
- Inspection: look around the bedside, observe for abnormal posturing or tremor; look at the skin and muscles
- Gait: look for spastic, scissoring or waddling gait
- Tone: assess by rolling the legs and gently lifting them at the knees; look for increased tone or hypotonia
- Power: assess the power in the different muscle groups and grade according to the MRC scale; compare both sides
- Reflexes: assess the knee, ankle and plantar reflexes
- Co-ordination: perform the heel-to-shin test
- Ask to perform an upper limb motor examination and examine the sensory system
- Thank the patient and conclude the examination

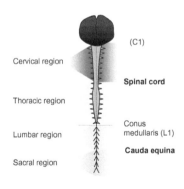

Fig 2.41 Spinal cord extending from C1 of the cervical region to L1 of the lumbar region.

Examining the motor system of the lower limb shares many of the same principles found in the upper limb motor examination (see *Chapter 2.7*). The motor system comprises the brain and spinal cord motor pathways as well as all the motor nerves and muscles throughout the body. The spinal cord extends from C1 (its junction with the medulla) to the vertebral body of L1 (*Fig 2.41*). Any cord compression (via cancer, TB, abscess) or dissectional trauma to the spinal cord between its uppermost point and its lowest (conus medullaris) may affect the motor function of the lower legs. Higher spinal cord lesions, i.e. cervical lesions, can result in paresis of all four limbs (tetraparesis), whereas lesions affecting the thoracic area or below result in paraplegia (legs only). Lesions affecting the lumbar area, particularly the L4/L5 or L5/S1, can result in cauda equina syndrome which is a medical emergency (see *Box 2.13*).

BOX 2.13 **Cauda equina syndrome**

Cauda equina syndrome is a medical emergency and requires immediate hospitalization for further investigations and treatment. It is most commonly caused by disc herniation at the level of L4/L5 or L5/S1 but may also be due to trauma, tumour or infection. It presents with rapid onset of back pain, saddle-shaped sensory loss, lower limb weakness and loss of reflexes, depending on the level of the lesion. Poor prognostic signs include faecal and urinary incontinence and reduced anal tone.

Table 2.2 Causes of muscle weakness		
Site of problem	**Motor neurons affected**	**Cause**
Motor cortex (pre-central gyrus of frontal lobe)	UMN	Ischaemia/haemorrhage or brain tumour
Corticospinal tracts	UMN	As above or demyelination (MS), spinal cord lesion
Anterior horn cells	LMN (motor neurone disease gives both UMN and LMN signs)	Polio, motor neurone disease, spinal muscular atrophy
Spinal nerve roots	LMN (patients may have motor, sensory and autonomic dysfunction)	Compression (e.g. root compression from disc prolapse)
Peripheral nerves	LMN (patients may have motor, sensory and autonomic dysfunction)	Compression, trauma, diabetes, demyelination
Neuromuscular junction	LMN	Myasthenia gravis (fatiguability)
Muscle fibres	LMN	Proximal myopathy due to drugs or endocrine disease, muscular dystrophy (e.g. Duchenne)

TOP TIP!

Remember that the spinal cord ends at L1/L2 so any spinal cord lesions below this point will give LMN (flaccid paralysis), not UMN signs. This is known as a cauda equina lesion. A common cause is central prolapse of an intervertebral disc at the lumbosacral junction. Lesions above T1 can cause UMN weakness of the arms and legs, lesions below T1 but above L1/L2 will cause paraplegia (UMN weakness of the legs only).

TOP TIP!

Lesions in the spinal cord will cause no signs above the lesion, LMN signs at the site of the lesion and UMN signs below the lesion. Also look out for a sensory level which will help determine the site of the problem.

Other patterns of muscle weakness that may present include (see *Fig 2.42*):
- monoplegia (single limb) – most commonly associated with diseases of the peripheral spinal nerves; it can be caused by a lacunar stroke, spinal root or plexus lesion
- hemiplegia (weakness of one side of the body) – the complete paralysis of the arm, leg and often the face of one side of the body; it is usually the result of a stroke, although any disease affecting the spinal cord or the cerebral hemispheres may also produce a similar state.

Myopathies are primary disorders of muscle (see *Table 2.2*). They tend to present with a gradual onset of proximal weakness, such as difficulty rising from a chair or brushing the hair. Although the muscles often appear wasted, they feel oddly firmer than the other muscles. The two most common types include Duchenne muscular dystrophy, which is an X-linked recessive condition mainly affecting young boys, and facioscapulohumeral muscular dystrophy, an autosomal dominant condition, presenting with weakness of the face, shoulder and pelvic girdles.

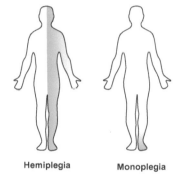

Hemiplegia   Monoplegia

Fig 2.42 Patterns of muscle weakness.

2.8.1 **Beginning the examination**

Ensure that you have washed your hands thoroughly and collected a tendon hammer for the examination. Introduce yourself to the patient, stating your name and job title. Establish their name and age before proceeding with the examination itself.

This examination involves you moving parts of the patient's limbs, so it is important to check that they are comfortable and not in any pain. Briefly explain to the patient the steps that you wish to carry out and obtain consent to proceed. You may wish to say: *'In view of the problem you presented with, I would like to perform a neurological examination of your lower limbs. This will involve observing you walking and then testing the strength of your legs. Before I proceed, can I just check if you are in any pain or discomfort?'*

Useful neurological questions to ask the patient before you begin the examination include establishing whether the patient is right- or left-handed, asking if they have noticed any weakness or stiffness in their limbs and enquiring whether their limbs become fatigued easily, especially after carrying out repetitive movements.

Patient exposure and position

Ensure that the patient has adequate privacy before asking them to undress to their undergarments. Ask the patient to lie comfortably on the couch and expose their legs. Offer the patient a sheet or blanket to maintain dignity.

2.8.2 Inspection

Stand back and observe the patient from the end of the bed. Look around the bed for any obvious walking aids or wheelchairs. Observe the patient's general posture, looking for signs of abnormal posturing such as a flexed upper limb and extended lower limb (hemiplegia). Also look out for any obvious tremors (resting or intentional) or choreiform movements. Then move closer to the patient and proceed in a systematic way to inspect the lower limbs in more detail.

Skin

Look closely at the skin for neurofibromas or café au lait spots consistent with neurofibromatosis.

Muscle

Observe the patient's general muscle bulk for evidence of any asymmetry. Move closer and inspect for signs of wasting, paying particular attention to the thigh muscles. Note the distribution of any wasting and whether it is proximal or distal; distal muscle wasting in the appearance of 'inverted champagne bottles' may be suggestive of Charcot–Marie–Tooth disease.

Note any foot deformities such as a claw foot (polio, Charcot–Marie–Tooth syndrome, Friedreich's ataxia) and Charcot foot (ankle deformity). Do not forget to look closely for fasciculation, which is a sign of an LMN lesion.

Gait

TOP TIP!

Assessing gait is not usually required as part of an OSCE lower motor neurological examination.

Testing for gait in the neurological examination is synonymous with assessing a patient's cerebellar system. However, it may also be relevant in the lower motor examination as different lesions may present with different gait patterns.

The best way to assess the patient's gait would be to ask them to walk to the end of the room, turn around and come back. However, not all patients would be able to do so. If the patient requires a walking aid, allow them to use it. Particular gaits that are relevant include:

- spastic – the spastic or hemiplegic gait appears as a patient with a stiff extended leg that requires it to be swung out to allow forward progression; it is often seen associated with a stroke
- scissoring – the scissoring gait is seen in patients suffering with spastic paraparesis whereby both legs are stiff and extended; the patient has to swing out each leg in turn, giving the appearance of a scissor-like motion
- waddling gaits – the myopathic or waddling gait is due to muscular disease of the pelvic girdle causing pelvic tilting upon walking, hence giving rise to the pathognomonic appearance of a waddle.

Tone

After inspecting the patient and asking them to walk, you must now assess the tone in their legs. Ask the patient to completely relax and lie flat on the couch. Next, with both your hands, gently roll the legs to and fro in turn before quickly flexing the knee and lifting it off the bed. In patients with normal tone the legs should roll freely with the foot following suit but subtly out of sync. Similarly, when lifting the knee the leg remains floppy with the heel dragging along the couch.

Observe for decreased (flaccid) or increased (rigid/spastic) tone suggestive of LMN and UMN lesions, respectively. If the patient's foot comes off the bed when you quickly flex it, this suggests increased tone.

Power

Test the strength of the different muscle groups in the arms by having the patient perform manoeuvres against resistance. Always compare one side to the other and start with the normal side first. Each joint should be tested in isolation and the strength should be graded on a scale from zero to five against the MRC scale (see *Medical Guidelines* box in *Section 2.7.2*).

When testing the power of a muscle group you should consider whether the strength of the muscle is typical for the patient's physique, if there are notable differences between the same group of muscles on either side, or if the weakness is present all the time or improves when the patient is rested (myasthenia gravis).

When testing different muscle groups you should try to explain clearly to the patient what posture they should hold. It may be an idea to demonstrate this first. Begin examining muscle power by assessing the proximal muscles first (thigh) before moving distally (foot).

Hip

Begin by examining proximally at the patient's hip joint. Start with hip flexion which is controlled by the iliopsoas muscles (L1/L2). Place your examining hand on the patient's thigh whilst applying downward pressure. Ask the patient to attempt to lift their leg off the couch. Move on to examine for hip extension, governed by the gluteus maximus muscle (S1). Place your hand underneath the patient's thigh and ask them to push their leg down into the bed.

Knee

Assess flexion and extension at the knee joint. Start by testing knee flexion which relies on the hamstring muscles (L5/S1). With the patient's knee partially flexed, place your left hand above their knee to stabilize the joint. With your right hand on their ankle, ask the patient to pull their heel towards their bottom. Apply gentle resistance to prevent them from doing so.

Knee extension should be assessed in a similar way, with the patient positioned as above but being instructed to kick out and straighten their leg. This will assess the strength of the quadriceps muscles (L3/L4).

Ankle

Move distally to assess the patient's ankles. Start with ankle dorsiflexion which relies on the tibialis anterior muscle (L4). Ask the patient to flex their ankle by pointing their toes towards their head. Stabilize the ankle using your left hand whilst pressing down with the ulnar part of your other hand against the dorsal aspect of the foot.

Check plantar flexion by placing the ulnar part of your examining hand against the sole of the patient's foot. Ask them to push down against your hand. Plantar flexion utilizes the gastrocnemius and soleus (S1) muscles.

With your left hand in the same position as above, this time place your other hand against the sole of their foot. Ask the patient to push down against your hand and then repeat the same test for the other side.

Foot

Finally, turn your attention to the patient's big toe. Examine dorsiflexion of the big toe by asking the patient to point their toe towards their face. With your examining hand apply pressure on the dorsal surface of the toe in an attempt to resist this motion. This will test the extensor hallucis longus muscle (L5).

Reflexes

With the patient in the supine position go on to assess their reflexes. It is important that the patient is lying completely relaxed and comfortable on the couch. Use an approved tendon hammer to elicit the reflexes, remembering that the force of the stimulus will determine the reflex response. Ensure that the patient understands what you wish to do and is happy for you to proceed.

Knee
Begin by assessing the knee reflex which is supplied by L3/L4. Lift the patient's knee so that it is held slightly flexed at a 60 degree angle so that it is supported underneath by your arm. Hold the tendon hammer at its end and briefly strike the patella tendon observing for any contraction of the quadriceps and extension of the knee.

Ankle
For the ankle jerk, position the patient such that their leg is abducted and externally rotated with the knee slightly flexed. Once you have obtained this position, use your non-dominant hand to dorsiflex the foot and with your examining hand strike the Achilles tendon to obtain the ankle jerk.

Make sure you test reflexes on both sides and compare. The knee jerk reflex tests L3/L4 and the ankle jerk tests S1.

All reflexes should be graded on a 0 to 4 or 'plus' scale (see *Box 2.12*). If the reflexes seem hyperactive, test for ankle clonus by supporting the knee in a partly flexed position and with the patient relaxed, quickly dorsiflex the foot. Observe for rhythmic oscillations of the foot; more than three beats are abnormal and this suggests a UMN lesion.

Plantar
Evaluating the plantar response is an important part of testing the motor system. This is elicited by stroking the outer part of the patient's foot from the heel to the big toe. In normal individuals the toes should curl downwards giving rise to the plantar reflex. If the big toe flexes upward and the other toes fan out, this is known as a Babinski reflex and is due to a UMN lesion. However, it is

TOP TIP!

If both legs appear weak, always remember to perform a rectal examination and ask about bladder and bowel function, as well as saddle anaesthesia. It may be due to spinal cord compression and this is a surgical emergency.

TOP TIP!

If you have difficulty obtaining the reflexes, you can use the reinforcement technique by having the patient clench their teeth as you strike the hammer.

TOP TIP!

In myopathies the tendon reflexes are often preserved, unlike in other LMN lesions.

important to note that a positive Babinski reflex is normal under the age of 2 years. Causes of a positive Babinski sign include multiple sclerosis, a brain tumour and meningitis.

Co-ordination

Co-ordination is evaluated by testing the patient's ability to perform point-to-point movements correctly.

Heel-to-shin test

Perform the heel-to-shin test by asking the patient to place one heel on the opposite knee and run it from the shin down to the big toe. Ask the patient to repeat this as fast as possible and then test the other side to compare. Abnormalities of the heel-to-shin test may occur if there is loss of motor strength, proprioception sense or a cerebellar lesion. If motor and sensory systems are found to be intact, an abnormal, unilateral heel-to-shin test is highly suggestive of an ipsilateral lesion in the cerebellum.

2.8.3 **Additional points**

In order to wrap up your examination, ask to perform a full sensory exam of the lower limbs and examine the sensory and motor systems of the upper limbs.

2.8.4 **Summing up**

Thank the patient for their co-operation, draw the curtain around them and give them time to get dressed. Make sure to wash your hands again once you have completed the examination. Whilst waiting you should collect your thoughts about what information you have gained from the examination before conveying it back to the patient.

2.8.5 **Common clinical scenarios**

The following are a list of common cases which you may encounter when undertaking a lower motor limb examination. For each one, consider:
- what the likely diagnosis is
- what key features you would look for
- what questions you would ask or further investigations you would order to refine or confirm your diagnosis

You could use role play with a friend, using the histories in the cases below as a framework.

CASE 1

A 75 year old man presents with weakness and heaviness in his left arm and leg, which have been progressively worsening over 3 days. He has atrial fibrillation and ischaemic heart disease. On inspection his left arm and wrist are flexed and his left leg extended. There is evidence of clasp knife rigidity in the left arm, and increased tone in the left leg with a positive Babinski sign. He has also noticed that the left side of his face was drooping more than usual and this was causing difficulty with speech and swallowing. The right side of the body was completely normal.

CASE 2

A 60 year old man with prostatic carcinoma has recently been complaining of lower back pain. This started a few weeks ago and since then he has also noticed some weakness in his legs and has been unable to walk. He has had a few episodes of urinary incontinence. On examination he has tenderness on palpation of the thoracic spine, with reduced power (4/5) in both legs. There were brisk reflexes with upward-going plantars bilaterally (positive Babinski sign).

CASE 3

A 30 year old woman who presented 2 years previously with painful loss of vision in her left eye, now presents with gradually increasing weakness of her right leg. This has been progressing over 2 weeks and she now uses a walking stick. The tone in her leg is increased and she has brisk reflexes on that side. She had a similar episode of weakness of her left arm 7 months ago, which has now resolved.

CASE 4

A 45 year old man has noticed that he has started dragging his leg when he walks and he tends to trip easily. He also becomes easily tired when climbing stairs, or when walking. His grip is less strong and he tends to drop things and has difficulty opening bottle tops. On examination, there is obvious wasting of the hands and legs with fasciculations; however, the tone is increased, reflexes are brisk and plantars are up-going (positive Babinski sign).

CASE 5

A 25 year old woman who has long-standing severe asthma has presented with difficulty brushing her hair or raising her arms above her head. When asked to stand up from the seated position and climb onto the examination couch, she uses the arm rests for support to get up. On examination she has wasting of the proximal muscles and numerous bruise marks over her lower limbs. She has been taking steroids for several months.

Chapter 2.9
Upper limb sensory examination

What to do . . .

- Introduce yourself to the patient – establish rapport and seek consent
- Appropriately position and expose the patient
- Inspection: look around the bedside, observe for abnormal posturing or tremor; look at the skin and muscles
- Light touch: apply cotton wool to the sternum and then each dermatome from distal to proximal; compare both sides
- Pain: apply the neurological pin to the sternum and then to each dermatome from distal to proximal; compare both sides; map out the distribution of abnormal sensation
- Proprioception: move the distal phalanx of the index finger up and down; compare both sides; move proximally if abnormal proprioception
- Vibration sense: use a 128 Hz tuning fork on the distal phalanx of the index finger; compare both sides; move proximally if abnormal vibration sense
- Ask to perform a lower limb sensory examination and examine the motor system
- Thank the patient and conclude the examination

The sensory exam is often the most difficult part of the neurological examination to interpret as it is the most subjective, relying to a large extent on the ability or willingness of the patient to report what they are feeling. Patients often complain of numbness, pins and needles (paraesthesia), pain or altered sensation, but have great difficulty in precisely localizing it. The purpose of the sensory examination is to determine the exact areas of sensory dysfunction, determine its modality (i.e. whether it is touch, temperature and proprioception) as well as establishing its origin (dermatomal level, peripheral nerve or sensory pathway). As with all neurological examinations, the key to success is a good working knowledge of the neuroanatomy. Once you have grasped these concepts, you will be able to determine the approximate site of any sensory lesion.

The sensory system

Peripheral nerves carry sensation from nerve endings to the spinal cord via the dorsal root ganglion. From there, two main pathways carry different sensory modalities relaying information to the thalamus and cerebral cortex. The first of these pathways is known as the dorsal column and this carries sensory information regarding vibration, proprioception (joint position sense) and pressure. As these fibres enter the spinal cord they ascend on the ipsilateral side and later decussate (cross over) in the medulla to form

TOP TIP!

A patient presenting with right-sided T5 sensory level with decreased pain sensation below the level will have a lesion at the spinal cord on the left side around T3 to T4 level.

TOP TIP!

Touch sensation consists of two modalities: discriminatory and non-discriminatory. The spinothalamic tract carries crude non-discriminatory touch whilst the dorsal column carries two point discriminatory or fine touch.

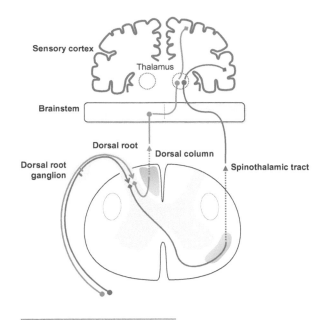

Fig 2.43 The position at which the spinothalamic tract and the dorsal column decussate.

TOP TIP!

Remember the mnemonic 'DISC': the **D**orsal columns affect the **I**psilateral side whilst the **S**pinothalamic tracts affect the **C**ontralateral side.

the medial lemniscus and from here onwards pass up to the thalamus (*Fig 2.43*). The second pathway is known as the spinothalamic tract which transmits impulses carrying pain and temperature information. The fibres of this tract run ipsilateral for a short distance (one or two vertebral levels) before crossing over and ascending in the contralateral side of the spinal cord until reaching the thalamus. This is particularly important when examining a patient with paraesthesia or loss of pain and temperature sensation because the dermatomal distribution elicited will in fact correlate with a spinal cord lesion a few levels higher than that which is perceived.

Both spinothalamic tracts and dorsal columns eventually terminate in the cerebral hemisphere on the opposite side of the body from where they originate. Thus a lesion affecting the cerebral hemisphere, such as a stroke or a space-occupying lesion, will result in a uniform hemisensory loss affecting all modalities on the contralateral side.

Dissociated sensory loss

A good example of a dissociated sensory loss is Brown-Séquard syndrome whereby trauma or a spinal tumour results in a hemisection of the spinal cord (*Fig 2.44a*). This usually causes a loss of vibration sense and proprioception on the ipsilateral side and loss of pain and temperature on the contralateral side below the level of the lesion (dissociated sensory loss). This is due to the fact that the spinothalamic tract and dorsal column cross the spinal cord at different levels, as described previously.

Another cause of dissociated sensory loss is syringomyelia. This is a disorder whereby a cyst or tubular cavity (syrinx) forms within the central canal of the cervical spinal cord. As fluid collects within the canal it affects structures that are in close proximity to it. Nerves from the spinothalamic tract are usually affected as they cross over near the central canal. This condition therefore presents with a loss of pain and temperature sensation in the arms and the trunk in a 'cape-like' distribution, but no loss of vibration or proprioception sense (*Fig 2.44b*).

Dermatomes

Dermatomes are specific well-defined areas of the skin that perceive sensory information and are supplied by a single spinal nerve root. Sensory fibres travel from the dermatome to the spinal cord and are grouped with other nerves (motor, automomic) to form peripheral nerves. As these nerves reach the spinal cord they separate out and travel to the brain along different tracts. There are 31 dermatomes in the body and they are divided up into 8 cervical, 12 thoracic, 5 lumbar and 5 sacral and 1 coccygeal nerves.

Peripheral nerves

Peripheral nerves, such as radial, median and ulnar, are located outside the spinal cord. They contain nerves that supply information regarding sensory, motor and autonomic function. Specific peripheral nerves can be affected by trauma or ischaemia. This will lead to a deficit in the sensory, motor or

Table 2.3 **Causes of polyneuropathy**	
Metabolic	DM, uraemia, amyloidosis, vitamin deficiencies: B_1, B_6, B_{12}
Toxic	Alcohol, lead poisoning
Drugs	Isoniazid, nitrofurantoin, metronidazole, phenytoin
Inflammatory	Guillain–Barré syndrome, sarcoidosis
Infections	HIV, syphilis, leprosy, Lyme disease
Malignancy	Paraneoplastic syndrome

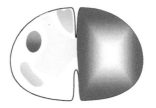

At the level of the lesion in Brown-Séquard syndrome, trauma causes a hemisection of the spinal cord. This results in loss of vibration and proprioception on the same side immediately below the lesion as well as loss of pain and temperature on the opposite side of the lesion a few levels below.

autonomic function that nerve was supplying. If a single nerve is affected this is known as a mononeuropathy whereas, if two or more separate peripheral nerves are affected asymmetrically, this is termed mononeuritis multiplex.

Polyneuropathy is used to describe a symmetrical sensory loss in peripheral nerves leading to a 'glove and stocking' distribution. It is often caused by a number of different processes that attack the Schwann cells of the nerves (*Table 2.3*). Longer nerves or axons contain larger numbers of Schwann cells and hence are more likely to be affected first. Thus for this reason the feet are affected before the hands. The most common causes for polyneuropathy in the UK are diabetes mellitus and alcohol abuse.

In polyneuropathy, vibration sense is the earliest sensory modality affected. Loss of pain and temperature, light touch and sometimes proprioception usually present later. Polyneuropathy can also involve motor function (LMN pattern) and autonomic function (arrhythmias, postural hypotension, impotence, constipation) depending on the nerve group affected (see *Table 2.4*).

2.9.1 **Beginning the examination**

Before you begin examining the patient ensure that you have the following equipment to hand: neurological pin, tuning fork and cotton wool. Thoroughly wash your hands and begin by introducing yourself to the patient, stating your name and job title. Confirm the patient's name, age and occupation.

You may wish to ask the patient some pertinent questions related to their neurological system before you begin the examination. Useful questions to ask may include establishing whether they are right- or left-handed, and whether or not they experience pain, numbness or pins and needles. If they have any symptoms, you should always ask the patient to indicate clearly the affected areas. Make sure you ask if they have any family history of disorders such as diabetes.

As the sensory neurological examination requires the use of a number of aids to perform correctly, it is important that you explain clearly each of the steps that you intend to perform. For example, you may wish to say to the patient: '*In view of the problem you have presented with, I would like to perform a neurological examination of your upper limbs today. This will involve testing the sensation in your arms by using both cotton wool and a pin and also checking that you can feel vibrations. I will also need to move the tips of your fingers up and down to check your joint position sense. Before I proceed, do you have any pain or discomfort at present?*'.

Treating patients kindly and gently and with appropriate respect helps put the patient at ease, and it can make them more helpful and compliant in the examination. Once the patient has understood what you have said, seek consent to proceed.

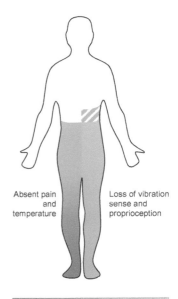

Absent pain and temperature

Loss of vibration sense and proprioception

Fig 2.44(a) Brown-Séquard syndrome.

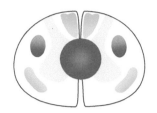

Syringomyelia usually affects the central canal and so dorsal columns are not affected. The spinothalamic tracts, on the other hand, decussate earlier and cross over the central canal and so bilateral loss of pain and temperature is usually noted.

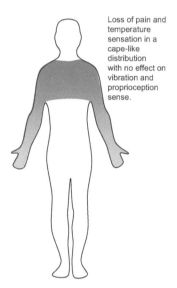

Loss of pain and temperature sensation in a cape-like distribution with no effect on vibration and proprioception sense.

Fig 2.44(b) Syringomyelia.

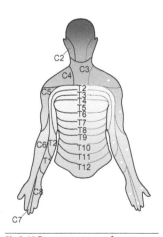

Fig 2.45 Dermatome map of upper limbs. White dots represent the optimum area to test each dermatome.

Patient exposure and position

Before beginning the examination and requesting the patient to undress, ensure that adequate privacy is maintained. Ask the patient to lie comfortably on the bed and expose their arms by asking them to remove their top. Offer the patient a sheet or blanket to maintain their modesty if relevant. Ensure that there is good lighting to observe the patient. You should always make a habit of washing your hands thoroughly before commencing your examination.

2.9.2 Inspection

Begin by performing a general inspection from the end of the bed. Look around the bed for any walking aids or wheelchairs. Observe the patient for abnormal posturing (for example, in hemiplegia there is often a flexed upper limb and extended lower limb, which may be accompanied by hemisensory loss), obvious tremors (resting or intentional) or choreiform movements. Inspect the arms more closely, looking at the skin and muscles (fasciculation).

Skin

Look closely at the skin for scars, neurofibromas and café au lait spots suggestive of neurofibromatosis. Other skin signs include ash leaf macules (areas of depigmentation), adenoma sebaceum (facial angiofibromas – small red nodules on cheeks and noses), shagreen patches (thickened skin with orange peel over sacrum).

Muscle

Observe for muscular asymmetry, wasting (pay particular attention to the hands) and fasciculation (visible contractions of single motor units). Carpal tunnel syndrome is the most common entrapment neuropathy resulting from pressure on the median nerve as it passes under the flexor retinaculum and the carpal tunnel. Patients often experience pain and paraesthesia in the lateral 3½ fingers of the hand, typically worse at night. This may be associated with wasting and fasciculation of the thenar muscles as well as sensory loss in the palm and palmar aspect of the same digits.

2.9.3 Examining sensory modalities

When examining a patient's sensory modalities you should always ask the patient to close their eyes when doing so. This will ensure that the patient's responses are not influenced by relying on visual stimulus or clues. Also test and examine both sides in turn to compare your findings and to establish whether there is a unilateral or bilateral deficit present.

Light touch

Request that the patient closes their eyes. Take a small piece of cotton wool and inform the patient that you will be touching this against their sternum. Touch the skin lightly with the cotton wool, ensuring that you do not do this in a stroke-like motion. Ask the patient if they can feel the cotton wool before progressing to examining the arms fully. Examine the dermatomes (*Fig 2.45*) with the cotton wool, comparing both sides of the body and tell the patient to let you know if they notice a difference in sensation between them.

Table 2.4 Peripheral nerve lesions				
Nerve affected (see *Fig 2.46*)	**Sensory loss**	**Motor loss**	**Nerve roots**	**Cause**
Median	Palmar aspect of thumb, index, middle and lateral half of ring finger; palm below these fingers	LOAF muscles in the hand (see *Chapter 2.7*)	C8, T1	Carpal tunnel syndrome: DM, sarcoidosis, acromegaly, pregnancy, hypothyroidism
Radial (wrist drop)	Dorsal aspect of thumb (anatomical snuff box), index, middle and lateral half of ring finger; back of forearm	Wrist extension	C6, C7, C8	Compressed by pressure on humerus: 'Saturday night palsy'
Ulnar (claw hand)	Palmar and dorsal aspect of medial half of ring finger and little finger	Intrinsic muscles of hand	C7, C8, T1	Elbow fracture

TOP TIP!

Sometimes patients get into a habit of saying yes even when you are not touching them. In order to avoid this, dab the cotton wool at irregular intervals.

Examine the arms by beginning distally before moving your way up proximally. This is useful in revealing a 'glove and stocking' distribution suggestive of polyneuropathy (see *Table 2.4*). With the palms facing upwards, touch the cotton wool lightly onto different areas of the hand. Start at the tip of the thumb (C6) before moving on to the middle finger (C7) and little finger (C8). Next move your attention to the medial aspect of the forearm (T1) and progress upwards to the lateral aspect of the upper arm (C5) and medial aspect of the upper arm (T2) before ending at the tip of the shoulder (C4).

Pain (spinothalamic tracts)

When examining the patient for their pain sensation, you should use a sterile neurological pin. Using the same technique as for light touch, ask the patient to close their eyes and then apply the pin over the sternal area as a reference: the patient should feel a sharp prick as you do so. Next turn the needle on its head and apply gentle pressure on the sternum. Make sure that the patient is able to distinguish between the blunt force and the sharp skin prick sensation.

Work your way with the pin from distal to proximal again in each dermatome and compare both sides. Ask the patient whether they can feel the pin prick and if it is felt as 'the same,' 'blunter' (hypoaesthesia) or 'sharper' (hyperaesthesia) than at the sternum. If at any point the patient describes an abnormality, go back and map out the distribution of sensory loss.

Temperature is rarely examined for, particularly if the pain sensation is found to be normal. If tested, a cold tuning fork or test tubes of hot and cold water are used in the same method described above.

Proprioception

In order to test the patient's joint position sense it is best to demonstrate it to them first. With the patient's eyes open take hold of the distal joint of their index finger (distal IPJ) and place it between your thumb and index finger. Use

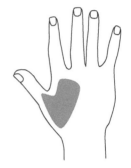

Radial nerve palsy

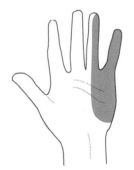

Ulnar nerve palsy

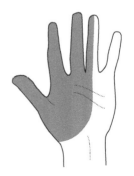

Median nerve palsy

Fig 2.46 Distribution of sensory loss in common neuropathies.

your other hand to move the distal phalanx up and down whilst describing its direction of travel, i.e. up or down. Take care not to move the finger by the nail bed because the patient may be able to sense the direction of movement from touch alone rather than from proprioception.

Next, ask the patient to close their eyes and repeat the test as you move the digit up or down. Ask the patient to inform you which direction they felt their finger move in. Repeat the process three times and compare both sides. The patient should be able to detect one degree of movement accurately. If they cannot detect the movement, you need to progressively test a more proximal joint, e.g. move to the proximal interphalangeal joint (PIPJ) then the metacarpophalangeal joint (MCPJ), then the wrist and elbow until they have correctly identified the movement.

Vibration sense (dorsal columns)

Test the patient's vibration sense using a 128 Hz tuning fork. Strike the fork to create a vibration and place the end upon the sternum. Once again use this as a point of reference.

With the patient's eyes closed, begin by placing the vibrating tuning fork over the sternum. Ask the patient if they are able to feel the presence of the vibrations and when they stop. Reapply the vibrating tuning fork upon the distal IPJ of the finger and establish if they can feel it. If the patient is unable to sense the vibrations move proximally to the PIPJ, MCPJ and wrist until the patient is able to correctly sense it.

2.9.4 Summing up

As you draw close to the end of the examination, request a full motor examination of the upper limb. You should also request a full sensory and motor neurological assessment of the lower limb. You may wish to consider examining the cranial nerves if it is deemed relevant to your clinical finding.

Thank the patient for their co-operation. Draw the curtain around them and give them appropriate time to get dressed. Make sure to wash your hands again once you have completed the examination.

2.9.5 Common clinical scenarios

The following are a list of common cases which you may encounter when undertaking an upper limb sensory examination. For each one, consider:
- what the likely diagnosis is
- what key features you would look for
- what questions you would ask or further investigations you would order to refine or confirm your diagnosis

You could use role play with a friend, using the histories in the cases below as a framework.

CASE 1

A 30 year old man presents with a 4 day history of numbness over the back of his right hand. He also notes that he cannot easily pick things up with this hand as he finds it difficult to bend it backwards. He denies any trauma or past medical history, but does remember that he fell asleep on a friend's chair five days ago after a night out and his right arm was hanging over the armrest. On examination you note a right wrist drop with numbness over the anatomical snuffbox of the right hand as well as inability to extend the right hand.

CASE 2

A 72 year old hypertensive, diabetic man presents to A&E with sudden onset slurred speech and weakness of the left arm and leg. He was watching television when the symptoms came on. On examination you note a left facial droop with sparing of the forehead and 2/5 power in the left leg and arm. On examination of the sensory system there is loss of all sensory modalities on the left side of the body. The right side has normal motor and sensory function.

CASE 3

A 30 year old woman presents with a 5 year history of bilateral hand weakness that has been progressing over the course of these years. On inspection you note numerous burn marks and wounds over the hands and up the arms associated with hand muscle wasting. On examination you note loss of pain and temperature in both hands with intact light touch, vibration and proprioception. The legs are unaffected.

CASE 4

A 60 year old man presents with a recent onset of numbness and tingling of his right middle finger. He has been suffering with neck and shoulder pain for years and has known osteoarthritis of his knee. On examination there is loss of sensation to light touch and pin prick of the middle finger of the hand. You also note weakness of elbow extension and loss of the triceps reflex. The remainder of the sensory examination is unremarkable.

CASE 5

A 55 year old homeless man presents with bilateral pins and needles in the hands and feet which is gradually worsening. He had a BM test in A&E which was 5.6. On examination he appears dishevelled and with a strong smell of alcohol. There is a reduced light touch and pin prick sensation in both hands and feet.

Chapter 2.10
Lower limb sensory examination

What to do . . .

- Introduce yourself to the patient – establish rapport and seek consent
- Appropriately position and expose the patient
- Inspection: look around the bedside, check for abnormal posturing or tremor; look at the skin and muscles
- Light touch: apply cotton wool to the sternum and then to each dermatome from distal to proximal; compare both sides
- Pain: apply a neurological pin to the sternum and then to each dermatome from distal to proximal; compare both sides; map out the distribution of abnormal sensation
- Proprioception: move the distal phalanx of the big toe up and down; compare both sides; move proximally if abnormal proprioception is present
- Vibration sense: use a 128 Hz tuning fork on the distal phalanx of the big toe; compare both sides; move proximally if abnormal vibration sense found
- Request an upper limb sensory examination and examine the motor system
- Thank the patient and conclude the examination

The lower limb sensory examination is conducted in a similar fashion to the upper limb examination (see *Chapter 2.9*) with knowledge of the underlying neuroanatomy and physiology playing a key role in localizing and identifying aetiologies and disease processes.

As seen in the upper limb, peripheral nerves carry sensory, motor and autonomic impulses to the spinal cord. Information relating to the sensory modality, such as pain and temperature, cross over to the contralateral side before passing onto the thalamus via the spinothalamic tract. Vibration, proprioception and two-point discriminatory touch moves up the ipsilateral side of the spinal cord within the dorsal column before crossing over at the medulla and then terminating at the thalamus.

Similar disease processes that affect the upper limb also influence the lower limb. A stroke or cerebral lesion will present with contralateral hemisensory loss of all the modalities, i.e. pain, temperature, touch and joint position sense. Syringomyelia will cause a reduced pain and temperature sensation but will preserve functions of the dorsal column such as vibration and proprioception.

Other conditions to be aware of include:
- acute spinal cord compression – this is a surgical emergency and can lead to bowel and bladder dysfunction (urinary retention and constipation or

TOP TIP!

Remember that a lesion of the spinal cord will lead to loss of pain and temperature sensation one or two vertebral levels below the site of the lesion.

incontinence); it presents with a loss of sensation below the level of the lesion and is usually accompanied with upper motor neuron signs

- cauda equina syndrome – this is a result of compression that occurs below the level at which the spinal cord terminates, i.e. L1; it presents similarly to cord compression although a 'saddle-shaped' sensory loss around the buttocks and back of the thigh area may be found, accompanied with lower motor neuron signs.

> **TOP TIP!**
>
> Lesions below the thoracic spine will often lead to sensory loss sparing the upper limbs.

2.10.1 Beginning the examination

Ensure that you have the necessary equipment, such as a neurological pin, tuning fork and cotton wool, to hand before commencing the examination. Introduce yourself to the patient, stating your name and job title. Establish the patient's name, age and occupation. Take a brief neurological history, asking about any changes in sensation noted in their legs. Enquire whether the patient has had any problems in passing urine or opening their bowels. Next explain to the patient what you intend to do and seek their consent to proceed.

Patient exposure and position

Ensure that adequate privacy is maintained before asking the patient to undress to their undergarments. Have the patient lie flat on a couch and offer them a sheet or blanket to maintain their modesty. Do not forget to wash your hands before examining them.

2.10.2 Inspection

Stand at the edge of the bed and observe the patient's lower limbs. Look around the bed for any walking aids or wheelchairs. Look for any abnormal posture, obvious tremors (resting or intentional) or choreiform movements. Move closer to the patient and inspect the legs in more detail.

Skin

Look at the skin for any stigmata of neurological disease such as café au lait spots or neurofibromas which are suggestive of neurofibromatosis. Look out for any obvious injuries, ulcers or disfigured joints (Charcot's joint) that may be indicative of neuropathic arthropathy.

Muscle

Observe the lower limbs from the anterior and posterior sides for muscular asymmetry, wasting and fasciculations (visible contractions of single motor units).

2.10.3 Examining sensory modalities

Move on now to examine the patient's sensory modalities in turn. Ensure that the patient closes their eyes as you examine them and compare each side as you go along.

> **TOP TIP!**
>
> Sometimes patients get into a habit of saying yes even when you are not touching them. In order to avoid this, dab the cotton wool at irregular time intervals.

Light touch

Using a wisp of cotton wool, lightly touch the sternum to demonstrate the type of sensation the patient should be feeling. Next, move the cotton wool over

TOP TIP!

If you forget the dermatomes of the lower limb, use 'knee L3' as your reference point and try to work your way from there.

the lower limbs and touch it at specific points that correspond to the body's dermatomes (*Fig 2.47*). Ensure that you progress proximally up the limb from a distal position.

Start at the tip of the big toe (L5) before progressing to the little toe (S1) and then onto the medial part of the lower leg (L4). Next, test light touch over the knee (L3), before moving up to the upper part of the lateral thigh (L2) and ending at the groin (L1). At each point check that the patient can feel the cotton wool and ask them if the sensation is the same as that of the sternum and whether there are any differences between the two sides.

Pain (spinothalamic tracts)

Test the patient's pain sensation using a neurological pin. As in the light touch examination, begin by lightly pricking the sharp end of the pin against the sternum. Confirm that they can feel the sharp prick and use this as your reference. Proceed to gently press the skin over the corresponding dermatomal areas as shown above, working your way proximally.

Ask the patient if they can feel the sharpness of the needle and if it is of a similar sensation to that of the sternum. If at any point there is an abnormal sensation, confirm whether it is 'blunter' (hypoaesthesia) or 'sharper' (hyperaesthesia) and then go on to map out the distribution of sensory loss. Remember to compare both sides.

Proprioception

Test the patient's proprioception sense by isolating the distal IPJ of the big toe. Place your thumb and index finger on either side of the joint to stabilize it and use your other hand to gently move the toe up and down, indicating to the patient the direction of movement. Once the patient understands what is required of them, ask them to close their eyes and repeat the process, this time asking them to tell you in which direction the toe is moving. Repeat this three times and compare both sides. If the patient is unable to detect the direction of movement at the toe joint then move your attention proximally to the ankle and then the knee if clinically indicated.

Vibration sense (dorsal columns)

Testing the vibrating sense of the lower limb is particularly important since this sense is often the first sensory modality to be lost in polyneuropathy. Ensure that you have a 128 Hz tuning fork to aid you in this part of the examination. First, confirm that the patient is able to sense the vibratory motions of the tuning fork by placing it over the sternum. Once the patient has done this, move the tuning fork to the MTPJ and establish whether they can sense the vibrations. If the patient is able to sense it then examine the other side. If the patient is unable to detect the movement of the tuning fork, move it proximally to the ankle joint and then the knee until they are able to identify the vibrations accurately.

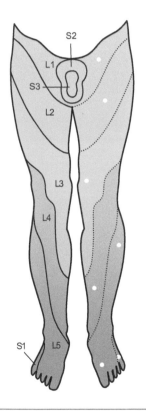

Fig 2.47 Lower limb dermatomes.

2.10.4 Summing up

As you draw close to the end of the examination, request a full motor examination of the lower limb as well expressing a desire to examine the sensory and motor elements of the upper limb. You may wish to consider examining the cranial nerves if it is deemed relevant to your clinical finding. If you suspect spinal cord compression offer to examine the anal sphincter tone by performing a digital rectal examination and also examine for saddle anaesthesia (loss of sensation in the perineum).

2.10.5 **Common clinical scenarios**

The following are common cases which you may encounter when undertaking a lower limb sensory examination. For both, consider:
- what the likely diagnosis is
- what key features you would look for
- what questions you would ask or further investigations you would order to refine or confirm your diagnosis

You could use role play with a friend, using the histories in the cases below as a framework.

CASE 1

A 54 year old man with type 1 diabetes presents with a painless foot ulcer and deformed joint with numbness in both feet. He has recently been constipated and gets dizzy when standing up quickly. On examination there is an obvious deformity of the right foot with two ulcers at the heel and the lateral part of the small toe. You note loss of sensation over both feet with reduced proprioception at the first MTPJ.

CASE 2

A 66 year old man presents with a 3 day history of severe lower back pain, which he states to be worse at night. He denies any history of trauma or heavy lifting. He has recently been diagnosed with prostate cancer and is awaiting his staging scans. On examination you note loss of all sensory modalities below L1 with power 3/5 in both legs. His anal sphincter tone is weak and he has loss of sensation over the perineum.

Chapter 2.11
Gait and co-ordination

What to do . . .

- Introduce yourself to the patient – establish rapport and seek consent
- Appropriately position and expose the patient
- Inspection: observe for abnormal posturing or tremor
- Ask the patient to stand: observe for instability and truncal ataxia
- Assess gait and comment on: initiation, rate, posturing, stride length, arms, stance and swing phase, turning and gait pattern; perform heel-toe walking
- Perform Romberg's test: ask the patient to stand with eyes closed and assess for instability
- Assess co-ordination:

    examine eyes for nystagmus

    examine speech for dysarthria

    examine arms for upward pronator drift, tone, fine finger movements, finger-to-nose test and dysdiadochokinesis

    examine legs for tone, heel-to-shin, past-pointing and pendular reflexes
- Request a full neurological assessment including upper and lower limb motor sensory examinations
- Thank the patient and conclude the examination

Testing the cranial nerves, motor and sensory systems of the upper and lower limbs is not always sufficient to localize pathology within the cerebellum and so a full neurological examination is never complete without examining the cerebellar function.

The cerebellum is the area of the hindbrain that helps to regulate motor function in conjunction with sensory information; one of its key functions is to fine tune motor movements and regulate posture and equilibrium. It also plays an important role in maintaining a normal gait and co-ordinating limb movements. Subsequently, disorders within the cerebellum may present with ataxia, tremor, loss of balance and loss of co-ordination of hand and leg movements.

The cerebellar and basal ganglia both play pivotal roles in motor control and gait co-ordination. The cerebellum consists of two lateral hemispheres and a midline vermis. Each hemisphere is responsible for controlling the movements on the ipsilateral side of the body, whereas the vermis is mainly concerned with the trunk muscles and maintaining posture. The basal ganglia are situated at the base of the forebrain and consist of the corpus striatum, pallidum, substantia nigra and the subthalamic nucleus. The basal ganglia act to receive and process neural motor signals from different parts of the brain before feeding the information to the thalamus.

Gait and co-ordination

Walking involves an interaction between different muscles, joints, peripheral nerves, corticospinal tracts, dorsal columns, extrapyradimal tracts and the cerebellum. Dysfunction in any one of these systems may lead to gait abnormalities that present with a distinct and recognizable pattern of movement. Identifying these patterns will allow you to predict where the underlying abnormality lies and assist you in determining the diagnosis.

Co-ordination is evaluated by testing the patient's ability to perform point-to-point movements and rapid alternating movements correctly. The motor cortex is involved in initiating voluntary movements via the descending motor pathways. After these movements are initiated they are adjusted by the cerebellum and the basal ganglia (extrapyradimal tracts) to ensure the movements are smooth and co-ordinated.

> **TOP TIP!**
>
> There is no definitive or logical order to assess the cerebellum. You should try to adopt a systematic approach that enables you test all areas without omission.

2.11.1 Beginning the examination

Begin by introducing yourself to the patient, stating your name and job title. Confirm the patient's name, date of birth and occupation. The gait and co-ordination examination involves getting the patient to undertake a number of tasks that vary in complexity and so it is important to give a clear explanation of what you intend to do before asking the patient for consent to proceed. You may wish to say to the patient: *'I would like to perform a neurological examination of your walking and the co-ordination of your arms and legs today. This will involve me observing you walk, moving your arms and legs and performing some special tests. Before I proceed, are you in any pain or discomfort at present?'*

Consider taking a brief focused history from the patient before commencing with your examination. Useful facts to determine include whether they are left- or right-handed, if they are able to walk independently or require the use of a walking aid. Enquire particularly about the presence of any family history of any neurological disorders such as benign essential tremor, Parkinson's disease, or autosomal dominant cerebellar ataxia.

Patient exposure and position

Before beginning the examination and asking the patient to undress to their undergarments, ensure that adequate privacy is maintained. Have the patient sit in a chair or on a couch with their arms and legs exposed.

> **TOP TIP!**
>
> Your examination starts when the patient walks into the room because this is the time they are less guarded and are less likely to act unnaturally.

2.11.2 Gait

Inspection

Start by noting whether the patient walks with a walking stick or Zimmer frame. Observe for the presence of orthotic devices such as a shoe raise or brace which may suggest that one leg is shorter than the other.

Observe the patient while they are sitting upright. Look for any abnormalities in their posture. A patient with a unilateral flexed upper limb and extended lower limb may have suffered a stroke. Look for further signs of postural instability, such as arching of the back and wriggling in the chair, which may be indicative of truncal ataxia due to a lesion of the midline vermis in the cerebellum.

Ask the patient to stand from the seated position without using the assistance of the arms of the chair. A patient standing using their hands to gain support will use their cerebellar system to co-ordinate the motion in addition to relying on their motor and proprioceptive pathways to achieve the desired movement. By asking the patient to stand independently this will help isolate the cerebellar pathways and may reveal dysfunction.

Difficulty standing from a sitting position may indicate truncal ataxia (midline cerebellar vermis lesion) or proximal myopathy (which would lead to a waddling gait). If the patient leans to one side, it may indicate a lesion in the ipsilateral cerebellar hemisphere.

Walking

Ask the patient to walk to the end of the room, turn around and walk back towards you. If you do not have sufficient space, then ask the patient to walk back and forth a number of times. If the patient requires the use of a walking aid, allow them to use it.

When observing the patient's gait note the following features:
- **Initiation:** this is the time it takes for the patient to go from the standing position to taking their first step. Observe for hesitancy or a delay in initiating the gait (Parkinson's).
- **Rate:** this describes the speed at which the patient is walking. Comment on whether it is normal or slow (bradykinesia).
- **Posturing:** note the patient's posture whilst they are walking. Are they able to walk with their back straight or are they stooped over?
- **Stride length:** comment on whether the steps are regular or if the stride length varies with each step. Also note if the steps are short and shuffling.
- **Arms:** observe the patient's arms when walking for normal bilateral arm swinging. Unilateral loss of arm swinging may be seen in spasticity (stroke).
- **Turning:** look at how the patient turns when they are walking back to you. Rotation of the body requires a significant amount of co-ordination and thought to achieve. Note for hesitancy, over-cautiousness or a wide turning angle. A wide turning angle or caution is observed in Parkinson's disease. In mild cerebellar disorders, the abnormality of gait may only become apparent on turning, where they may stagger or even fall.
- **Gait patterns:** whilst observing the patient's gait you may notice a particular pattern of movement emerging. Such patterns of movement may often be pathognomonic to a specific underlying cause (*Table 2.5*).

Heel-to-toe walking

Once you have observed the patient's gait, ask them to walk in a straight line with one foot in front of the other as if walking a tightrope. For patients with cerebellar lesions this type of walking will be extremely difficult and the individual will veer towards the side of the lesion. If, however, the lesion is located in the midline cerebellar vermis, the patient may present with general unsteadiness and imbalance.

Romberg's test

The Romberg's test assesses proprioception sense in the lower limbs as well as cerebellar function. Ask the patient to stand up straight with their feet together and arms by their sides. Once they are comfortable they should close their eyes

TOP TIP!

Make sure that you position yourself close to the patient such that you can offer your assistance if they are too unstable.

TOP TIP!

When undertaking a Romberg's test, stand by the side of the patient with your arms outstretched in case the patient becomes unsteady.

Table 2.5 Gait patterns and their possible causes

Gait	Pattern	Associated signs	Possible cause
Antalgic	Appears to limp, with limited stance phase on affected side	Muscle wasting due to lack of use	Cause of leg pain, e.g. osteoarthritis, trauma
Hemiparetic/ scissoring (spastic)	Affected leg held in extension with inturned foot. *Hemiplegia:* one leg affected; pelvis tilts upwards on affected side to swing leg off floor (circumduction) *Paraplegia (scissoring):* hips and thighs cross over during gait with knees and hips slightly flexed	UMN signs. Hemiplegia, arm is also affected Paraplegia: both legs affected, with sensory level (this represents the lowest possible level where the injury can be located and is established by examining the sensory system)	Hemiplegia: stroke, demyelination, space-occupying lesion Paraplegia: spinal cord compression, demyelination
Cerebellar ataxia	Wide-based gait to maximize stability, veering towards side of lesion. Appears giddy and drunken	Cerebellar signs	Alcohol, cerebellar stroke, MS, cerebellar space-occupying lesion
Sensory ataxia (stomping)	High steps bilaterally; stomps feet with each step	Abnormal proprioception and vibration sense in lower limbs, sensory loss. Positive Romberg's test	Subacute combined degeneration of the cord, tabes dorsalis, peripheral neuropathy
High stepping	Usually unilateral foot drop. The patient lifts the affected leg high to clear the foot off the floor. Cannot stand on heel on affected side	Weak dorsiflexion, common peroneal nerve palsy (on the ipsilateral side)	Trauma, L4/L5 radiculopathy
Parkinsonian	Stooped posture, no arm swing, short shuffling steps as if chasing centre of gravity (festinating)	Resting tremor, bradykinesia, lead-pipe and cogwheel rigidity: signs of Parkinson's	Parkinson's disease
Waddling/ myopathic	Pelvis tilts down on the side where the leg is off the ground, due to weakness of proximal muscle. Pelvis shifts side to side	Signs of underlying cause, i.e. hypothyroidism	Alcohol, Cushing's disease, hypothyroidism, vitamin D deficiency, steroids

for around a minute. Make sure that you are well positioned in case they lose their balance.

Balance relies on input to the cerebellum from the visual, proprioception and vestibular systems. By closing the eyes, the visual input is removed and so the Romberg's test will help identify a sensory ataxia or abnormalities in proprioception. Patients with sensory ataxia will begin to sway or may even fall over, whereas normal individuals will be able to maintain their balance.

TOP TIP!

Romberg's test is positive if the patient is more unsteady with the eyes closed than open; this occurs in proprioceptive loss and not in cerebellar disease.

TOP TIP!

Examining co-ordination involves attempting to elicit all the cerebellar signs, remembered by the mnemonic DANISH: **D**ysdiadochokinesia or **D**ysmetria, **A**taxic gait, **N**ystagmus, **I**psilateral intention tremor, **S**lurred speech (dysarthria) and **H**ypotonia.

TOP TIP!

If a patient has weakness of grade 3/5 or less, there is no point testing co-ordination on that side.

Romberg's test is said to be positive only if the patient is more unsteady with the eyes closed than open. A negative Romberg's sign may be seen in cerebellar disease, where the patient will feel unsteady even when the eyes are open.

2.11.3 **Co-ordination**

Co-ordination is a complex task that relies on intact visual, proprioception, motor and cerebellar pathways. The cerebellar system plays a unique role in modulating each of these systems to achieve a refined movement. A disorder of cerebellar function will therefore result in abnormal co-ordinated movements, slurred speech, nystagmus, ataxic gait and an intention tremor. Such disorders are usually ipsilateral in nature because the spinocerebellar tracts that carry unconscious proprioception do not generally cross the midline (see *Fig 2.48*). Those that do cross the midline eventually return to the ipsilateral side before entering the cerebellum.

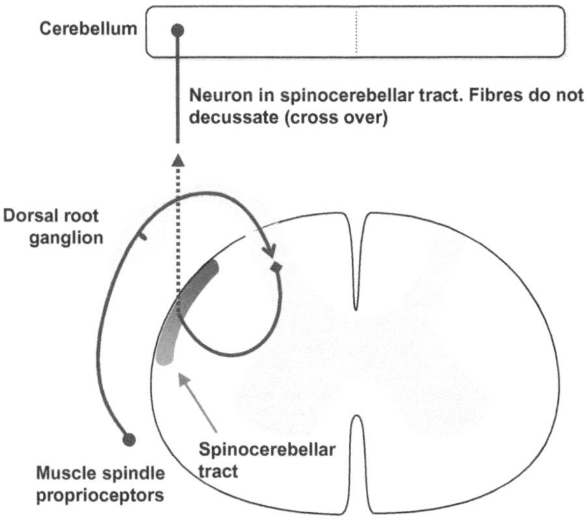

Fig 2.48 The spinocerebellar tract.

Normal performance on the tests assessed when examining for co-ordination also depends on integrated function of joint position sense pathways, motor systems and the basal ganglia as well as the cerebellum. Therefore, to accurately determine that the abnormality lies in the cerebellum, all the other systems must be confirmed as functioning well.

Inspection

Inspect the patient, looking for titubation of the head or a resting tremor. Titubation of the head is a rhythmic postural tremor of the head found in cerebellar disease and which is indicative of Parkinson's disease. An intentional tremor is seen when the patient is seated at rest and improves when the patient performs an action. This is also a sign of Parkinson's disease.

Eyes

Look at the patient's eyes for any signs of nystagmus. Ask the patient to follow your finger with their eyes as you move it in the horizontal and then vertical planes with their head fixed. In cerebellar disease horizontal nystagmus will occur with the fast component towards the side of the lesion.

TOP TIP!

Patients will often move their head as you move your finger; prevent this by lightly resting the finger of your non-examining hand underneath the patient's chin.

TOP TIP!

Dysarthria usually suggests bilateral or cerebellar vermis lesions.

Speech

Speech is affected in cerebellar disorders because the cerebellum is responsible for co-ordinating and modifying both planned and ongoing speech movements. Dysarthria usually occurs with bilateral or cerebellar vermis lesions. The patient may present with difficulty in pronunciation and articulation of words but the content and syntax of the speech is intact. The patient's speech may sound slurred or staccato and scanning in nature, which is typically jerky, explosive and loud with irregular syllables. To check if the patient suffers from dysarthria ask them to say either 'baby hippopotamus' or 'British constitution' – in dysarthria the words will sound slurred and will be separated into syllables. Also note any low volume monotonous speech, which may indicate Parkinson's disease.

Arms

Assess the cerebellar function in the arms by performing a number of specific tests:

- check for pronator drift by asking the patient to hold their arms in front of them with their palmar sides facing upwards; then ask them to close their eyes and observe for any drift of the upper limbs. In cerebellar dysfunction the arms will drift upwards due to hypotonia, whereas in UMN lesions the arm will drift down and inwards; this is because the pronator muscles have an increased tone compared to the supinator muscles.

- check for tone in the upper limbs; in cerebellar disease, hypotonia may be elicited. Stiffness with increased muscle tone felt throughout when moving the upper limbs is known as lead-pipe rigidity. An associated resting tremor will present with cogwheel rigidity. Both signs are features of Parkinson's disease.

Fine finger movements

Ask the patient to touch the tip of each finger with the thumb of the same hand as if they are counting digits. Patients with cerebellar disease will find this difficult because they will not have fine finger co-ordination on the side of the lesion.

Finger-to-nose test

To test for dysmetria or past-pointing, hold your finger at approximately arm's length from the patient. Ask the patient to touch the tip of their nose with the tip of their index finger and then ask them to touch the tip of your finger; finally, get them to retouch the tip of their nose. Then get them to repeat the process as fast as possible – make sure that you keep your own finger in the same place so as not to confuse the patient. Once you have tested one side, repeat the test on the other side, comparing your findings. Look out for any past-pointing, which is when the patient's index finger overshoots the target, as well as the emergence of an intentional tremor as they approach your finger.

Dysdiadochokinesis

Dysdiadochokinesis, typically found in cerebellar disease, is the inability to perform rapid alternating movements and can be checked as follows. Ask the patient to repeatedly tap one hand onto the palm of the other in a clapping motion. Once they are able to do this, ask them to supinate the tapping hand and begin to tap over the same area with the dorsal surface of the hand. Next, ask them to rapidly alternate between the two motions as they continue to tap. Repeat the test on the other side. Clumsiness in doing so indicates an ipsilateral cerebellar lesion. Patients with Parkinson's disease and other movement disorders may also be unable to perform rapid alternating movements due to akinesia or rigidity.

Legs

Having assessed the upper limbs, move your attention to the lower limbs. Ask the patient to lie down on the couch in the supine position. Test for tone in the same way that you would in the lower limb motor examination, remembering to check that the patient is not in pain before doing so. With their legs extended on the couch, put your hands over the patient's knee and gently roll the leg back and forth, observing the movement of the foot. Next briskly lift the leg off the couch at the knee and look for reduced tone as the ankle or foot drops straight away. Repeat this on both legs.

Heel-to-shin

Test for co-ordination in the lower limbs by employing the heel-to-shin test. This is the equivalent of the finger-to-nose test in the upper limb. The heel-to-shin test is useful as it tests dysmetria and the presence of an intentional tremor, both signs seen in cerebellar disease. The test may be difficult to interpret, particularly if there is evidence of spasticity or weakness of grade 3/5 or less in the legs. The heel-to-shin test relies on the motor, proprioception and cerebellar neural pathways being intact and so an abnormal test should not immediately be assumed to be a unilateral cerebellar lesion unless the other systems are fully functioning.

Ensure that the patient has a pillow beneath their head that gives them a full view of their legs so that any abnormalities noted can be accurately attributed to cerebellar disease rather than due to poor joint positional sense. Ask the patient to lift their leg up and touch the knee of the contralateral leg with their heel. If the patient is unable to do this, then this may be a sign of dysmetria. Next ask them to run the heel down the shin until it reaches the ankle. Whilst the patient is performing this movement make sure you observe for an intentional tremor as the heel slides down. Finally, ask the patient to lift the leg back up into the air and repeat the previous steps as fast as they can. Repeat the test on the other leg and compare your findings.

Past-pointing

In similar fashion to the finger-to-nose test in the upper limb you should carry out the toe-to-finger test in the lower limb. This involves you holding your index finger at a point approximately one metre above the patient's feet as they lie flat. Have them raise their leg off the couch and use their big toe to touch your finger. Assess both legs in turn.

Reflexes

It is usually best to leave this test to the end of the examination as it requires the patient to sit up on the edge of the bed. Use a tendon hammer to try to elicit the reflexes in both the upper and lower limbs. Damage to the cerebellum may often present initially with areflexia and later on with hyporeflexia and pendular reflexes; these are reflexes that are not brisk but involve less damping of limb movement than normal reflexes. This response is best observed in the knee with the lower legs hanging freely and will appear as the leg swings backwards and forwards for several beats.

2.11.4 **Additional points**

TOP TIP!

If you have elicited obvious unilateral cerebellar signs, ask to examine cranial nerves V, VII, and VIII for evidence of cerebellopontine angle lesion.

Before completing your examination you should go on to perform a full motor and sensory examination of both the upper and lower limbs. In addition, if you found abnormalities suggestive of an obvious unilateral cerebellar problem, ask to examine cranial nerves V, VII and VIII for evidence of a cerebellopontine angle tumour. Do not forget to examine the patient's fundi for papilloedema due to raised intracranial pressure from a space-occupying lesion.

2.11.5 **Summing up**

Thank the patient for their co-operation. Draw the curtain around them and give them appropriate time to get dressed. Whilst waiting you should collect your thoughts about what information you have gained from the examination before conveying it back to the patient. Make sure you wash your hands again once you have completed the examination.

2.11.6 **Common clinical scenarios**

The following are a list of common cases which you may encounter when undertaking a gait and co-ordination examination. For each one, consider:

- what the likely diagnosis is
- what key features you would look for
- what questions you would ask or further investigations you would order to refine or confirm your diagnosis

You could use role play with a friend, using the histories in the cases below as a framework.

CASE 1

A 65 year old man presents with a limp in his right leg which has been progressively worsening over the past 2 months. On further questioning he tells you he has stiffness of his right hip and pain which worsens on exercise. On examination he has no tenderness on palpation of the right hip, but has reduced internal rotation and evident crepitus. There is no muscle wasting, no weakness and no sensory deficit. On examination of his gait, he has reduced stance phase on the right leg but no difficulty initiating, starting and stopping.

CASE 2

A 34 year old woman presents to you 3 weeks after being hit by a car on the left side of her body while crossing the road. She states that since the accident she keeps dragging her left foot along the ground and it is damaging her shoes. On examination you find weakness of dorsiflexion of the left foot and loss of sensation over the outer aspect of the lower leg. There are no abnormalities on the right. When examining her gait you notice that she bends her left knee high up into the air, otherwise her left foot drags along the floor.

CASE 3

A 72 year old man presents complaining of 'shakiness' of his left hand for the last few weeks. On further questioning you find that he feels like he has slowed down in his activities and is falling over at home a lot more often. On examination you note a resting tremor of his left hand and lead-pipe rigidity of his arms and legs. When examining gait you notice that the patient has difficulty initiating, his feet are close together and he shuffles forward with a stooped posture. When it comes to turning, he almost falls over and you have to support him.

CASE 4

A 45 year old man comes to see you because his family have noted that he has become deaf in his left ear. He tells you that he also experiences a high-pitched ringing noise in his left ear which is really starting to trouble him. He is a non-smoker and drinks alcohol only occasionally. He has no other medical problems and does not take any medication. On examination of his cranial nerves you note that he has sensory loss, loss of corneal reflex in addition to weakness of the left side of the face. He has nystagmus with the fast component to the left. His upper and lower limb motor and sensory examinations are insignificant, but you elicit dysdiadochokinesis and past-pointing on the left. On examining gait, you notice that his base is wide and he veers to the left side, but has no difficulty initiating, turning or stopping.

CASE 5

A 50 year old man who does not drink complains of unsteadiness on his feet as well as difficulty pronouncing words. On examination he sits uneasily in the chair and is unintentionally nodding his head rhythmically. On assessing his gait he is found to have an unsteady wide-based gait. When performing the heel-to-toe test he finds it impossible to walk in a straight line. The rest of the examination is normal.

Chapter 2.12
Eye examination

What to do . . .

- Introduce yourself to the patient – establish rapport and seek consent
- Appropriately position and expose the patient
- Inspect the patient's eyes for asymmetry, ptosis or protrusion
- Assess visual acuity with Snellen and Jaeger charts
- Assess visual fields using the confrontation method; check for visual inattention
- Check pupillary reflexes including direct, consensual, swinging light reflex and accommodation
- Test ocular movements and observe for nystagmus; ask about double vision
- Use ophthalmoscope to elicit the red reflex and inspect the optic disc, periphery and macular region
- Repeat the process in the other eye
- Thank the patient and conclude the examination

The eye is one of the most complex of the body's organs and it plays a vital role in helping to appreciate and understand the surrounding environment. Its primary role is to detect changes in light and convert these into electrical signals that can be interpreted and understood by the brain.

Anatomy

The eye is a globe-like structure that is divided broadly into two compartments: the anterior and posterior chambers. In the anterior chamber, light is captured through the pupil and then the cornea and lens focus the image and project it onto the retina in the posterior chamber. The retina is a light-sensitive layer (comprising rods and cones) that lines the posterior wall of the eye. Using a combination of cones and rods, light can successfully be converted into electrical impulses that are conducted through the optic nerve:

- rods help detect contrast between light and dark shades – they are distributed mainly in the periphery and function best in low light
- cones are able to discern colour and spatial resolution – a high concentration of cones, that provide sharp central vision, are found in the fovea (an area that is located in the middle of the central macula region of the retina).

The blind spot is a small area, adjacent to the macula, which contains neither rods nor cones because it is where the optic nerve exits the globe of the eye.

Eye movements

A range of muscles help co-ordinate the movement of the eye, working in tandem to ensure that a single clear image is obtained and allowing the individual to fix and track an object in an uninterrupted, smooth and effortless motion. Each eye is attached to six muscles which, when contracted, move the eyeball in a

> **TOP TIP!**
>
> In the medical school examination setting, it is unlikely that you would be requested to take a patient history as well as to examine the patient's eyes. However, it is good practice to try to elicit a brief history from the patient prior to examining them.

> **TOP TIP!**
>
> If tropicamide is used, be aware that it may take up to 10 minutes for its effects to take place. In an examination, the patient may have already had eye drops applied.

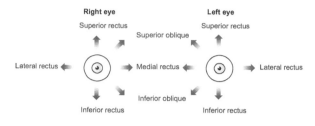

Superior rectus
Superior oblique
Lateral rectus
Medial rectus
Inferior oblique
Inferior rectus

Left eye
Superior rectus
Lateral rectus
Inferior rectus

Fig 2.49 Muscles used to cause a range of eye movements.

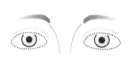

Normal
Normal reactive pupils

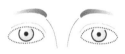

Small / pin-point pupils
(opiates, pontine lesion)

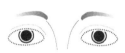

Large fixed dilated pupils
(TCAs, sedatives, eye drops)

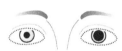

Left Holmes–Adie pupil
Unilateral dilated pupil

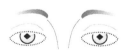

Argyll Robertson pupils
Bilateral ptosis and small irregular pupils

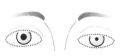

Left Horner's syndrome
Unilateral ptosis and miosis

Fig 2.50 Typical eye signs.

particular plane or direction (*Fig 2.49*). There are four rectus muscles, lateral, medial, superior and inferior, that move the eye in the horizontal and vertical planes. The superior and inferior oblique muscles rotate the eye towards the nasal bridge, allowing the individual to look up and inwards and down and inwards. The lateral rectus works in conjunction with the superior rectus and inferior rectus muscle to permit the eye to look up and out and down and out.

The extraocular muscles are innervated by three cranial nerves, the oculomotor (III), trochlear (IV) and abducens (VI). The lateral rectus is only supplied by the abducens nerve, whilst the superior oblique muscle is connected to the trochlear nerve. The remaining muscles are innervated by the oculomotor nerve. Damage to one or a group of these nerves may limit the range of eye movements achievable and lead to double vision when the eye moves in certain directions.

When examining the eye it is important to test each of its functions separately and in a systematic way. Start off by examining the patient's visual acuity, colour vision, visual fields, and presence of a blind spot before moving on to the pupillary reflexes and eye movements. Finish your examination by using an ophthalmoscope to examine the retina located at the back of the eyes.

2.12.1 **Beginning the examination**

Before beginning your examination you should introduce yourself to the patient, stating your name and job title. Ask the patient their name and age and also how they are currently feeling. Explain to the patient the nature of the examination you wish to perform and gain their consent before commencing.

Ask the patient about common eye symptoms such as itchiness, discharge, redness, change in vision, pain, double vision (diplopia), presence of scotomas and floaters. Also ask if the patient suffers from any chronic disease that may affect the eye such as diabetes, hypertension, migraine or glaucoma. It may be also useful to ask whether or not the patient requires glasses or contact lenses.

Patient exposure and position

Ask the patient to sit upright in a chair. Be prepared to turn off the lights and draw curtains round to help darken the room when examining the back of the eye. Have all necessary equipment ready before commencing the examination: you should have access to a Snellen chart, Jaeger charts (variable sized prints for reading), Ishihara colour plates, red-topped pin and ophthalmoscope. It may also be useful to have some mydriatic eye drops available, such as tropicamide 1%, to facilitate fundoscopy examination.

2.12.2 **Inspection**

Stand back from the patient and check whether the patient appears well or in any pain and note if there is any obvious facial asymmetry. Observe the eye lids for any ptosis (drooping eyelid) which may be caused by oculomotor nerve (III) palsy, Horner's syndrome (interruption of sympathetic chain caused by an apical lung tumour, trauma) or myasthenia gravis. Look at the eyeball to see whether it is protruding (exophthalmos – thyroid eye disease, orbital metastases) or sunken (enophthalmos – congenital, trauma).

Ensure that there are no inflammatory changes in the eye. Redness and itchiness in the eye may be caused by conjunctivitis, scleritis, uveitis or blepharitis (inflammation of the eyelid margin). Look closely for the presence of corneal deposits such as Kayser–Fleischer rings seen in Wilson's disease, corneal arcus in hyperlipidaemia and senile arcus in old age.

Next assess the shape, size and symmetry of the pupils (see *Fig 2.50*). Bilateral irregular pupils that constrict on convergence but not in response to light may be caused by Argyll Robertson pupils present in neurosyphilis. A large unilateral irregular pupil that responds poorly to light may be due to Holmes–Adie pupil.

Visual acuity

This tests the patient's ability to see objects up close and far away. Ask if the patient wears any spectacles or contact lenses and, if so, ask them to use them. If they do not have access to their corrective lens then consider offering them a pin hole to correct for any refractive error.

Far vision

Visual acuity should be formally assessed using a Snellen chart (*Fig 2.51*), at a distance of 6 m from the patient. Snellen charts consist of rows of random letters that decrease in size as you go down. Each row is attributed a number that corresponds to the distance at which a normal eye should be able to read the figures (i.e. 6/60, 6/36, 6/18, 6/12, 6/9, 6/6). For example a figure of 12 means that a patient with normal vision should be able to read that row from a distance of 12 m (the first number, usually 6, simply indicates the distance away from the chart).

Ask the patient to cover one eye with their hand and read the chart from the top row downwards. A patient with normal vision should be able to read the letters on the row that is numbered 6 (this usually corresponds to the second last row on the chart). Establish the lowest line that the patient is able to read comfortably. Determine the number attributed to this row and express it as a fraction. For example, a patient that can read down to the row corresponding to 12 at 6 m has a visual acuity of 6/12 in that eye.

If the patient's visual acuity is worse than 6/60, i.e. they cannot read even the top line, then you should bring the Snellen chart forward to a distance of 3 metres and retest. Record visual acuity as 3/X where X represents the number attributed to the row they can reach. If their acuity is worse than 3/60 then you should stand in front of the patient and get them to count your fingers from a distance of 1 m; if they are unable to do this then consider testing whether they are able to note hand movements and, if not, test for light perception.

Near vision

For near vision testing, you may wish to employ specialist Jaeger charts that should be held approximately 30 cm away from the patient. Again, if the patient uses corrective glasses or contact lenses for reading then they should use them during the test. If these are not readily available you may wish to consider asking the patient to read a newspaper or a book. This should be done with each eye being assessed individually.

TOP TIP!

In smaller examination rooms the Snellen chart should be placed immediately behind the patient with a mirror positioned 3 m in front of them. The patient should read the chart through the mirror and this will reproduce results at an ideal 6 m distance.

TOP TIP!

In the UK a person who has a visual acuity of 3/60 or worse is registered blind, whereas a person whose acuity ranges from 3/60 to 6/60 is considered partially sighted.

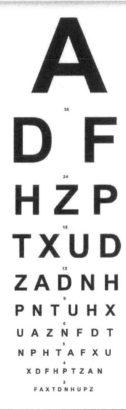

Fig 2.51 Example of a Snellen chart.

TOP TIP!

The Jaeger chart utilizes different sizes of text to determine the patient's near visual acuity. It contains a series of 11 paragraphs with each paragraph written in an increasingly larger sized font. An average person should experience no difficulty in reading any of the paragraphs in good lighting.

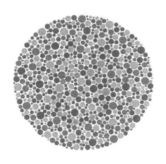

Fig 2.52 An example of number 8 in an Ishihara plate.

Colour vision

Colour vision can be tested using Ishihara plates (see *Fig 2.52*). These are a collection of coloured spots that are arranged to make up a number within a larger circle. In the absence of any colour vision defect all the plates should have a number that is readable. However, in presence of red and green colour blindness a number of plates will appear blank.

Visual fields

Visual fields refer to the area that one can visualize when the pupils are fixated at a particular point. In a normal adult the visual field should extend across 160 degrees horizontally, stopping 10 degrees short of the parallel on either side, and across 130 degrees vertically. All patients have a physiological scotoma, known as the blind spot, located 15 degrees lateral to the point on which the eye is focused at any given time; this corresponds to the head of the optic nerve.

Information is collected by the retinas in the posterior wall of the eye and is transmitted through the optic nerve to the brain. When describing visual fields, the fields of the eye should be divided vertically in half, with the outer region known as the temporal hemifield and the inner region known as the nasal hemifield. Light from the temporal hemifield is projected onto the nasal half of the retina which in turn is carried along the nasal fibres of the optic nerve. Likewise, the nasal hemifield is served by the temporal half of the retina with information transmitted along temporal axons of the optic nerve. These fibres make up the optic nerve as it passes through the orbit before entering the cranium through the optic canal. Optic nerves from both eyes converge at the optic chiasm, with nasal fibres from each nerve crossing over to the other side. These fibres combine with the remaining non-decussated temporal fibres to form the optic tract.

The optic tracts eventually terminate at the lateral geniculate bodies of the thalamus. From here, axons continue as the optic radiations, passing through the parietal and temporal lobes to the occipital cortex. Knowing this optic nerve anatomy, you can begin to localize any lesion by examining the patient's visual fields (see *Fig 2.53*).

Confrontation

Examine the visual fields using a technique known as confrontation. This involves sitting approximately 1 m away from the patient and facing them. Ask the patient to focus on your eyes and then ask them to cover their left eye with their left hand whilst you cover your right eye. Examine the visual fields of their right eye using a hat pin or the tip of your moving index finger. With the patient maintaining focus on your eyes bring the object or your finger from the periphery to the centre and test each of the four quadrants (upper, lower nasal and temporal areas). Ensure that you always keep your finger at an equal distance between yourself and the patient so that you can accurately compare your own visual field with that of the patient. Ask the patient to tell you when they first notice the object in their peripheral field of their vision. Ensure that you repeat the whole process for the contralateral eye.

To test the patient's central vision you should ideally use a red-topped hatpin. Move it across a horizontal plane through the centre of the patient's visual field using the confrontation technique as described above. Ask the patient to tell you when they first notice the pin being red and compare this to when you first

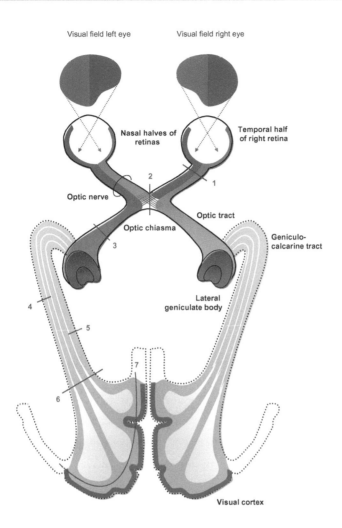

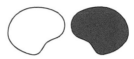

1. Blindness of the right eye from a complete lesion affecting the optic nerve

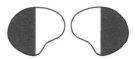

2. Bitemporal hemianopia from a lesion of the optic chiasm

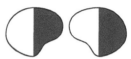

3. Right homonymous hemianopia from a complete left optic tract lesion

4. Right homonymous inferior quadrantopia from a partial lesion of the optic radiation in the left parietal lobe

5. Right homonymous superior quadrantopia caused by partial involvement of the optic radiation in the left temporal lobe

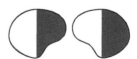

6. Right homonymous hemianopia from a complete lesion of the left optic radiation

7. Right homonymous hemianopia (macular sparing) from a posterior cerebral artery occlusion

noticed it; colour desaturation is often an early sign of optic neuritis or an optic chiasm lesion. Continue moving the pin along until it disappears completely from the patient's vision. Once you have located the blind spot, move the pin slowly horizontally and then vertically to attempt to map out its approximate size. An enlarged blind spot may be seen in papilloedema and optic neuritis.

Finally, assess the patient for visual inattention. The patient should have both eyes open and be facing forwards looking at you. Hold both your index fingers such that each is located in the upper parts of the patient's visual field. Gently wiggle each finger in turn and then both at the same time to test whether the patient has any signs of visual neglect (this can be seen where a stroke has affected the parietal lobe region); a patient with visual neglect will correctly identify when each finger is individually moved, but will report movement only in the contralateral field to their lesion when both are wiggled at the same time. Repeat the process, this time with your index fingers held in the lower quadrants.

Pupillary reflexes

The pupillary light reflex controls the size of the pupil in response to the amount of light that falls upon it. It depends upon both the optic nerve (CN II) and the

Fig 2.53 Lesions of the visual fields.

The numbers correlate to the location of the damage to the nerves as they travel from the eye to the visual cortex.

oculomotor nerve (CN III) to operate. The optic nerve is the afferent limb of the reflex that is triggered by the detection of light upon the retina. It sends impulses to the Edinger–Westphal nuclei (EWN) within the midbrain where it synapses with the oculomotor nerve, the efferent limb, that innervates the pupillary constrictor muscles of both eyes, causing pupillary constriction.

Intense light causes the pupils to constrict, allowing less light in, whereas dim light will cause the pupils to dilate, allowing more light to shine on the retina. When a bright light is pointed at the eye it causes pupillary constriction in that eye, known as the direct light reflex, as well as constriction in the contralateral pupil, known as the consensual light reflex.

Shine a light in one pupil and observe the pupillary response in the ipsilateral and then the contralateral pupil. Ensure you test both eyes in succession. In the presence of optic nerve damage to one of the eyes you will notice a loss of the direct pupillary reflex in the ipsilateral eye as well as the consensual light reflex in the other eye. For example, in a lesion affecting the left optic nerve, shining a light in the left eye will result in an absence of pupillary constriction in both the left and right eyes. However, if a light is shone into the right eye, both pupils will constrict as normal. This is because the left optic nerve is damaged and is unable to carry sensory impulse to trigger a response within the efferent limb (oculomotor nerve) to both pupils.

However, in the case of unilateral oculomotor nerve (CN III) damage, because the motor supply to that eye is interrupted, regardless of whether light is shone into it or into the contralateral eye, there will be no pupillary constrictor response. Hence, in left-sided oculomotor nerve damage you will notice a loss of the direct reflex in the ipsilateral eye; however, the consensual reflex of the other eye will still be present. When light is then shone into the right eye, the right eye will constrict but there will be an absence of the left consensual reflex.

Swinging light test

The swinging light test (*Fig 2.54*) utilizes the principles described above regarding the direct and consensual light reflexes. In a normal eye, if you were to swing a light source from one eye to another repeatedly, both eyes would remain constricted. However, when the optic nerve is damaged, the afferent stimulus sent to the midbrain is reduced, the pupil responds less than it should and therefore *appears* to dilate when the light is shone onto it. As the light is moved to the other eye, both pupils will begin to constrict because the healthy eye has intact direct and consensual reflexes. This response is known as the relative afferent pupillary defect and is commonly seen in multiple sclerosis.

Convergence and accommodation

The accommodation reflex is governed by both the optic and oculomotor nerves. It allows the pupil to focus on near objects and is accompanied by pupillary constriction of both eyes. Ask the patient to focus on a distant object, then place another object 10 cm away from the patient's nose and ask them to quickly fixate on it. Whilst doing so, examine the pupils for signs of bilateral constriction.

Eye movements

Explain to the patient that you will now be testing the movements of their eyes. Inform them that they should keep their head still whilst tracking your moving finger. Whilst sitting in front of the patient ask them to focus on the tip of your index finger and then slowly move it across a horizontal and vertical plane,

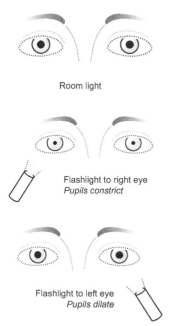

Room light

Flashlight to right eye
Pupils constrict

Flashlight to left eye
Pupils dilate

Fig 2.54 The swinging light test.

The left optic nerve is not functioning properly and displays paradoxic dilation when light is shone on it (left relative afferent pupillary defect).

TOP TIP!

The relative afferent pupillary defect is also known as the Marcus Gunn pupil and may be seen in MS or in a large retinal detachment.

making a 'H' sign. This should enable you to effectively assess the full range of ocular movements. Ask the patient to report any double vision or pain when doing so. Observe the eyes carefully for signs of nystagmus (the involuntary repetitive rotary movements of the eyes moving to and fro) and the direction it occurs in.

- Pendular nystagmus, in adults, could be a sign of an underlying brainstem or cerebellar lesion
- Jerk nystagmus is described as having a slow phase and subsequent fast corrective phase, hence giving a jerky appearance
- Unidirectional nystagmus produces a fast phase away from the side of the lesion (vestibular system lesions)
- Bidirectional nystagmus is where the direction of the nystagmus changes with direction of gaze.

Causes of nystagmus include drug (benzodiazepines, lithium, SSRIs) or alcohol toxicity, or a central lesion in the brainstem or cerebellum.

If the patient complains of any double vision during the examination, spend some time establishing which particular direction exaggerates it. This will help determine the muscle groups that are involved and ultimately the nerve root that is implicated.

Horizontal diplopia would imply a problem with either the medial or lateral recti, whereas vertical diplopia is due to a problem with either the superior or inferior recti or obliques. The direction of gaze at which there is maximal distance between the two 'images' represents the muscles which are weak. Of course, if there is maximal diplopia looking horizontally right, this could be caused by the medial rectus of the left eye or the lateral rectus of the right eye. Ask the patient to cover each eye in turn and to tell you which image disappears; if the outermost image disappears, the covered eye contains the weak muscle.

The oculomotor (III) nerve supplies the levator palpebrae superioris, superior rectus, medial rectus, inferior rectus, inferior oblique, as well as the parasympathetic branch, to the constrictor pupillae in the pupil. A palsy in the oculomotor nerve would therefore cause the patient to suffer with ptosis, dilated pupil and misalignment of the pupil, with it held in the classical 'down and out' position (*Fig 2.55*). This is because the superior oblique and lateral rectus muscles will act unopposed. Causes include diabetes, posterior communicating artery aneurysm, brain tumour and MS.

The trochlear (IV) nerve only supplies the superior oblique muscle and so injury to this nerve will cause reduced downward ocular movements with subsequent diplopia in the vertical plane (*Fig 2.56*). Trochlear nerve palsy occurs in head trauma, diabetes, MS and hydrocephalus.

The abducens (VI) nerve innervates the lateral rectus, thus causing diplopia on lateral gaze. You may notice on examination that the affected pupil lies slightly medially due to the unopposed action of the medial rectus muscle. In addition, when requesting the patient to look laterally, the affected eye remains stationary and cannot pass the midline (see *Fig 2.57*). This can be seen in brain tumours as well as aneurysm.

Ophthalmoscopy

An eye examination will be incomplete without spending some time looking at the back of the eyes using an ophthalmoscope. The ophthalmoscope is essentially a barrel-shaped device that has a light source on one end and a magnifying

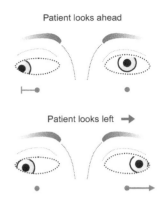

Fig 2.55 Right oculomotor nerve (III) palsy.

The affected right eye is abducted and tilted downwards regardless of direction of gaze.

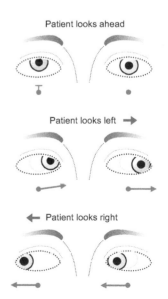

Fig 2.56 Right trochlear nerve (IV) palsy.

The affected right eye is elevated on forward gaze and in adduction but elevated to a lesser extent in abduction.

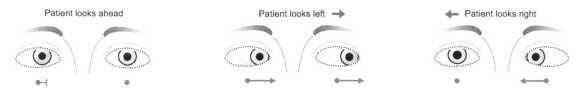

Patient looks ahead   Patient looks left →   ← Patient looks right

Fig 2.57 Right abducens nerve (VI) palsy.

The affected right eye is slightly adducted at rest and cannot abduct when looking right.

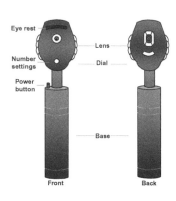

Fig 2.58 Parts of an ophthalmoscope.

viewfinder on the other side with a rotary dial on the side to adjust for refractive errors (*Fig 2.58*). It allows for the examination of the eye chambers including the health of the retina, optic disc and vessels as well as the vitreous humour. Signs within the eye may point towards an underlying systemic illness such as raised intracranial pressure, diabetes and hypertension.

When using an ophthalmoscope you should bear in mind that you will have to get quite close to the patient and will invade the patient's personal space – warn the patient about this and ensure that they are happy to proceed. Ideally, you should give the patient mydriatic eye drops beforehand in order to dilate the pupils. Ask the patient to focus on a point somewhere behind you, preferably above your shoulder. Switch the ophthalmoscope light on and reset it to 0. Remove your own glasses as well as the patient's unless you have a significantly large refractive error. You should try to correct for the refractive index of both your own eyes as well as the patient's if known. If you know the refractive error of your glasses then dial this in to the ophthalmoscope before adjusting it to compensate for the patient's.

When examining the patient's right eye, hold the scope in your right hand. Rest your left hand on the patient's forehead, gently retracting their upper eyelid. This will prevent you from inadvertently knocking the patient's forehead with your own.

Do not immediately rush towards the patient's eye. Hold the ophthalmoscope approximately 30 cm away from the patient's pupil whilst looking through the viewfinder for the presence of the red reflex in both eyes. An occlusion to the red reflex may signify a cataract in an older patient or retinoblastoma in the young.

Approach the eye slowly at an angle of around 15 degrees – this should ideally have you looking at the patient's optic disc. If you find yourself away from the optic disc, locate a vessel in the peripheral retina and track it back to the disc.

Optic disc

The optic disc is an orange–pink oval-shaped disc with well-defined margins that represents the exit point of the optic nerve. It measures approximately 1.5 mm by 2 mm with a slightly paler central depression known as the optic cup. When examining the disc you should note its size, colour, margins, as well as the cup to disc ratio.

Isolated optic disc pallor is associated with optic atrophy where there is loss of nerve fibres at the optic nerve head; this may be caused by ischaemic optic neuropathy, optic neuritis or central retinal artery occlusion. Blurring of the disc margins may be due to papilloedema (see *Box 2.14* for causes) as seen with raised intracranial pressure; because the subarachnoid space of the brain is continuous with the optic nerve sheath, pressure within the cranium is transmitted to the optic disc.

TOP TIP!

Having the room dimmed and asking the patient to fixate at a distant point will promote pupillary dilatation and aid your view of the retina.

BOX 2.14 **Causes of papilloedema**

Cerebral abscess, brain tumour, intracerebral haemorrhage
Subarachnoid haemorrhage
Guillain–Barré syndrome
Malignant hypertension
Idiopathic intracranial hypertension

TOP TIP!

The dial has a set of numbers that range from −20 to +20 including the number 0 as the reset value. They are usually coloured with green numbers representing positive or convex lens and red signifying concave lens and negative values.

Look for vascular neogenesis around the disc margins as a sign of advanced diabetic retinopathy. Approximate the length of the optic cup compared with that of the optic disc (see *Fig 2.59*). A normal healthy ratio would be between 0.3 and 0.5: a ratio above 0.5 may occur in glaucoma, while an absent ratio may be indicative of papilloedema.

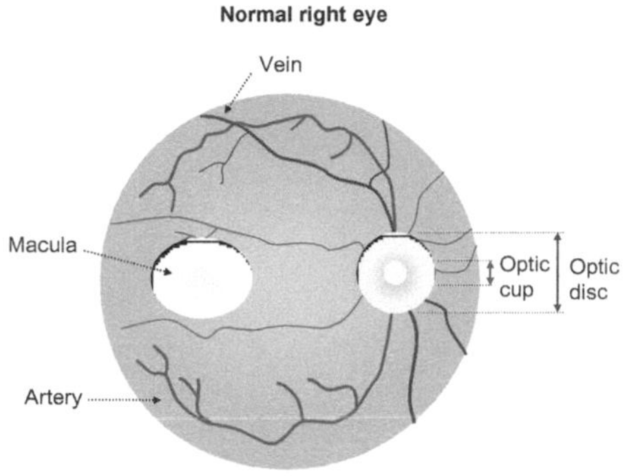

Periphery
Move your attention away from the optic disc and follow each of the retinal vessels out into the periphery. The retinal arteries and veins often run in tandem with one another, with the veins appearing wider and darker in colour then their counterparts. Look out for any AV nipping which is when the thickened small arteries push onto the veins as they cross over, making them appear as if they have been 'nipped'; this is a common sign in hypertensive retinopathy (see *Box 2.15*). Other signs to look out for in hypertension are copper and silver wiring. Arteriosclerotic changes in the vessel wall give a copper-like appearance, whilst extensive thickening and hyperplasia give it the appearance of silver wiring.

Normal right eye

Fig 2.59 Location of macula in relation to the optic disc.

Systematically inspect the four quadrants of the retina looking for signs of disease:
• cotton wool spots – ischaemic fluffy creamy-white discolorations in the retina usually caused by branch retinal artery occlusion; if present you should consider diabetes or hypertension as a possible aetiology

BOX 2.15 **Hypertensive retinopathy**

The 3-year survival of a person with Grade 1 hypertensive retinopathy is 70%.

Grade 1
Mild generalized arteriolar narrowing

Grade 2
More severe generalized narrowing (copper/silver wiring)
Focal areas of arteriolar narrowing
Arterio-venous (AV) nipping

Grade 3
Grade 1 and 2 signs plus:
    retinal haemorrhages
    micro-aneurysms
    hard exudates
    cotton wool spots

Grade 4
Grade 1, 2 and 3 signs plus:
    papilloedema
    macular oedema

BOX 2.16 **Diabetic retinopathy**

Mild non-proliferative diabetic retinopathy
Micro-aneurysms
'Dot and blot' haemorrhages
Hard exudates

Moderate–severe non-proliferative diabetic retinopathy
The above lesions plus:
    cotton wool spots
    venous beading and loops
    intraretinal microvascular abnormalities (IRMA)

Proliferative diabetic retinopathy
Neovascularization of the retina, optic disc or iris
Fibrous tissue adherent to vitreous face of retina
Retinal detachment
Vitreous haemorrhage
Preretinal haemorrhage

- micro-aneurysms – small dark red dots in the retina which can bleed, causing 'dot and blot' shaped haemorrhages; they are commonly seen in diabetes (see *Box 2.16*)
- haemorrhages – branch retinal vein occlusion presents with large flame-shaped haemorrhages, caused by rupture of the superficial precapillary arterioles, which give the fundus a 'stormy sunset' appearance; can be caused by diabetes, raised blood pressure and raised intraocular pressure (glaucoma)
- exudates – collections of fat and protein that have leaked from the capillaries; they tend to have a yellow–white appearance and are usually found in diabetes as well as in hypertensive retinopathy
- scars – may be seen in diabetics who have had laser treatment for neovascularization.

Finally, ask the patient to look directly into the light so that you can examine the macula (see *Fig 2.59*). The macula is the most important area for high acuity vision and hence any haemorrhages, exudates or other abnormalities in this area can have serious consequences for the patient's vision. Pigmentation that can be seen in the macula may be caused by senile macular degeneration.

Once you have completed your examination of the back of the eye, remember to examine the other eye and repeat the whole process.

2.12.3 **Summing up**

Thank the patient and acknowledge any concerns they may have. Based upon your findings you may wish to investigate further for signs of raised blood pressure, diabetes or glaucoma. In the case of glaucoma, the patient should be referred to a specialist to have their intraocular pressures measured formally by tonometry.

If the patient had eye drops placed in the eyes, you should remind them that the possible side effects of itchy eyes, blurred vision and light sensitivity may persist for approximately four hours. In such cases they should neither drive nor operate any machinery during this period.

2.12.4 **Common clinical scenarios**

The following are a list of common cases which you may encounter when undertaking examination of the eye. For each one, consider:

- what the likely diagnosis is
- what key features you would look for
- what questions you would ask or further investigations you would order to refine or confirm your diagnosis

You could use role play with a friend, using the histories in the cases below as a framework.

| CASE 1 | A 56 year old man with known renal disease presents with headache, nausea and vomiting, and visual disturbances. On examination of the eyes, visual acuity was reduced with intact visual fields. Fundoscopy revealed bilateral retinal haemorrhages and exudates. The patient's blood pressure was 220/150 mmHg. |

| CASE 2 | A 38 year old obese man presents complaining of fatigue and increased urination; he is found to have micro-aneurysms and dot and blot haemorrhages. HbA1C was found to be 8.3. |

| CASE 3 | A 65 year old female patient complains of deterioration in vision, headaches, halos around light and nausea. On examination she is found to have a tender firm eye on palpation and an oval-shaped pupil with a sluggish response to light. The optic disc has an enlarged cup with a cup to disc ratio of 0.7. |

| CASE 4 | An 18 year old man with a family history of polycystic kidneys complains of sudden onset of severe headache described as the 'worst headache of his life'. The headache is associated with nausea and vomiting. On examination he is found to have mild photophobia and an enlarged blind spot. There is bilateral blurring of optic margins. The rest of the examination is unremarkable. |

| CASE 5 | A 75 year old woman with known diabetes complains of a gradual cloudiness to her vision over several years which has significantly affected her quality of life. On examination there is absence of a red reflex in the right eye. |

Chapter 2.13
Ear examination

What to do . . .

- Introduce yourself to the patient – establish rapport and seek consent
- Appropriately position the patient
- Inspect the outer ear looking for sinuses, skin changes, skin tags and discharge, etc.
- Inspect the middle ear with an otoscope looking at the canal and the tympanic membrane; comment on its colour, integrity and presence of light reflex
- Perform the additional tests (on both ears) including:

   whisper test: whisper a sequence of number and letters into each ear

   Weber test: place tuning fork on the patient's head and check for any lateralization

   Rinne test: place a vibrating tuning fork against the mastoid process until it is no longer heard before immediately positioning close to the opening of the ear canal

- Thank the patient and conclude the examination

The primary function of the ear is to collect sound waves from the person's surrounding environment and convert them into electrical impulses that are later interpreted by the brain. It also plays an important role in maintaining the body's equilibrium and balance. Ear disorders usually present with symptoms that are easily identifiable such as ear pain, discharge, tinnitus and hearing loss. On occasion, however, disease of the ear may present with non-specific symptoms such as nausea and vomiting, dizziness and vertigo. If a patient presents with such complaints you should always examine the ear as a possible cause.

Anatomy

The ear can be conveniently divided into three sections, each of which plays an important role in the performance of its overall function: the outer, middle and inner ear.

Outer ear

The external portion of the ear is known as the outer ear and runs from the cartilaginous appendage, the pinna, through the external auditory canal and ends at the tympanic membrane. Its primary function is to help gather, filter and then transmit sounds into the inner ear. The pinna acts as a funnel which amplifies sounds from the external environment and channels them into the auditory canal; the auditory canal is a narrow tube, part cartilaginous and part bone, which contains hair follicles and apocrine glands. These glands secrete a yellow waxy substance known as cerumen that protects the ear canal and provides lubrication. However, the collection of such material in large quantities may impact and hinder normal sound conduction. The tympanic membrane is a thin membrane that occludes the medial end of the auditory canal and converts sound waves into vibrations that are transmitted through the bony ossicles within the middle ear.

Middle ear

The middle ear describes the air-filled space immediately behind the tympanic membrane. It contains important structures including the ossicles and the Eustachian tube. There are three ossicles found in this chamber which include the malleus, attached to the tympanic membrane, the incus that acts as a bridge between the other two bones and the stapes that attaches to the oval window of the inner ear. Together these bones act to amplify sounds gathered at the tympanic membrane and transmit them accurately into the cochlea. The Eustachian tube is a tube that runs from the middle ear to the throat and helps equalize the pressure of the middle ear with the outside environment – this allows the tympanic membrane to vibrate without hindrance.

Inner ear

The inner ear comprises the main organs for hearing and balance: the bony labyrinth, cochlea and vestibular systems. The cochlea is a fluid-filled spiral structure that receives vibration from the stapes bone at the oval window. As the vibrations enter the cochlea, fluid is displaced triggering hair cells to produce an equivalent electrical impulse that is transmitted along the auditory nerve (VIII) to the brainstem. The vestibular system contains three semicircular canals that help to regulate balance. Each canal contains fluid known as endolymph that moves depending on the position of the body. As the fluid moves, cilia lining the walls of the canal transmit electrical signals to the vestibular portion of the auditory nerve, indicating the position of the individual.

2.13.1 **Beginning the examination**

Introduce yourself to the patient, stating your name and job title. Ask the patient for their name, age and occupation and how they are currently feeling. A patient's age and occupation may play an important role in the cause of hearing loss. Elderly patients are prone to develop presbycusis, age-related hearing loss particularly affecting high frequency sounds. Musicians, or labourers who work using pneumatic drills, may expose themselves to excessively loud sounds for prolonged periods of time and this may eventually lead to hearing loss or tinnitus.

Before examining the patient's ear, you should ideally take a brief focused history to try to establish the characteristics of the presenting problem (see *Chapter 1.14* for full details of history taking for hearing loss). If the patient presents with hearing loss, ask whether the problem affects one ear or both, if it started suddenly or developed over a period of time, and whether it affects high-pitched or low-pitched sounds. Establish if there are any associated symptoms such as tinnitus, ear discharge or pain in the ear (otalgia). Then try to elicit any risk factors that may be implicated in the patient's symptoms. Ask about recent medication use (NSAIDs, aspirin, gentamicin, loop diuretics), and previous ear operations or infections.

If the patient complains of dizziness, clarify whether this is true vertigo where the room is perceived to be spinning around despite them being stationary. Ask how long the dizziness lasted for and over what period of time. Determine what triggers or precipitates an episode (e.g. movement) and if they feel nauseous or have vomited. The following are all causes of vertigo:

- Acute labyrinthitis is usually caused by a viral infection of the inner ear, particularly the labyrinth. Patients present with acute onset of vertigo and nausea and vomiting lasting from a few days to weeks. There may be nystagmus with no hearing loss.
- Ménière's disease is a disorder of the inner ear due to excessive endolymph production. Often presents in middle-aged adults with recurrent attacks of vertigo, tinnitus and progressive hearing loss. Symptoms may be associated with nystagmus and vomiting.
- Benign positional vertigo is one of the most common causes of true vertigo. It is when the otoliths are displaced from their normal position into the semicircular canals. It presents with short-lasting episodes (up to 30 seconds) of vertigo associated with head movements. There is usually a feeling of nausea but not vomiting or hearing loss. Causes are usually unknown, although it may be associated with a previous head injury or following an episode of vestibular neuronitis.

Patient exposure and position

Ask the patient to sit upright in a chair and inform them that you wish to examine their ears. Tell the patient that this will require you to pull back on each ear to get a better look inside. Also mention that you intend to insert an otoscope into their ear canal to try to visualize their ear drum. Obtain consent before proceeding.

2.13.2 Examining the ear

Examining the ear is best performed in stages, focusing on the three sections of the ear, i.e. outer, middle and inner ear. The bulk of the examination involves inspecting the ear using an auroscope to help magnify the structures contained within. The inner ear is examined using an array of special tests that help discern between conductive and sensorineural hearing defect.

Outer ear

Stand back and observe the patient's ears, checking for symmetry, alignment and any obvious abnormalities. Patients with low-set ears may be suffering from a congenital disorder such as Down syndrome.

Pinna

Move closer to the patient and inspect the pinna more closely. Look for any abnormalities in size and shape and for signs of trauma or injury (a 'cauliflower' ear may indicate a haematoma of the pinna). Look for any congenital defects such as a pre-auricular sinus, usually found above the level of the tragus, and the accessory auricle, found below the tragus. Note any skin tags or skin changes: eczema or psoriasis may be seen in and around the ear and may be missed if the pinna is not gently lifted away from the skin.

> **TOP TIP!**
>
> Do not forget to look behind the ears when inspecting because pre-auricular and post-auricular swellings caused by enlarged lymph nodes may be present.

Auditory canal

Inspect the opening of the external ear canal for signs of discharge. If there is a discharge present, note its consistency, colour, presence of blood and its smell:
- a mucopurulent discharge may be found in otitis media and otitis externa
- a brown–yellowy discharge with a cheesy smell is synonymous with cholesteatoma
- a watery discharge with a background history of a head injury may indicate the serious possibility of CSF leakage

- a bloody discharge may also be seen after trauma or possibly from an underlying cancer

Next move on to examine the inner part of the auditory canal using an otoscope (*Fig 2.60*).

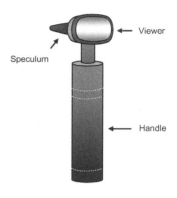

Choose an appropriately sized speculum for your otoscope depending on the size of the patient's canal, remembering that the speculum should ideally lie in the middle of the canal rather than touching its walls.

Fig 2.60 An otoscope.

Gently insert the speculum into the ear canal after warning the patient of a possible feeling of discomfort as you do so. Pull the patient's pinna backwards and upwards as this will straighten the ear canal's natural curve and improve viewing of the ear drum. If the patient is very apprehensive as you insert the speculum and complains of pain it is likely they are suffering with otitis externa, an inflammatory condition of the ear canal due to dermatitis or microbial infection; symptoms include ear pain, discharge, itchiness and conductive hearing loss.

The normal auditory canal is approximately 2 cm long, contains small hairs, and should be of a similar colour to the patient's own skin. Observe the canal for dry flaking skin, as seen in eczema, for ear wax and for any foreign bodies such as cotton buds. Although cerumen may be a normal finding in the canal, excessive accumulation may lead to impaction, resulting in conductive hearing loss and an inability to visualize the tympanic membrane.

Middle ear

The whole of the tympanic membrane should be visible from the end of the otoscope (see *Fig 2.61*). It should appear as a pinkish–grey membrane that is translucent and demonstrates a light reflex. The handle of the malleus can be seen though it with the umbo being the lowest depressed point. Above the malleus is an area of membrane that is known as the pars flaccida and is the slackest and most mobile portion of the ear drum. The pars tensa represents the main area of the drum where the membrane is held taut. A cone of light should be seen emerging from the umbo and pointing in an anterior–inferior direction. When examining the tympanic membrane note its colour, its integrity, presence of the cone of light and the shape of it, i.e. whether it is convex or concave in position.

If the tympanic membrane is red and inflamed this is likely to be due to otitis media, a middle ear infection. A bulging membrane may be seen along with other features such as fever, otalgia and coryza. It is often caused by a viral infection but occasionally may be bacterial in origin. A retracted membrane can be present in both Eustachian tube dysfunction and chronic serious otitis media.

If the tympanic membrane loses its natural colour and adopts a darker greyish–blue tinge, with air bubbles or a visible fluid level, it may mean that the patient is suffering from acute secretory otitis media (glue ear). This is where mucoid secretions collect

> **TOP TIP!**
>
> Hold the otoscope as you would a pen, with the index finger resting just below the head of the otoscope. Use your right hand to examine the patient's right ear, and left hand to examine the left ear. This allows you to rest the ulnar border of your hand against their face, providing stability, as well as angling the speculum in the direction of the canal.

> **TOP TIP!**
>
> In order to straighten the ear canal in an adult, pull backwards, upwards and outwards on the pinna. In children, pull the pinna backwards and downwards.

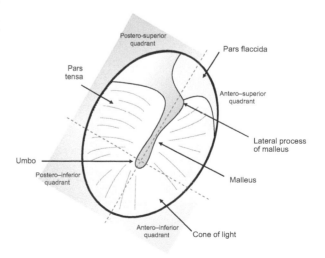

Fig 2.61 Right tympanic membrane.

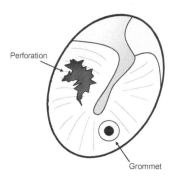

Fig 2.62 Typical position for a grommet.

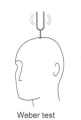

Weber test

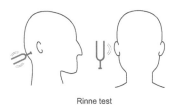

Rinne test

Fig 2.63 Positioning of tuning forks for Weber and Rinne tests.

in the middle ear due to Eustachian tube dysfunction. Milky, non-transparent spots on the membrane suggest tympanosclerosis, caused by hyaline deposits and calcification.

When examining the integrity of the tympanic membrane, note whether it is continuous or has any perforations. A perforation is a tear in the membrane, usually occurring after trauma, such as from a cotton bud when clearing the ear, or after a middle ear infection. These usually heal by themselves after 4–6 weeks. A healed perforation would appear as a whitish grey area.

Also look at the tympanic membrane for a grommet (see *Fig 2.62*) which is a small plastic tube, usually inserted in the anterior–inferior quadrant to help equalize the pressures between the two chambers. If present, it may indicate that the patient is suffering with glue ear and the grommet is being used to drain it.

Inspect the upper part of the pars flaccida, also known as the attic area, for a keratinized lesion. This may represent a cholesteatoma and present with unilateral hearing loss, recurrent offensive ear discharge (often with blood present), vertigo, tinnitus and occasionally with a facial nerve palsy (Bell's palsy).

Inner ear

Although the components of the inner ear cannot be visualized directly, their function can be assessed by taking a thorough history in addition to performing a set of special hearing tests using tuning forks.

The whisper test

This is a simple yet effective test to discern if there is a gross hearing loss in one or both ears. In order to perform this test correctly you need to position yourself behind the patient (so that your lips cannot be read) and at arm's length from them. Create a masking sound in the ear not being tested by gently massaging the tragus whilst whispering a set of numbers and letters in the other ear, e.g. '5, M, Q'. Ask the patient to repeat the sequence – if the patient correctly repeats the set then the hearing in this ear is considered grossly normal. If, however, the patient makes a mistake, then repeat the process using a different sequence. The patient has failed the test if they are unable to repeat at least 3 out of a possible 6 numbers or letters.

Tuning fork tests

These are used to try to distinguish between a conductive hearing loss and a sensorineural deficit. A 512 Hz tuning fork is recommended, although a 256 Hz fork can be used instead.

- Conductive hearing loss is usually a result of impairment of sound transmission from the environment to the inner ear. This may be due to an obstruction in the ear canal by wax, fluid or foreign body, damage to the middle ear such as drum perforation, or damage to the stapes bone due to otosclerosis or trauma.
- Sensorineural deafness describes hearing loss that originates in and beyond the inner ear. This could be due to prolonged exposure to loud sounds, ototoxic drugs (gentamicin, loop diuretics), congenital infections (mumps, German measles), Ménière's disease, acoustic neuroma or presbycusis.

Weber test

This involves placing a vibrating tuning fork onto the midline of the skull, equidistant from both ears (*Fig 2.63*). The patient is asked to state where the

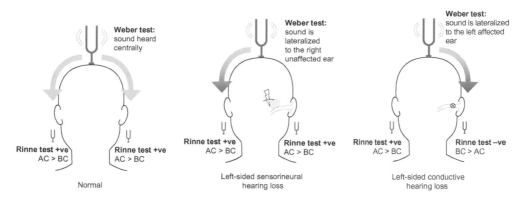

Fig 2.64 Typical results of Weber and Rinne tests.

AC = air conduction; BC = bone conduction.

sound is heard loudest, i.e. left or right, or whether it is equally loud on both sides. If the sound lateralizes to one side then this raises the possibility of a conductive deafness on the same side or a sensorineural hearing loss on the other side.

The Weber test in isolation cannot distinguish between the conductive and sensorineural hearing loss but, used in conjunction with the Rinne test (*Fig 2.64*), it can help determine which of the disease processes is present.

Rinne test

The Rinne test (see *Fig 2.63*) utilizes the principle that air conduction is superior to bone conduction. Take a vibrating tuning fork and place the base of it against the patient's mastoid bone. The patient should be able to sense the vibrations being transmitted through the bone and into the cochlea. Ask the patient to inform you when they can no longer 'hear' the vibration and, as soon as they do, hold the fork a few centimetres away from the opening of the external auditory meatus and ask if they can hear anything. If the patient is able to hear a sound (via air conduction) then the Rinne test is positive and the ear is considered normal. However, if bone conduction is found to be better than air conduction then this is known as a negative Rinne test and suggests the presence of conductive hearing loss on that side. In conductive hearing loss, sound transmitted through the auditory canal is impeded by an obstruction, resulting in bone conduction being heard better than air conduction.

> **TOP TIP!**
>
> To mimic the effects of a conductive deafness, simply insert a finger into the auditory canal and carry out Rinne and Weber tests.

2.13.3 **Summing up**

Before completing your examination ensure that you have repeated all tests on both ears. You should also consider carrying out a full ENT examination, including examining the nose and throat, because pathologies in these areas may provide supportive evidence to your working diagnosis.

Thank the patient for their co-operation and address any concerns that they may have. Dispose of any used speculum heads.

You may wish to consider organizing a pure tone audiogram to fully test the range of frequencies the patient can hear. Such a test may delineate any 'air–bone gaps' or sensorineural loss over a range of frequencies. A tympanogram assesses the compliance of the membrane and ear volume.

2.13.4 **Common clinical scenarios**

The following are a list of common cases which you may encounter when undertaking examination of the ear. For each one, consider:

- what the likely diagnosis is
- what key features you would look for
- what questions you would ask or further investigations you would order to refine or confirm your diagnosis

You could use role play with a friend, using the histories in the cases below as a framework.

CASE 1

A 65 year old man complains of slowly deteriorating hearing in both ears. On examination the tympanic membrane is pearly grey. The whisper test reveals poor recognition in both ears. The Rinne test is positive for both ears and the Weber test was heard equally in both ears. An audiogram performed in the ENT outpatient clinic reveals loss of high frequency sounds.

CASE 2

A 17 year old woman presents with right-sided ear pain, coryzal symptoms and a raised temperature for 4 days. No ear discharge is noted. On examination, the patient has a slight temperature, the tympanic membrane is red, bulging and inflamed. Rinne and Weber tests are normal for both ears.

CASE 3

A 28 year old lifeguard complains of unilateral pain, itchiness and mild hearing loss in the right ear. On examination, there is creamy discharge with debris noted in the ear canal. The patient complained of significant pain on insertion of the otoscope. The Weber test localized in the right ear, with a Rinne test being negative in the same ear.

CASE 4

A 52 year old man presents with recurrent smelly ear discharge that is unresponsive to antibiotic therapy. More recently he has developed vertigo, tinnitus and noted a bloody discharge in the same ear. On examination a crusty lesion is noted in the attic region of the ear. A Weber test localized in the left ear, whilst a Rinne test was negative in the same ear.

CASE 5

A 35 year old woman complains of pain in her right ear. She admits attempting to clear her ears with cotton buds when the pain acutely came on. On examination of the right ear, a small tear is noted in the pars tensa region with clear visualization of the malleus bone.

Chapter 2.14
Peripheral vascular examination: arterial

What to do . . .

- Introduce yourself to the patient – establish rapport and seek consent
- Take a focused history, noting the site, onset and character of the leg pain and the claudication distance
- Risk stratify the patient
- Appropriately position and expose the patient
- Inspection: look at the limbs for colour, trophic changes and presence of ulcers
- Palpation:
    bilaterally for temperature and capillary refill time
    the dorsalis pedis, posterior tibial artery, popliteal and femoral artery
    ask to palpate the radial, brachial and carotid arteries
    ask to palpate the abdomen for a palpable aortic aneurysm
- Auscultation: listen over the large vessels for the presence of a bruit
- Perform Buerger's test looking for Buerger's angle; hang the leg over the side of the bed looking for reactive hyperaemia
- Consider performing a full peripheral vascular examination
- Thank the patient and conclude the examination

Peripheral arterial disease (PAD) refers to the narrowing of the peripheral blood supply, primarily due to atherosclerosis. Whilst it can occur anywhere in the arterial system it is more commonly found in the lower limbs. Due to its pathophysiology, PAD has a greater prevalence with increasing age: studies have shown that up to 10% of those over 65 years suffer with vascular disease, increasing to 25% in the over 75s.

PAD is caused by deposition of fat within the intima layer of the artery walls forming an atherosclerotic plaque (see *Fig 2.65*). This narrows the patency of the arterial lumen, thereby restricting blood flow to the distal limbs. Initially early narrowing is usually insufficient to cause symptoms in the patient. However, as the atherosclerotic plaque builds, moderate stenosis may present itself with pain and fatigue on activity, i.e. intermittent claudication. When such patients are resting, despite there being restricted blood flow, oxygen supply is sufficient to match the demand generated by the low level muscular activity, and so aerobic respiration is maintained. During exercise, however, the demand for oxygen-rich blood dramatically exceeds supply and the muscles are forced to resort to anaerobic respiration to generate the energy needed to continue with activity. The increasing reliance on this type of respiration creates unwanted by-products, such as lactic acid, that accumulate to cause a cramp-like pain in the muscle. The pain typically decreases when the patient

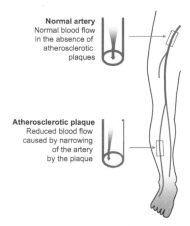

Normal artery
Normal blood flow in the absence of atherosclerotic plaques

Atherosclerotic plaque
Reduced blood flow caused by narrowing of the artery by the plaque

Fig 2.65 The effects of an atherosclerotic plaque.

Medical Guidelines
Risk factors for PAD

Diabetes mellitus   Optimal glycaemic control is recommended

Smoking   Cessation advice is strongly encouraged

Dyslipidaemia   Lipid-lowering therapy is considered if total cholesterol >3.5 mmol/l

Hypertension   Good blood pressure control should be achieved

Obesity   Patients with a BMI >30 should be given advice and treatment

Family history   Patient may have a strong history of previous arterial disease

SIGN Guidelines: Diagnosis and management of peripheral arterial disease (2006)

TOP TIP!

Intermittent claudication often presents with a dull cramp-like pain in one or both legs. It is usually brought on after walking a set distance and relieved after a short period of rest. A shortening of distance may suggest worsening symptoms.

rests for a few minutes because the muscle activity diminishes and so demand for oxygenated blood drops; this produces the characteristic comment from patients that the pain occurs on exercise and is relieved by rest. The pain is often described as originating from the calf. However, pain can be noted in the thigh or buttock, which may suggest that the obstruction is more proximal.

In severe forms of PAD (see *Box 2.17* for a classification scale), where the arterial narrowing is greater than 80%, tissue hypoxia may be so marked that the pain occurs even at rest. Such patients usually complain of pain in their foot which can be so severe that it awakens them from sleep. Some find benefit in hanging their foot over the edge of the bed, whilst others may find getting up and walking around helps to ease their symptoms.

Acute arterial insufficiency

Acute arterial ischaemia is a surgical emergency that can occur following an embolic event. The arterial plaque can rupture, partially dislodging itself from the arterial wall before completely occluding an artery at a more distal point. Blood supply beyond the point of occlusion is interrupted and leads to symptoms including severe pain, pallor, pulseless limb and paraesthesia.

Risk factors

Because of the nature of PAD and the severity of its complications, it is important to determine the risk factors that contribute to this condition; they are in fact very similar to those seen in ischaemic heart disease due to the common pathology, i.e. atheroma formation.

2.14.1 Beginning the examination

Introduce yourself to the patient, stating your name and job title. Check the patient's name and age and ask if they are in any discomfort. Explain to the patient what you intend to do and gain consent to proceed.

Before starting the examination it is useful to take a brief focused vascular history to elicit the patient's symptoms as well as to perform a risk assessment. Ask if the patient has any leg pain and, if they do, elicit the site and the character of the pain, its onset and any exacerbating or relieving factors. Ask the patient how far they can walk before experiencing the pain and whether this distance has recently shortened. If the patient complains of pain at rest, try to establish whether it occurs during the day or at night and what they do to try to relieve it.

BOX 2.17 **Classification of PAD**

PAD is classified according to the severity of symptoms and is subdivided according to the Fontaine classification:
I   Asymptomatic
II   Intermittent claudication
   a   Pain-free, claudication when walking >200 metres
   b   Pain-free, claudication when walking <200 metres
III   Pain while resting / nocturnal pain
IV   Necrosis / gangrene

Establish whether the patient has any of the risk factors listed in the *Medical Guidelines* box above.

Patient exposure and position

Ensure adequate privacy and then ask the patient to undress to their undergarments to expose their legs for examination. Ask if they would like a chaperone if the patient is of the opposite gender. It is important that the examination room is warm as excessive coldness may lead to vasoconstriction and reduced peripheral pulses.

Ask the patient to lie fully supine on the couch with their head resting on a pillow. Offer them a sheet or a blanket to maintain their modesty when they are not being examined. Make sure that you wash your hands thoroughly before commencing your examination.

TOP TIP!

Night pain is a poor prognostic indicator for PAD and suggestive of significant stenosis in the artery as well as multi-level disease. Patients complain of burning, typically in the feet, that can wake them from sleep. They may hang their legs over the edge of the bed or go for a brief walk to try to alleviate their discomfort.

2.14.2 Inspection

Observe the patient from the end of the bed. Assess their general appearance, noting whether the patient appears to be comfortable at rest and well-perfused. Look more closely at their lower limbs, noting their general colour. Look for scars from previous surgery (e.g. femoral popliteal bypass) and evidence of surgical amputation.

Colour

Note whether the colour of the skin is white, blue, dusky red or even black, each representing a different degree of ischaemia. A white leg may suggest early ischaemic changes whilst a black sooty colour at the peripheries may indicate cell and tissue death (necrosis).

In Raynaud's disease the tips of the fingers or toes may undergo a cyclical change in colour from white to blue and finally to red. The areas of colour change are well demarcated compared to the rest of the limb. The majority of Raynaud's disease is idiopathic and is due to excessive vasomotor constriction of the arteries.

Trophic changes

Poor perfusion may cause visible trophic changes including hair loss, thin shiny skin, thickened nails and skin breakdown. These usually represent longstanding ischaemia. Other features include gangrenous patches, necrosis and auto-amputation of toes and fingers.

Pressure points

Inspect more closely over the most common pressure point areas on the foot because ulcers tend to occur here. Specifically check the heel, both the lateral and medial malleoli, the head of the first metatarsal, the lateral aspect of the feet and between the toes. Pressure ulcers tend to have undefined edges.

If you see an ulcer, note its location and shape. Ulcers caused by arterial insufficiency are often painful, coin-shaped with a well-defined border or 'punched out' appearance. They can be found anywhere on the leg but are usually seen in between the toes, heels or bony prominences of the foot. They tend to be deep, sometimes to muscle and even bone and are extremely painful. Poor perfusion can lead to peripheral neuropathy and resultant neuropathic ulcers. These appear much the same as arterial ulcers, except that they are usually painless.

Palpation

Palpation is an important part of the arterial examination. You should palpate for the temperature of both limbs, check for the presence of oedema, assess the patient's capillary refill and finally palpate each of the arterial pulses.

Temperature

Using the dorsal surface of your hands, run them simultaneously down the patient's arms and legs, feeling for any temperature change or discrepancy between the two sides. Ischaemic limbs are usually pale and cold to touch. Bilateral cyclical change in temperature with accompanying skin changes may indicate Raynaud's phenomenon.

Capillary refill

Assess capillary refill in both legs by pressing on a toe for at least 5 seconds while waiting for it to blanch. Release it and then note the time in seconds it takes for the colour to return. A capillary refill time of more than 2 seconds is a sign of poor perfusion. Increased capillary refill time can also be due to peripheral vasoconstriction caused by cold or hypovolaemia.

Pulses

Palpating the pulse, if done accurately, allows the doctor to locate the approximate level where an obstruction or stenosis is present in the arterial system. It is fair to say that if a distal pulse is absent and the next more proximal pulse is present, then the lesion should lie between these two points.

When palpating for a pulse use the pulps of your fingers to gently compress the artery against the underlying structures, i.e. bone. Feel the pulse and determine whether it is normal, diminished or absent. Ensure that you compare both sides to see if there is any disparity. Finally note the presence of any dilated vessels or aneurysms.

Begin in the upper limbs, palpating the radial, brachial and carotid pulses before moving down to feel the arteries in the lower limbs (see *Fig 2.66* for locations). Palpate for the dorsalis pedis artery, posterior tibial artery, popliteal artery, common femoral artery and finally the abdominal aorta.

Radial pulse. Palpate the patient's radial pulse which is located between the styloid process of the radius and the flexor carpi radialis tendon, just proximal to the wrist joint.

Brachial pulse. Locate and palpate the brachial artery which is medial to the biceps tendon and best felt under the belly of the biceps muscle.

Carotid pulse. Observe for any obvious pulsations which may be caused by a carotid pulse. Use your thumb to assess the carotid pulse. The pulse is located between the anterior border of the sternocleidomastoid muscle and the larynx around the level of the cricoid cartilage.

Dorsalis pedis pulse. Examine the patient's dorsalis pedis pulse by placing three fingers longitudinally between the first two metatarsals just lateral to the tendon of the extensor hallucis longus.

> **TOP TIP!**
>
> When palpating, try to avoid using your thumbs as this may lead you to believe that you are palpating a pulse when in fact you are feeling your own pulse.

> **TOP TIP!**
>
> In an OSCE examination, make sure that you carefully read the vignette to ascertain which limbs should be examined – it may be that you are only expected to examine the lower limbs!

> **TOP TIP!**
>
> In 10% of patients the dorsalis pedis artery may be congenitally absent.

Posterior tibial pulse. Palpate the posterior tibial pulse located approximately 2 cm posterior and inferior to the medial malleolus just in front of the Achilles tendon.

Popliteal pulse. This is very often the hardest pulse to palpate. Flex the knee to a 15 degree angle and with both thumbs on the tibial tuberosity, reach around to the popliteal fossa with your fingers. Feel the pulse with your eight fingertips, pressing the popliteal artery against the tibial plateau. In obese patients the popliteal pulse may be very difficult to palpate.

Femoral pulse. Palpate the femoral pulse which is located just below the mid-inguinal point, halfway between the anterior superior iliac spine and the pubic symphysis.

Abdominal aorta pulse. Finally, check for an abdominal aorta which may be located in the lower epigastrium or umbilical area. It can normally be palpated in thin individuals but is often impalpable in muscular or obese patients. Use the edge of your fingers to locate the border of the palpating mass. Establish its size and whether it is expansile or not. This can be done by placing your two index fingers either side of the mass and observing if they are being pushed apart in an upwards and outwards direction. An expansile mass could indicate an aortic aneurysm. If the mass is greater than 5 cm in size, surgical intervention may be required. A pulsatile mass suggests a non-aneurysmal abdominal aorta. In this case your fingers will be pushed only in an upward direction.

Auscultation

After palpating the arteries, auscultate over the larger- to medium-sized arteries for a bruit. Place the diaphragm of the stethoscope over the brachial, carotid, femoral and abdominal aortic areas. A bruit is the sound generated from turbulent blood flow occurring though narrowed vessels; it is often described as a swishing washing sound.

Buerger's test

The Buerger's test assesses for arterial sufficiency of the lower limbs, with a positive test suggestive of critical limb ischaemia.

Check that the patient is comfortable at rest and does not suffer from any back or hip pain. Lay them supine on the couch and note the colour in their legs. Elevate the patient's leg slowly until the blood drains (usually occurs with the leg held at a 15 degree angle). In an ischaemic limb, the low arterial pressure cannot overcome gravity and the veins collapse – this is known as venous guttering.

Continue to elevate the legs until the leg becomes very pale. The angle at which this occurs is known as Buerger's angle (*Fig 2.67*). The more acute the angle, the more severe is the state of disease. An angle of less than 20 degrees represents severe ischaemia; in a normal healthy patient this angle should be greater than 90 degrees, or there may be no loss of colour.

Complete the test by quickly getting the patient to sit up and hang their legs over the edge of the bed. In ischaemia, the leg will slowly fill with blood causing a flushed purple–red colour to be displayed in the distal limb. This is known as reactive hyperaemia (positive Buerger's test) and is due to hypoxia-induced vasodilation.

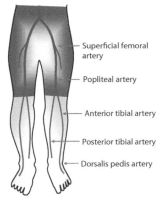

TOP TIP!

If the popliteal pulse is felt very easily, suspect a popliteal aneurysm.

- Superficial femoral artery
- Popliteal artery
- Anterior tibial artery
- Posterior tibial artery
- Dorsalis pedis artery

■ Occlusion in femoral or common inguinal artery
☐ Occlusion in popliteal or tibial arteries
☐ Occlusion in posterior tibial or dorsalis pedis artery

Fig 2.66 Area of pain representing location of occlusion.

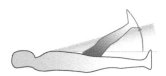

Buerger's angle: the angle at which the leg becomes pale, < 20 degrees suggests severe disease

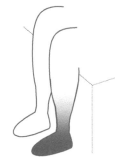

Reactive hyperaemia: deep red colour change to the lower leg noted upon swinging the raised leg over the edge of the couch (positive Buerger's test)

Fig 2.67 Buerger's test.

2.14.3 **Summing up**

After you have completed your examination, to form a working diagnosis it may be necessary to undertake some further investigations depending on the signs elicited. Ask to perform a full peripheral vascular exam, including the venous system, a cardiovascular and abdominal examination, and check their ankle-brachial pressure index (ABPI).

Thank the patient for their co-operation and offer to cover them with a blanket to maintain their dignity. Draw the curtain around them and give them appropriate time to get dressed.

2.14.4 **Common clinical scenarios**

The following are a list of common cases which you may encounter when undertaking an examination of the peripheral arterial system. For each one, consider:

- what the likely diagnosis is
- what key features you would look for
- what questions you would ask or further investigations you would order to refine or confirm your diagnosis

You could use role play with a friend, using the histories in the cases below as a framework.

CASE 1

A 62 year old man complains of intermittent calf pain when walking more than 100 metres. He notices that the pain settles after resting for 5 minutes. He is a heavy smoker, smoking 1 packet a day, and also suffers from hypertension. On examination his lower limbs are shiny with some hair loss and are cool to touch. On palpation he is found to have a weak dorsalis pedis but intact posterior tibial pulses.

CASE 2

A 82 year old man, who is a known diabetic and hypertensive, attended his GP 1 day ago complaining of severe night pain affecting his buttock and calf. He attends today in A&E with severe left-sided leg pain. On examination, you find a pale cold left leg with absent pulses throughout.

Chapter 2.15
Peripheral vascular examination: venous

What to do . . .

- Introduce yourself to the patient – establish rapport and seek consent
- Take a focused history, noting the site, onset and character of any leg pain or swelling
- Ask the patient about any recent trauma, surgery, pregnancy or DVT
- Appropriately position and expose the patient
- Inspection: look at the legs for any varicose veins along the long and short saphenous distribution; look for signs of chronic venous insufficiency, i.e. lipodermatosclerosis, venous ulcers, stars and eczema
- Palpation: palpate down the leg feeling for temperature change; palpate the varicose vein for tenderness and the gaiter area for lipodermatosclerosis
- Auscultation: listen over any varicosities for bruits
- Special tests:

  perform the tap test looking for fluid thrill

  perform the Trendelenburg test by emptying the superficial veins with the patient lying down and then asking them to stand up whilst applying pressure to the sapheno–femoral junction

  ask to perform the tourniquet test to assess for incompetent perforators

  ask to perform Perthes' test to assess for deep vein occlusion
- Consider performing a full arterial examination
- Thank the patient and conclude the examination

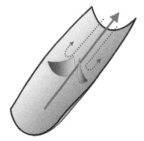

Normal vein
Blood flowing in a unilateral direction (one way); valve prevents reflux

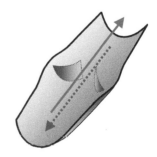

Varicose vein
Damaged valve with swelling of the vein permits bilateral blood flow

Fig 2.68 Pathology of varicose veins.

The examination of the peripheral venous circulation focuses primarily on examining for varicose veins and venous insufficiency. Varicose veins are visible dilated tortuous veins of the superficial venous system (*Fig 2.68*). They usually result from valvular incompetence causing venous congestion and backflow (*Box 2.18*). They are often seen in the superficial veins and more commonly present within the distribution of the long or short saphenous veins. Varicose veins are common, with around 20% of people having had them at some point in their life. They are more prevalent in women with a two to one ratio compared to men.

There are a number of risk factors that can predispose you to developing varicose veins such as previous trauma, prolonged standing, obesity, pregnancy and a strong family history.

Anatomy

Blood is pumped through the closed circulatory system via a network of arteries and veins. Arteries take blood away from the heart under high pressure and

BOX 2.18 **Causes of varicose veins**

Primary	Idiopathic or valve defect
Secondary	Pregnancy (hormonal factors and obstruction of venous outflow)
	Pelvic mass (fibroids, ovarian cancer, colorectal cancer) preventing venous return
	Previous DVT, trauma

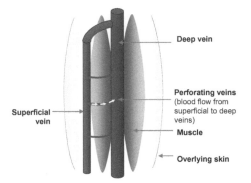

Fig 2.69 Anatomy of the venous system in the legs.

transmit oxygenated blood to the peripheral cells and tissues. The veins return deoxygenated blood to the heart and lungs under low pressure for reoxygenation. Because blood is returned under low pressure, the veins consist of numerous one-way valves that assist venous return to the heart against gravity and prevent reflux.

Venous drainage is conducted through the deep and superficial venous systems (*Fig 2.69*):

• deep system – the large veins that are found deep within the fascia of the lower limb; they handle the vast majority of blood flow back to the heart

• superficial veins – these are located just beneath the surface of the skin and handle less than 10% of venous return; they drain into the deep system at two major points (sapheno–femoral and sapheno–popliteal junctions) and via a number of perforator veins primarily located in the calf muscles (perforator veins are a set of small one-way intersecting veins that drain blood from the superficial to the deep system)

The calf muscles play an additional role in ensuring blood is returned to the heart. The deep veins that pass through the calf muscles are compressed when the muscle contracts, thus pushing blood upwards through the venous system to the right atrium against gravity. When the muscle relaxes, negative pressure is created in the deep system that encourages blood to fill from the superficial veins.

2.15.1 Beginning the examination

Introduce yourself to the patient, stating your name and job title. Check the patient's name and age and ask if they are in any pain. Explain to the patient the nature of the examination you wish to perform and gain their consent before commencing.

Take a focused history regarding their vascular complaint and any associated symptoms. Enquire if the patient has any leg pain and, if they do, elicit the site, character of the pain, its onset and any exacerbating or relieving factors. Also try to establish any risk factors that can predispose to varicose veins.

Patient exposure and position

Ensure that the patient is adequately exposed (undressed to their undergarments so that their legs can be examined) whilst maintaining their privacy and dignity. Ask patients of the opposite gender if they would like a chaperone.

Ask the patient to stand in front of you as this will aid venous filling and make the task of inspection easier. Make sure that you wash your hands thoroughly before commencing your examination.

TOP TIP!

Varicose veins present with a dull ache that worsens towards the end of the day. The pain often originates from the distribution of the varicosities. Patients may note that the pain worsens on standing and improves when lying down with legs elevated. They may also be associated with ankle oedema.

TOP TIP!

Patients with varicose veins may present solely because of unsightly veins and have no other complaints.

TOP TIP!

Reflux from venous valvular incompetence accounts for most chronic venous disease.

2.15.2 **Inspection**

Stand in front of the patient, inspecting their legs anteriorly before looking at them from behind. Look for evidence of any scars from previous varicose vein operations or venous graft procedures used in coronary bypass operations. Look for any obvious tortuous superficial dilated varicose veins in the long and short saphenous vein distribution. Next pay particular attention to the gaiter area of the legs looking for signs of chronic venous insufficiency.

> **TOP TIP!**
>
> During an OSCE examination, it is useful when inspecting for varicose veins to inform the examiner that you are looking for them within the saphenous veins. Be prepared to describe the course that the long and short saphenous veins run along.

Distribution of long and short saphenous veins

Varicose veins often occur within the long and short saphenous veins of the lower leg, with the long vein being more commonly affected. Understanding their distribution will aid in your ability to locate them (*Fig 2.70*). The long saphenous vein starts from the medial malleolus running up the medial aspect of the leg. The vein travels through the medial border of the knee and thigh before terminating in the femoral vein at the sapheno–femoral junction.

The short saphenous vein commences behind the lateral malleolus running up the lateral aspect of the calf, before draining into the popliteal vein via the popliteal fossa.

Chronic venous insufficiency

Inspect the patient's gaiter area (extends from the mid-calf down to and including the malleoli) for signs of chronic venous insufficiency (*Fig 2.71*). Chronic venous insufficiency that has been present for a number of years presents with a range of skin changes including the following:

- Lipodermatosclerosis – the inflammation and thickening of the underlying layers of the skin. The overlying skin becomes fibrosed and scaly and the patient shows the appearance of 'inverted champagne bottle' shaped legs.
- Skin discoloration – this is a classical sign in chronic venous insufficiency and results from the rusty brown appearance caused by haemosiderin deposition. Haemosiderin is a breakdown product of haemoglobin and is caused when venous pooling leading to chronic venous hypertension forces red blood cells into the interstitial tissues. As these blood cells accumulate, the body begins to break them down, leading to the deposition of haemosiderin.
- Venous ulcers are usually found around the medial malleolus in the gaiter area because of pooling of blood within the venous system. They have a classic flat and shallow appearance with an irregular sloping edge. They are usually painless but can on occasion penetrate deep into the underlying structures.
- Venous stars – small dilated veins surrounded by a number of micro-venuoles giving the appearance of stars. Unlike spider naevi, they do not blanch on compression.
- Venous eczema – may present with localized inflammation with scaling and crusting of the skin.
- Atrophie blanche – a patchy white lesion seen on the skin where the underlying veins have been atrophied.

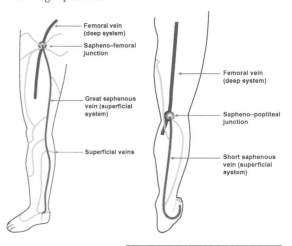

Femoral vein (deep system)
Sapheno–femoral junction
Great saphenous vein (superficial system)
Superficial veins

Femoral vein (deep system)
Sapheno–popliteal junction
Short saphenous vein (superficial system)

Fig 2.70 Distribution of the long (left) and short (right) saphenous veins.

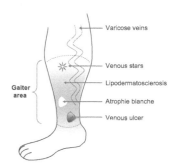

Varicose veins
Venous stars
Lipodermatosclerosis
Gaiter area
Atrophie blanche
Venous ulcer

Fig 2.71 Signs of chronic venous insufficiency.

Palpation

After completing the inspection you should now begin to palpate the legs. Run the dorsal surface of your hands down both the patient's legs, feeling for any change in temperature. In varicose veins the overlying skin may be warm to touch due to venous dilatation. However, if the vein is also tender, this may indicate the presence of an infection (thrombophlebitis).

Feel the gaiter area for the presence of lipodermatosclerosis and pitting oedema: lipodermatosclerosis has a hard ropey texture to the overlying skin, whilst in pitting oedema a thumb indentation may be left once palpated.

Palpate the sapheno–femoral junction for the presence of a saphena varix. The junction is located 4 cm inferior and lateral to the pubic tubercle and represents the point at which the long saphenous vein of the superficial system drains into the femoral vein of the deep system. The saphena varix is a venous dilatation of the sapheno–femoral junction due to valvular incompetence. Due to its location it can easily be confused with a femoral hernia. It presents with a bluish soft compressible lump in the groin that has a positive expansile cough impulse. Unlike a femoral hernia, a saphena varix disappears once the patient lies flat. Elicit a cough impulse by asking the patient to cough whilst palpating over the junction. Also check for a cough impulse over the sapheno–popliteal junction, which is located in the popliteal fossa, for signs of incompetence.

> **TOP TIP!**
>
> Venous disease pre-disposes to superficial thrombophlebitis – feel for hard, inflamed and tender veins in an area of overlying erythema and swelling.

Auscultation

Use the bell of the diaphragm to listen over any areas where there is a clustering of veins. Listen for a bruit, a machine-like sound that could suggest the presence of an underlying arteriovenous fistula.

Special tests

Up to this point much of the examination has focused on collecting evidence of varicose veins and their sequelae. A series of special tests should now be performed that try to localize the level of the vascular incompetence.

> **TOP TIP!**
>
> The varicose veins may refill slowly despite the sapheno–femoral junction being compressed. This may suggest that there is an incompetence at the sapheno–femoral junction as well as at a point below the junction, i.e. perforator veins.

Tap test

Place a finger along the lower regions of the varicosity. Using the finger of the other hand, gently tap over the superior part of the same varicose vein. If the vibrations (fluid thrill) are felt in the lower finger then this suggests that there is valvular incompetence at that level, i.e. in the superficial system.

Trendelenburg test

For this test, ask the patient to lie supine on the couch. Ask the patient to lift their leg off the couch and rest their heel on your shoulder. Gently empty the engorged varicosities towards the groin area. Once you have emptied the varicosities, compress the sapheno–femoral junction with two fingers in order to occlude it. Keeping your fingers in place, ask the patient to stand up so that their legs can be examined. With your fingers still in place, note whether the varicosities in the legs refill immediately. If, by maintaining pressure over the sapheno–femoral junction, the varicose veins remain collapsed, the level of the incompetence must be above the sapheno–femoral junction. If the veins simply refill immediately, then you can conclude that there is incompetence at a level below this point, probably originating from one of the perforating veins.

Tourniquet test

The tourniquet test (*Fig 2.72*) involves using a tourniquet over the leg to assess for the presence and level of incompetent perforators. As for the Trendelenburg test, ask the patient to lie down and then raise their leg to empty their varicose veins. Apply a tourniquet around the upper part of the thigh and then ask the patient to stand up. Inspect the legs and note whether the veins have refilled. With the tourniquet in place, filling of varicose veins below this level suggests that there are incompetent perforators below the level of the tourniquet. Repeat the test and each time move the tourniquet down the thigh until the superficial veins remain collapsed; the level at which this first occurs suggest the approximate site of the incompetent perforators.

TOP TIP!

It is unlikely that you would be expected to perform all the special tests together; however, you should be able to explain to the examiner how to perform each one and what they are testing.

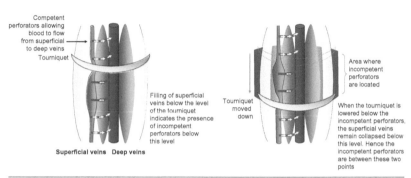

Fig 2.72 Tourniquet test.

Perthes' test

Ask to perform the Perthes' test to check for deep vein compromise. With the patient lying down and superficial veins emptied, fasten the tourniquet around the upper third of the thigh. Ask the patient to stand up on their feet and then onto tiptoes, repeating this process at least ten times. Observe the superficial veins for signs of swelling or to see if they remain unfilled. If the deep veins are occluded, then the superficial veins will begin to fill, resulting in them becoming more tense.

2.15.3 **Summing up**

Once you have completed the examination of the venous system, you should ask to perform a full abdominal, pelvic and scrotal examination, as relevant, to rule out any intra-abdominal or pelvic pathology. You should ask to perform a full arterial examination, including palpating the peripheral pulses, because the patient could be suffering from mixed arterial and venous disease.

Before finishing off, confirm your findings by requesting a venous duplex ultrasound to pinpoint the area of valvular incompetence or to look for a deep venous thrombosis.

Thank the patient for their co-operation and offer them a blanket to maintain their dignity before giving them appropriate time to get dressed.

2.15.4 **Common clinical scenarios**

The following are a list of common cases which you may encounter when undertaking an examination of the peripheral venous system. For each one, consider:

TOP TIP!

Do not forget that an abdominal or pelvic mass can cause inferior vena caval obstruction.

TOP TIP!

Using duplex ultrasound it is possible to map out valvular incompetence at the common and superficial femoral, long and short saphenous, popliteal, posterior tibial, and perforator veins.

- what the likely diagnosis is
- what key features you would look for
- what questions you would ask or further investigations you would order to refine or confirm your diagnosis

You could use role play with a friend, using the histories in the cases below as a framework.

CASE 1

A 52 year old school crossing monitor complains of a dull ache over her leg. It is worse towards the end of the day. On examination she has evidence of lipodermatosclerosis as well as a rusty brown discoloration to the gaiter area of the right leg. She also has an obvious superficial vein running along the back of her leg and terminating in the back of the knee.

CASE 2

A 29 year old woman, who is 36 weeks pregnant, complains of unsightly veins in her legs. On examination you note mild pedal oedema as well as dilated superficial veins running from the medial maleollus up to the inner thigh. When performing the Trendelenburg test you note that by maintaining pressure over the sapheno–femoral junction the vein remains collapsed.

Chapter 2.16
Examination of a lump

What to do . . .

- Introduce yourself to the patient – establish rapport
- Appropriately position and expose the patient's lump
- Inspection: look generally at the patient to see if there is one lump or multiple; describe the lump's site, size, shape, colour and surroundings
- Palpation: feel the lump for its temperature, tenderness, edge, surface and consistency; press the lump to assess compressibility, pulsatility and fluid thrill fluctuance
- Move the lump in two planes and attempt to move the skin above it
- Percussion and auscultation: check the lump for the presence of bruits or bowel sounds
- Transilluminate the lump
- Assess and examine regional lymph nodes
- Thank the patient and conclude the examination

Lumps or swellings may present almost anywhere in the body. They usually arise from localized underlying structures of the skin and are commonly benign. Despite this they usually cause much concern in the patient because of the fear that they may be cancerous or due to their unsightly appearance. A good knowledge of the anatomy of the skin and underlying structures as well as a comprehensive clinical examination should lead you to the correct diagnosis of the lump.

This chapter focuses on the general approach to be adopted when examining a lump but, depending on its location, a more focused and complete examination may be required, such as for the neck or an inguinoscrotal lump (see *Chapters 2.17* and *2.4*, respectively, for more information).

TOP TIP!

The most common lumps seen in exams include sebaceous cysts, lipomas and fibromas.

Anatomy of the skin

The skin is the largest organ of the body and consists of three layers including the epidermis, the dermis and the subcutaneous layer. The epidermis is the thin outer layer of the skin containing mainly keratinocytes which help protect the skin as well as melanocytes that secrete melanin. It acts as a physical barrier against heat, injury and infections. The dermis is the layer that is between the epidermis and subcutaneous tissue. It contains blood and lymph vessels, hair follicles and sweat glands. Also located in this layer are the sebaceous glands that produce sebum and lubricate the skin. The subcutaneous layer is the deepest layer of the skin and is primarily made up of fat cells and collagen. It helps to conserve the body's heat and provides structure for the overlying layers.

TOP TIP!

Remember that common things are common; the most likely types of lumps (see *Box 2.19*) you will be faced with in an examination are sebaceous cysts, lipomas, ganglions, dermatofibromas, neurofibromas, lymph nodes and perhaps boils or carbuncles (although these may be too painful to examine).

BOX 2.19 **Common causes of lumps**

Sebaceous cysts
Also known as epidermal cysts, these are usually found within the dermis of the skin. They are derived from the outer sheath of the hair follicle following obstruction of the mouth of the sebaceous duct within the dermis and not from the sebaceous gland as the name suggests. In some cases they are caused by swollen hair follicles, or following trauma, and usually contain a thick cheesy protein called keratin. The cysts classically have a punctum on the surface and cannot be transilluminated. They may have a foul malodorous discharge, particularly if they are infected.

Fibromas
These are benign tumours derived from fibrous tissue. Although they are usually found under the skin they may appear anywhere in the body. They have a white rounded appearance with a firm texture. They are often painless and freely mobile because they are not fixed to any underlying structures; examples include dermatofibromas and neurofibromas.

Lipomas
These are the most common form of soft tissue tumour that arise from adipose tissue located in the subcutaneous layer of the skin. They are often felt as small, soft, semi-fluctuant, circular structures that are mobile within the skin layer. They can be found almost anywhere in the skin although they rarely present on the palms of the hand or the soles of the feet.

Boils and carbuncles
These are skin lesions that originate from the hair follicle and are usually caused by staphylococcal skin infection. Patients may present with a hard, red, warm lesion that is often painful. Boils occur more superficially on the skin and are seen as a single abscess, whereas carbuncles are often a collection of boils extending to the subcutaneous tissue. Both lesions can exude pus and form sinuses. Patients presenting with recurrent boils or carbuncles should always be investigated for diabetes or immunocompromised states.

Although visually a lump may appear to be coming from the skin, it may well originate from structures beneath it. With this in mind, when making a diagnosis it is important to consider the range of tissues and underlying structures that lie below the lesion, such as muscle, fat, nerve, or even tissues specific to a particular location such as the thyroid, parotid gland or breast.

2.16.1 **Beginning the examination**

Introduce yourself to the patient, stating your name and job title. Ask the patient's name and age, and ask whether they are in any pain or discomfort.

Explain clearly to the patient what you intend to do when examining the lump, especially if it is in a part of the body that the patient is not comfortable exposing. In such cases you may need a chaperone. Once the patient has understood what you have said, seek consent to proceed with the examination. You may say to the patient, *'In view of the swelling you have noticed, I wish to examine the area to determine the cause of it. Before I proceed may I ask if the swelling is causing you any pain or discomfort?'*

Before starting the physical examination you should ask the patient a few questions pertaining to their lump which should focus the examination and help produce a list of potential diagnoses. Ask where the lump is, when it was first noticed and if it has recently changed in size. Ask if there was any trauma, such as fall or direct injury, prior to the lump appearing. Establish if the lump is painful or restricts the patient's range of movement. Ask if the patient has

TOP TIP!

Always ask the patient if they have more than one lump.

lost any weight, or suffers from night sweats because this may highlight more systemic causes for the lumps such as lymphoma or tuberculosis.

Patient exposure and position

Ensure that adequate privacy is maintained before beginning the examination and asking the patient to expose the swelling. Ask the patient to remove any clothing around the swelling to expose it and its surroundings sufficient for inspection. Depending on the location of the swelling, ask the patient to sit on a chair or lie on a couch, whichever is more comfortable for them. Make sure that you wash and warm your hands before palpating the patient.

2.16.2 Inspection

Begin by standing at the edge of the bed or chair and ask the patient to point to the lump in question; also note whether there is a single lump or multiple. Move closer to the patient, kneeling down if necessary, and begin to inspect the swelling in the following systematic manner.

Site

Note the location of the lump, the region in which it is found (e.g. head, scalp, arm, leg, chest wall, abdomen), the side (right or left), the surface (dorsal, ventral, palmar, anterior, posterior) and its relation to the nearest anatomical landmark (usually the distance from a bony prominence).

Lumps such as sebaceous cysts are found in hairy areas such as the scalp, neck or face and rarely occur on the palms or soles of the feet. Lipomas can be found anywhere that adipocytes exist, but commonly occur on the back or the shoulders. Ganglions are small fluid-filled cysts that are commonly seen at the wrist joint or dorsum of the hand.

Size

Ensure that you measure both the width and length of the lump with a ruler or tape measure, describing it in centimetres or millimetres. It is important to determine whether the lump has recently changed in size and when the patient first noticed it. For example, an abdominal aortic aneurysm may rapidly increase in size, with lesions greater than 6.5 cm requiring surgical intervention.

Shape

Occasionally the shape of the mass may help discern its aetiology. Swellings can be circular, oval or irregular; lipomas are almost universally hemi-spherical in shape, whereas ganglions are commonly circular or oval.

Colour

Note whether the lesion is pigmented, red, black, white or of normal skin colour. Lesions that are red in colour may suggest an infection or inflammatory process taking place, such as an abscess or infected sebaceous cyst. A purple–red discoloration may indicate the presence of a vascular tumour, i.e. a haemangioma, whilst a dark brown colour may represent a haematoma. A black lesion may be a mole or melanoma.

Surroundings

Conclude the inspection by looking around the lump for adjacent changes which can be seen in the skin, muscle and joints. Patients presenting with multiple small, smooth, firm skin-coloured lumps with adjacent café au lait rashes may be caused by neurofibromatosis, which is benign tumours of nerves.

Palpation

Before palpating the swelling, ensure that your hands are adequately warmed and that the patient is aware that you now intend to feel the lump. While examining the lesion, check the patient's face at regular intervals to make sure that they are not in any discomfort. Feel the lump before attempting to compress and move it to check for mobility.

Temperature

Run the back of your hand over the lump to check if there is any change in temperature compared with the surrounding areas. A warm and red lump may indicate infection or strangulation in hernias.

Tenderness

Check if the lump is tender when palpating. A tender lump may be caused by an underlying infective or inflammatory process such as in abscesses or infective cysts. A strangulated hernia will also be acutely painful.

Edge

When assessing the swelling, note whether its edge is regular or irregular. Lesions which have well-defined smooth edges are usually benign, such as lipomas and sebaceous cysts, whereas lesions with irregular indistinct borders may be cancerous in nature.

Surface

Comment on whether the surface of the lump is smooth, rough, irregular or bosselated. A lipoma has a bosselated surface (meaning that it has many protuberances), sebaceous and ganglion cysts have smooth surfaces, whereas arterio-venous malformations or fistulas usually have irregular edges. Gently feel the surface of the skin which may give vital clues to the cause. Breast cancers may demonstrate a 'peau d'orange' effect whereby the lesion has the appearance of orange peel dimpling of the skin. A depression felt within the centre of the swelling may be a punctum found in a sebaceous cyst.

Consistency

Feel the lump between your thumb and index finger and determine its consistency. Lumps can be described as being soft, firm, hard or rubbery. Lipomas usually feel soft, whereas enlarged lymph nodes can have a rubbery consistency to them. Sebaceous cysts tend to be firm but may exhibit some fluctuance to them. Hard lesions represent solid structures such as rheumatoid nodules, gouty tophi or osteoarthritic nodes (Heberden's, Bouchard's).

Pressing the lump

Once you have felt and described the lump, you must assess it for compressibility, pulsatility and fluctuation by pressing it in different directions.

Compressibility

Assess compressibility by pressing firmly downwards over the top of the swelling. If the lump is compressible it should reappear spontaneously after you remove your finger. If the lesion fails to reappear when the pressure is removed then it is said to be reducible. Lipomas and saphena varix can exhibit compressibility, whereas some hernias may be reducible.

> **TOP TIP!**
>
> The term 'soft' describes a similar consistency to that of touching a lip, 'firm' is similar to touching the tip of a nose and 'hard' is similar to touching the forehead.

Pulsatility

Test for pulsatility of the lump by placing the index finger of both your hands on either side of it. If you feel that your fingers are being pushed upwards and away from each other then the lump exhibits expansile pulsation, such as in a vascular aneurysm. On the other hand, if your fingers are simply pushed upwards in only one plane then the lump demonstrates transmitted pulsations; these may be seen in lumps of a vascular origin such as a carotid body tumour, or may simply be due to a swelling overlying an artery.

Fluid thrill

Check the lump for a fluid thrill. For small lesions place your middle finger and thumb on either side of the swelling and depress the top of it. When doing so, if you feel pressure being transmitted to your fingers, this may suggest a fluctuant lesion as seen in lipomas and ganglions.

For grossly enlarged swellings, ask the patient to place the ulnar edge of their hand in the centre of the lump and gently flick one side whilst you feel the other side for transmitted vibrations. If demonstrated, this is known as a fluid thrill and is used to confirm the presence of abdominal ascites.

Move

The purpose of assessing the moving of a lump is to determine whether it is attached to any underlying structure, is tethered to the overlying skin, or moves freely. Attempt to move the lump in two planes that are perpendicular to one another and note the degree of manœuvrability. Carotid body tumours only move in one plane because they are vertically fixed. Breast fibroadenomas are also commonly known as 'breast mice' due to their ability to be freely mobile.

Check whether the lump is attached to any underlying structures such as muscle or bone. A swelling attached to a muscle may move when it contracts (leiomyosarcomas), whereas lesions fixed to the bone are often immobile (osteomas).

Check for skin tethering by observing the overlying skin when the lump is moved. Dimpling of the skin may occur when an attempt to reposition the lump is impeded by the attachment to the superficial skin. If the skin moves freely over the lump then the mass probably arises subcutaneously, such as a lipoma. On the other hand, if the skin cannot be rolled over the lump then it can be assumed that it arises from the dermis or epidermis (sebaceous cyst).

Percussion and auscultation

Although percussion is not a vital part of examining a lump it can, on occasions, be carried out to provide useful information. Place your middle finger over the lump and gently tap it with the other hand, trying to elicit a percussion note. Lumps that originate from the skin or subcutaneously, i.e. lipomas, will be dull, whereas any lumps that involve bowel loops, such as a hernia, are likely to be resonant.

Auscultate over the lump using the diaphragm of the stethoscope, listening out for bruits or bowel sounds. An arterio-venous fistula (used for dialysis) or AV malformations will generate a continuous murmur or bruit on auscultation. Bowel sounds may be heard over a hernia.

TOP TIP!

Do NOT forget that transmitted pulsations can be felt when a lump overlies an artery!

TOP TIP!

When examining an AV fistula, inspect for needle stick marks which may suggest recent use. Palpate, feeling for thrill and finally auscultate it, listening out for a buzzing machine-like murmur (bruit).

Transillumination

Place a pen torch on one side of the lump and an opaque tube on the other which will help eliminate as much external light as possible. Switch the torch on and observe the swelling for transillumination (when the lump glows bright red in colour which indicates a fluid-filled swelling). Lumps that transilluminate include ganglions, hydroceles and very large lipomas. Sebaceous cysts and solid lumps do not transilluminate.

Lymph node involvement

An examination of a lump is not complete without examining the surrounding areas for sensation, motor deficit and regional lymph nodes. These checks will identify whether the lump is completely benign or whether it has affected other structures in the local area.

Complete your examination of the lump by examining the surrounding lymph nodes. If you find any enlarged lymph nodes, this may suggest that the swelling is inflammatory or infectious in nature or possibly malignant.

2.16.3 Summing up

Thank the patient for their co-operation. Draw the curtain around them and give them appropriate time to get dressed. Whilst waiting you may wish to collect your thoughts about what information you have gained from the examination before conveying it back to the patient. Make sure that you acknowledge the patient's concerns. Remember to wash your hands again at the end of the examination.

2.16.4 Common clinical scenarios

The following are a list of common cases which you may encounter when undertaking a lump examination. For each one, consider:
- what the likely diagnosis is
- what key features you would look for
- what questions you would ask or further investigations you would order to refine or confirm your diagnosis

You could use role play with a friend, using the histories in the cases below as a framework.

CASE 1

A 45 year old man presents with a painless, slowly enlarging lump on his back that has been present for about 7 months. On examination there is a single, soft swelling 2 cm below the inferior border of the right scapula. It measures 2 by 3 cm, and there are no obvious abnormalities of the overlying skin. The lump is not tender and feels soft and lobulated with well demarcated edges. It is freely mobile with no tethering to skin nor to the underlying muscle and there was no associated lymphadenopathy.

CASE 2

A 50 year old man presents with a hard painless lump on his scalp. On examination there was a single, skin-coloured, round swelling with well demarcated edges about 1 cm above the left mastoid process. On the upper surface of the lump appeared to be a central punctum. The lump measured 1 by 2 cm, was non-tender and felt firm. The lump was semi-fluctuant and did not transilluminate. It was not possible to move the overlying skin but the lump was not fixed to any underlying structures. There was no associated lymphadenopathy.

CASE 3

A 30 year old woman presents with a recurring lump over the dorsum of her right wrist. On examination, there was a single 1 by 1 cm lump adjacent to the right radial styloid process. The lump appeared to be smooth, hemispherical, skin-coloured and had well demarcated edges. It was firm, non-tender, slightly fluctuant and weakly transilluminable. It was not tethered to the overlying skin but fixed to the underlying structures. There was no associated lymphadenopathy.

CASE 4

A 16 year old diabetic youth presents with a 3 day history of a painful lump in his back. On examination there was a tender red, 3 by 4 cm erythematous fluctuant lump in the posterior margin of the axilla. The lump had a discrete border and was very tender and warm to palpation. Due to the pain, fluctuance and transillumination were not examined.

CASE 5

A 47 year old diabetic who attends dialysis regularly describes a lump in his arm. On examination he has a 2 by 5 cm pulsatile mass over his right forearm. On auscultation you hear a distinct bruit.

Chapter 2.17
Thyroid examination

What to do . . .

- Introduce yourself to the patient – establish rapport and seek consent
- Appropriately position and expose the patient
- Inspect the neck for any lumps
- Ask patient to swallow and protrude their tongue
- Palpation: palpate the neck and lump and describe its location and consistency; check for lymph nodes and tracheal position
- Percuss over the thyroid gland down to the sternal angle for retrosternal extension
- Auscultate over goitre for bruits
- Assess for thyroid dysfunction: inspect nails and hands; feel for pulse; check for tremor; inspect for eye signs of Graves' disease
- Thank the patient and conclude the examination

Lumps in the neck often cause a significant amount of distress and concern in patients, not only because they are often unsightly, but also because of the possibility of their being cancerous. In reality, the majority of lumps that arise from the neck area are benign with more than half being simply an enlarged thyroid gland. However, when examining a lump in the neck one must pay particular attention to its location, its qualities and associated symptoms to exclude the possibility of more sinister causes.

Anatomy of the neck

The neck describes the area between the chest inferiorly and the head anteriorly. It contains a number of important structures including the thyroid gland, carotid artery, internal and external jugular veins, larynx, trachea, oesophagus and the cervical lymph node chains. For examination purposes the neck is further divided into two triangles separated by the sternoclavicular muscle (*Fig 2.73*):

- the anterior triangle describes the area bound superiorly by the mandible, medially by the midline of the neck and laterally by the sternoclavicular muscle
- the posterior triangle has the trapezius muscle forming the lateral margin, the clavicle as the inferior border and the sternoclavicular muscle as the medial margin.

Thyroid gland

The thyroid gland is a butterfly-shaped organ located in the midline of the neck. It comprises two lobes divided

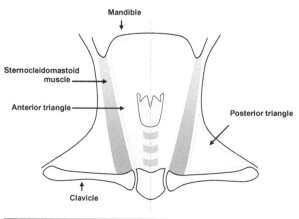

Fig 2.73 Triangles of the neck.

by an isthmus and is found in front of the trachea just below the cricoid cartilage. The thyroid is supplied by branches of the external carotid artery and thyro-cervical trunk.

The thyroid is one of the largest endocrine glands in the body with its primary function being to control the body's metabolism. It operates in conjunction with the hypothalamus and the pituitary to form the hypothalamic–pituitary–thyroid axis. The hypothalamus secretes thyrotrophin-releasing hormone (TRH) that stimulates the pituitary to release thyroid-stimulating hormone (TSH). This in turn acts on the thyroid gland to secrete thyroxin (T_4) and triiodothyronine (T_3). These hormones go on to affect the body's growth and metabolism.

2.17.1 Beginning the examination

Introduce yourself to the patient, stating your name and job title. Ask the patient for their name and age and how they are currently feeling. Explain to the patient the nature of the examination you wish to perform and gain their consent before commencing.

Take a focused history about the patient's lump. Ask where the lump is, when they first noticed it, and if it has recently changed in size. Also try to establish if there are any associated symptoms such as an intolerance to cold or warm environments, change in appetite, weight or bowel habits.
- Hypothyroidism is caused by an underactive thyroid gland. It usually causes a number of symptoms over a period of time including weight gain, profound fatigue, constipation, hair loss, hoarseness of voice and cold intolerance.
- Thyrotoxicosis, also known as hyperthyroidism, is due to an overactive thyroid secreting high levels of thyroid hormones. Patients usually present with symptoms that directly contrast with hypothyroidism, such as weight loss, increased appetite, heat intolerance and diarrhoea. Other symptoms include palpitations, tremor, sweating, amenorrhoea and irregular heart beat (AF).

> **TOP TIP!**
>
> It is important to remember that a neck lump with night sweats, weight loss and decreased appetite may also be attributed to cancers originating from the neck, lymphoma or TB.

Patient exposure and position

Ask the patient to sit upright in a chair. Ensure that there is ample space behind the chair so that you can position yourself here later on in the examination. Ask them to remove any clothes that may obscure your view of their neck. Ensure that you can also visualize the upper chest as some neck lesions can extend down towards this area.

2.17.2 Inspection

Stand back and undertake a general observation of the patient. Note their general appearance, their clothing (whether it is appropriate for the current season or climate), the condition of their skin, as well as for any obvious hair loss or thinning. Note the character of their voice, weight (obese or cachectic) and general demeanour, i.e. are they agitated, irritable or showing poor concentration?

Stand directly in front of the patient looking for any obvious swelling in the neck before inspecting from the side. A normal healthy thyroid is neither visible nor palpable. An enlarged thyroid goitre may present as a swelling, often in the midline below the level of the cricoid cartilage. Other features to look out for include evidence of scars, such as a thyroidectomy, and distended neck veins indicating thoracic outlet obstruction from retrograde extension of the goitre blocking venous drainage.

Swallowing and tongue protrusion tests

If there is a neck lump in the midline a few further simple tests will help to establish a possible cause. Have the patient take a small sip of water in their mouth and hold it. Observe the lump and then ask the patient to swallow. If the midline lump moves upwards on swallowing then it may be a thyroid goitre or a thyroglossal cyst; this helps differentiate it from other midline lesions such as lymph nodes, lipomas or dermoid cysts that remain static on swallowing.

To help distinguish a goitre from a thyroglossal cyst ask the patient to stick their tongue out whilst you observe the lump. A thyroglossal cyst will move when the patient sticks their tongue out whereas a goitre will remain still. This is because a thyroglossal cyst represents a remnant of the thyroglossal tract which arose during embryology when the thyroid migrated from the back of the tongue to its final location in the lower neck.

Finally, ask the patient to open their mouth and then use a pen torch to inspect the oral cavity. Look for a lingual thyroid (undescended thyroid), enlarged tonsils and macroglossia (hypothyroidism).

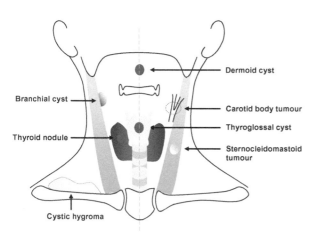

Fig 2.74 Location of lumps in the neck.

Palpate

Examining the neck in some patients may be an uncomfortable process as they may be unduly sensitive. Give them clear information about what you intend to do before palpating the neck.

Position yourself behind the patient and examine the neck area with the pulp of your fingers. If you have already visualized a lump palpate and assess it immediately. However, if you have not, then check the neck in a systematic way, examining the anterior and posterior triangles as well as the midline of the neck.

A palpable lump should be assessed for a number of characteristics which help differentiate it from other possible aetiologies (see *Figs 2.74* and *2.75*). First determine the lump's location, i.e. anterior or posterior triangle, and its proximity to any anatomical landmarks. Feel for its consistency and note whether it is soft, spongy, rubbery or firm in texture. Check whether it is a solitary nodule or if multiple nodules are found. Note its temperature, whether it is painful or not, and if it is fixed to underlying structures or freely mobile.

Goitres are usually found in the midline of the neck and are often soft, diffusely large or multinodular in nature. Occasionally a single thyroid nodule may be palpated unilaterally within the gland itself. This can simply be an adenoma or single distinct nodule within a multinodular goitre. If a goitre is suspected, repeat the swallowing test and the protusion of the tongue test whilst palpating over the gland feeling for any movement.

A hard irregular thyroid gland with an indistinct edge may be a thyroid carcinoma. A tender warm thyroid gland may suggest an inflammatory process such as thyroiditis.

Other lumps that can be found within the anterior and posterior triangles include a branchial cyst, which is a smooth painless swelling found beneath the

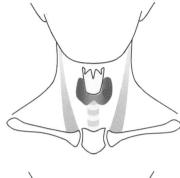

Thyroid nodule

A thyroid nodule is a growth found within the thyroid gland. They may occur singularly or with other nodules in a multinodular goitre. Although most are benign some may be cancerous. Most patients have no symptoms. The nodule may present as a firm swelling in otherwise smooth thyroid gland.

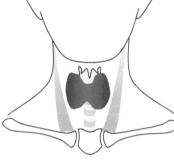

Thyroid goitre

A goitre refers to an enlarged thyroid gland that can be diffusely enlarged or have an enlarged lobe. Goitres are usually painless and may present with symptoms such as difficulty breathing and swallowing problems if there is a retrosternal extension. Presents as a palpable enlarged mass within the midline that moves on swallowing but not on protruding the tongue.

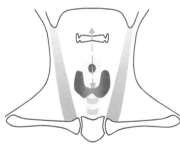

Thyroglossal cyst

Thyroglossal cysts are caused by non-obliteration of the thyroglossal tract during embryonic descent of the thyroid from the foramen caecum to its final position. They are attached to both the tongue and the thyroid and will move on swallowing and tongue protrusion.

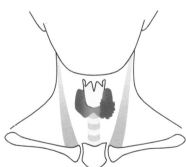

Thyroid carcinoma

Thyroid cancer is a malignancy of the thyroid gland. It may present fairly conspicuously as a solitary thyroid nodule or more overtly as a hard craggy thyroid mass. The most common thyroid cancer is the papillary form which affects young females particularly but has a good response to treatment.

Fig 2.75 Lumps on the thyroid.

anterior border of the upper third of the sternoclavicular muscle. A carotid body tumour is a hard ovoid swelling usually found at the level of the bifurcation of the common carotid just beneath the sternoclavicular muscle in the anterior triangle; it is painless and mobile predominantly in the horizontal plane.

Certain lumps in the neck may transilluminate brightly with light. These include cystic hygromas which are multiloculated lymphatic congenital lesions that are soft and cystic in quality and usually found in the posterior triangle of the neck.

Lymph nodes

Whilst behind the patient, you should also examine the lymph nodes in the head and neck (see *Chapter 2.18* on lymph node examination for full details). Any enlarged lymph nodes should warrant a full examination to look for generalized lymphadenopathy.

A swollen lymph node may be a reaction to a simple infection and so may resolve after a short period of time. Persistent lymph nodes that are rubbery and occur with a background of weight loss and night sweats may be due to lymphoma, TB or metastasis.

Trachea

Palpate the trachea to establish if it resides in the midline or is deviated to one side. A grossly enlarged thyroid with large retrosternal extension may distort the tracheal position.

Percussion

Using your dominant hand percuss down from the goitre to the sternal angle. Normally the percussion note should be resonant. However, a dull note may suggest the presence of retrosternal extension of the goitre. The goitre may expand downwards behind the sternum invading the underlying structures and causing compression symptoms such as breathlessness and the feeling of choking. Percuss the sternum and check for retrosternal extension of the goitre, if present; retrosternal goitres can interfere with breathing and cause hoarseness of the voice.

Auscultate

Use the diaphragm of your stethoscope to check both sides of the thyroid gland for a bruit. Make sure that the patient takes a deep breath in and holds it when auscultating. Bruits suggest increased blood flow typically seen in Graves' disease.

2.17.3 Assessing thyroid function

If a thyroid goitre (see *Box 2.20*) was palpated during the examination, clinical evidence of thyroid dysfunction should be established. As mentioned earlier, thyroid hormone has wide-reaching effects on the body and so any dysfunction in hormone secretion (whether the result of an overactive or underactive thyroid gland), will usually show signs and symptoms outside the neck area. Look to the nails and hands, pulse, and the eyes for evidence of thyroid disease.

Nails and hands

Inspect the nails and hands for thyroid disease. Look at the nails for thyroid acropachy which causes clubbing and painful swelling of the fingers and toes, characteristically seen in Graves' disease. Also look out for onycholysis which describes dehiscence of the nail from the nail bed, also seen in Graves' disease.

BOX 2.20 **Causes of goitre**	
Diffuse smooth goitre	Graves' disease, hyperthyroidism, thyroiditis, iodine deficiency, lithium, pregnancy, puberty
Nodular goitres	Cyst, adenoma, cancer

Inspect the palms of the patient's hand looking for palmar erythema, a sign of hyperthyroidism. Then palpate the palms feeling to assess skin texture as well as hydrosis. In hypothyroidism you would expect to find dry coarse skin whilst in hyperthyroidism sweaty moist hands are more common.

Ask the patient to hold their hands outstretched before you and look for a resting tremor. This sign can be exaggerated by placing a plain piece of paper on the dorsal surface of their hands and observing for a tremor which is seen in hyperthyroidism.

Pulse

Move on to palpate the patient's radial pulse, assessing its rate, rhythm and character. In hypothyroidism one may find a slow heart rate with a low volume pulse whereas in hyperthyroidism you may note tachycardia or atrial fibrillation with a bounding pulse.

Eyes

Move your attention to the patient's eyes to observe for a number of signs associated with Graves' disease (see *Box 2.21*). In Graves' disease one may see chemosis (swelling of the conjunctiva), exophthalmos (protrusion of the eyeballs, best seen by standing behind the patient and looking down) and ophthalmoplegia (weakness in the eye muscles causing double vision). In severe cases periorbital oedema may occur resulting in optic nerve compression with reduction in visual acuity and a relative afferent papillary defect sign (RAPD).

You should also test for lid lag. This can be done by asking the patient to follow your finger as you move it through the vertical plane fairly rapidly. You should notice that the upper eyelid lags behind the upper edge of the iris as the eye moves downward. Lid retraction as well as lid lag are both features of Graves' disease.

Hair

Briefly look at the patient's hair, observing for its general state. Thin and brittle hair as well as loss of hair in the outer third of the eyebrow is often seen in hypothyroidism.

> **TOP TIP!**
>
> Both exophthalmos and proptosis are protrusion of the eyeball from the socket, with exophthalmos being reserved for protrusion with an endocrine aetiology.

> **TOP TIP!**
>
> Pretibial myxoedema, also known as thyroid dermopathy, is a red–purplish swelling over the lateral malleoli and anterolateral aspect of the shins, caused by lesions resulting from the deposition of hyaluronic acid. It is almost always associated with Graves' disease and is not to be confused with myxoedema of hypothyroidism, in which there is non-pitting oedema of eyelids, hands and feet.

> **TOP TIP!**
>
> Other signs of hypothyroidism include proximal myopathy (seen by asking the patient to stand up) as well as slow relaxing reflexes.

BOX 2.21 **Signs of Graves' disease**

Thyroid acropachy
Pretibial myxoedema
Exophthalmos
Ophthalmoplegia

2.17.4 **Summing up**

Having completed the examination, thank the patient for their co-operation and allow them to get dressed. You may wish to consider performing a number of other investigations to confirm your working diagnosis. Simple requests such as the following may be useful:

- thyroid function tests (TFTs)
- thyroid antibodies (for Graves' disease)

- FBC (for iron-deficient anaemia in hypothyroidism)
- CRP (for signs of infection seen in thyroiditis)

An ultrasound of the neck will help determine the difference between cystic and more suspicious solid nodules. A fine needle aspiration cytology helps take a sample from a solitary nodule and may identify malignancy.

2.17.5 **Common clinical scenarios**

The following are a list of common cases which you may encounter when undertaking an examination of the thyroid. For each one, consider:
- what the likely diagnosis is
- what key features you would look for
- what questions you would ask or further investigations you would order to refine or confirm your diagnosis

You could use role play with a friend, using the histories in the cases below as a framework.

CASE 1

A 29 year old pregnant woman presents with painless fullness around the neck. On examination she has a diffusely enlarged swelling located in the midline below the level of the cricoid cartilage. The lump moves with swallowing. There is no lymphadenopathy or retrosternal extension.

CASE 2

A 39 year old clinically obese woman known to suffer with diabetes and depression presents with tiredness, thinning of hair and constipation. She also notes a number of lumps in her neck area. On examination she has dry coarse skin, bradycardia and sluggish reflexes. You note a diffusely enlarged swelling in her lower neck.

CASE 3

A 19 year old man complains of a long-standing lump in his neck. On examination he is euthyroid with a small 4 mm midline neck lump that moves on swallowing and when he sticks his tongue out.

CASE 4

A 48 year old woman presents complaining of weight loss, change in voice and a neck lump. On examination you notice a small irregular hard craggy lump inferior to the cricoid cartilage. You also notice enlarged cervical chain lymph nodes.

CASE 5

A 15 year old student presents with smooth swelling in his neck that he has had for a number of years. On examination, he has a soft 2 cm lump that is cystic in nature and found behind the upper portion of the right sternocleidomastoid muscle. It does not transilluminate and is mobile in both planes.

Chapter 2.18
Lymph nodes examination

What to do . . .

- Introduce yourself to the patient – establish rapport and seek consent
- Appropriately position and expose the patient
- Inspection: look for scars, masses and lymphoedema
- Palpation: feel all lymph node regions for the presence of lymphadenopathy
- Describe enlarged lymph nodes in terms of site, size, number, shape, consistency, tenderness, matting and fixation
- Palpate both sides of the body, comparing like with like
- Examine for hepatosplenomegaly
- Thank the patient and conclude the examination

The lymphatic system plays an important role in the body's defence against infections. It produces antibodies and provides a drainage system to remove dead cells, proteins and other waste products. The average human being has up to 700 lymph nodes spread across the body.

Lymph nodes are groups of small pea-shaped structures of the immune system that are linked together via lymphatic vessels. They fulfil two functions: the production of lymphocytes (B, T, and other immune cells) and the removal of toxic products from the systemic circulation. In the presence of pathology, individual lymph nodes or groups may become swollen and clinically palpable. This process in known as lymphadenopathy and is largely due to B cell proliferation in the germinal centres priming the defence system against possible infection.

Lymph nodes may become inflamed or enlarged in various conditions and in certain diseases they can have a characteristic consistency and location. When lymph nodes are involved in metastatic disease their distribution and size may indicate the potential severity of the disease and can be useful in the staging process of cancers.

Lymph and the lymphatic drainage system

Lymph originates from plasma and circulates slowly in a one-way system throughout the body. Nodes that first receive lymph from a specific part of the body are known as regional lymph nodes. From here they communicate with secondary and then tertiary lymph nodes in a typical pattern. Lymphatic drainage is organized into two unequal drainage areas which cover the right and left sides of the body.

- The right drainage area involves the right lymphatic duct which receives lymph from the right side of the head and neck, right arm and right upper

TOP TIP!

When lymph nodes are removed or damaged, lymph is prevented from draining normally from the affected region, leading to accumulation of excess lymph and lymphoedema.

quadrant of the body. The right lymphatic duct then empties the lymph into the right subclavian vein.

- The left drainage area involves the lower body and the left side of the upper body. Lymph from the lower trunk and both legs moves upwards and is temporarily stored in the cisterna chyli. The thoracic duct transports this lymph upwards towards the left lymphatic duct which also drains the left arm, left upper quadrant and the left side of the head and neck. The left lymphatic duct then empties the lymph into the left subclavian vein.

2.18.1 **Beginning the examination**

Ensure that you introduce yourself to the patient, stating your name and job title. Ask the patient for their name, date of birth and how they are feeling.

TOP TIP!

It is unlikely that you will be expected to examine all of the lymph node groups in one examination; however, you will be expected to be competent in performing a general screening examination involving the head and neck, axillary and inguinal areas.

Make sure that you clearly explain to the patient what you intend to do when examining the lymph nodes of a specific region. If you are going to be exposing and examining the genital or breast area, it is particularly important that you seek explicit consent to do so. If you are exposing the genital region during your examination it will be necessary to seek the assistance of a chaperone.

If the patient presented with a lump you should ask when they first noticed it and whether it is tender. Painful lymph nodes usually indicate a local infective cause, whereas enlarged painless lymph nodes may point to a more sinister diagnosis of cancer. Ask the patient if they have noticed any changes to the lump since they first noticed it. Check whether they found just one lump or more and, if more than one, are they in the same region or elsewhere? This will help you in deciding whether the lymphadenopathy is due to a local or systemic cause.

Ask the patient whether they have had any infections recently. Ask about systemic symptoms such as night sweats, fevers, weight loss and general malaise. This will highlight causes for concern such as tuberculosis, malignancy or lymphoma.

Patient exposure and position

TOP TIP!

When you are examining the axilla, women can leave on any undergarments.

Before beginning the examination and asking the patient to undress, ensure that adequate privacy is maintained; you should draw curtains around the cubicle or close any doors. If you are examining the genital region, ask the patient to remove all outer clothing below the waist, leaving on any underwear.

Ensure the patient is in an appropriate position for the examination: this may require them to be sitting, lying down or standing, depending on which region you are examining. Offer the patient a sheet or blanket to maintain their modesty if required. Wash your hands thoroughly before starting your examination.

2.18.2 **Inspection**

If you have been asked to examine a patient with generalized lymphadenopathy, work from the top downwards in a systematic fashion in order to inspect the whole body for enlarged lymph nodes without missing out any areas.

TOP TIP!

If you are asked to examine a specific region, begin with that region before stating that you would like to examine other areas.

If you notice any enlarged lymph nodes then describe them as you would any lump, stating their site, size, shape, surface appearance and surroundings as well as the colour of the skin above the swelling. Erythematous, red, inflamed skin may indicate infection, also known as lymphadenitis which can be caused by a local infection, such as with *Staphylococcus aureus*, or systemic infection such as in HIV, herpes simplex or infectious mononucleosis.

Inspect for the presence of any surgical scars that may indicate previous biopsy or lymph node excision. Note if there are any obvious masses, sinuses or ulcers in the region drained by the lymph nodes you are inspecting. Do not forget to comment on evidence of skin breakdown or trauma. Also remember to state if you see obvious lymphoedema, which may indicate that the lymph nodes have either been damaged or removed secondary to cancerous invasion.

Observe for signs of lymphangitis, which is an inflammation of the lymphatic channels occurring due to an infection distal to the site of the channels. If this is present you will see thin red lines, running along the course of the affected lymph vessels. This is usually accompanied by lymphadenitis of nearby lymph nodes.

Palpation

Ensure that your hands are warm prior to palpating the lymph nodes and ask the patient if they are in any pain. If you are examining the head and neck lymph nodes (see *Fig 2.76*) remember to palpate from in front of and then behind the patient.

Use the pads of the index and middle fingertips to palpate the lymph node regions by moving the skin in a circular fashion over the underlying tissue. When palpating the neck, make sure both sides are palpated at the same time in order to compare like with like.

If you feel a swelling or an abnormal node, describe it in terms of site, size, shape, surface, surroundings, tenderness, temperature, consistency, edge and whether it is mobile or fixed. Also comment on the number of abnormal nodes that you can feel. If there are many abnormal nodes comment on whether they feel matted together or are distinct and separated. Matting is used to describe lymph nodes that adhere to each other and this may be seen in tuberculosis, lymphadenitis, lymphomas or malignancy.

During the examination, measure any palpable nodes with a ruler. Small nodes that are less than the size of the distal phalanx of your little finger may be normal unless they are in an unusual location. If the nodes are small (< 1 cm), mobile and hard, these are known as 'shotty' and are of little clinical significance. In very slim individuals it is often easy to feel the lymph nodes. Nodes greater than 1 cm are considered significant particularly if associated with red flag features (see *Box 2.22*). Fixed, non-mobile enlarged lymph nodes usually suggest malignancy as opposed to a benign process.

Lymph nodes are usually oval or round in shape. If they are irregular it suggests that the lymph node capsule has been invaded in some way, possibly by

---

BOX 2.22 **Red flag symptoms for lymphadenopathy**

Nodes lasting for > 4 weeks associated with
- nodes > 2 cm
- non-mobile or fixed
- non-tender
- weight loss
- night sweats
- multiple sites

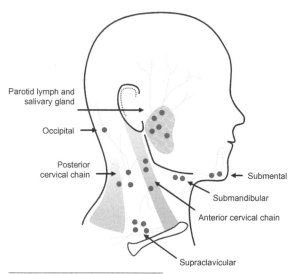

Parotid lymph and
salivary gland

Occipital

Posterior
cervical chain

Submental

Submandibular

Anterior cervical chain

Supraclavicular

Fig 2.76 Lymph nodes in the head and neck.

malignancy. In infection, lymph nodes are classically soft, tender and warm, whereas in malignancy they are very hard and non-tender. In Hodgkin's lymphoma they are usually described as rubbery whereas in leukaemia they are firm.

Site

As previously stated, lymphadenopathy can be local or systemic. Localized lymphadenopathy occurs if there is a disease process affecting only the lymph node that drains a specific region, such as cervical or axillary chains. General lymphadenopathy on the other hand affects lymph nodes of different areas which may be due to a malignant or infective process. In order to correctly classify lymphadenopathy a good understanding of which lymph nodes drain particular regions is needed (see *Table 2.6*).

Cervical

When examining the lymph nodes of the cervical chain (*Fig 2.76*), ensure that the patient is seated whilst you stand behind them. Use the fingertips of all four fingers of each hand to palpate both sides of the head and neck at the same time.

Begin with the submental nodes (under the chin), then move either side under the jaw to feel the submandibular group. Move upwards in front of the ear to palpate the pre-auricular region that contains the parotid gland and then behind the ear for the post-auricular set. Next, move down the anterior border of the sternocleidomastoid (SCM) muscle to palpate the superficial (on top of the SCM) and deep (below the SCM) anterior cervical chain. Move your fingers just along the superior border of the clavicle for the supraclavicular nodes, then

TOP TIP!

Enlargement of the supraclavicular and epitrochlear nodes are signs that may indicate the presence of malignancy.

Table 2.6 **Lymph node groups and their drainage region**	
Lymph node group	**Drainage region**
Cervical:	
Submental	Floor of the mouth, lower lip
Submandibular	Oral cavity, nose, maxillary sinuses, buccal mucosa, lips
Pre-auricular	Eye (conjunctiva), temporal scalp, pinna
Post-auricular	Ear, temporal and parietal scalp
Occipital	Outer ear, mastoid region, posterior scalp
Anterior cervical	Pharynx, tonsils
Posterior cervical	Pharynx, tonsils
Supraclavicular	*Right side:* mediastinum and lungs
	Left side: abdomen, breast, thyroid, oesophagus
Axillary:	
Lateral	Arm
Central, anterior	Anterior chest wall and most of breast
Posterior	Posterior chest wall and upper arm
Epitrochlear	Medial arm below the elbow
Para-aortic	Ovaries and testes (gonads)
Inguinal	Pelvic viscera, deep perineum, genitalia, urethra, buttock, posterior thigh, abdominal wall below the umbilicus
Popliteal	Lower leg

back up the neck between the posterior border of the SCM and anterior border of the trapezius muscle for the posterior cervical chain. Finally examine the base of the skull posteriorly by feeling the occipital lymph node group.

Localized cervical lymphadenopathy is most commonly caused by either a bacterial or viral infection of the ear, nose or throat. Scalp, outer ear infections, rubella and toxoplasmosis often cause occipital lymphadenopathy whereas orbital cellulitis and middle ear infections can cause pre-auricular lymph node enlargement.

Other rare causes of cervical lymphadenopathy include malignancy. A persistent unilateral firm, painless cervical mass should raise the suspicion of nasopharyngeal carcinoma. Enlargement of the supraclavicular nodes is also a possible sign of malignancy. The left supraclavicular node, otherwise known as Virchow's node, is most commonly caused by gastric carcinoma, but may also arise due to secondary metastatic obstruction of the thoracic duct. Right supraclavicular lymphadenopathy may be due to lung cancer, oesophageal cancer and lymphoma.

Generalized causes of cervical lymphadenopathy can be classified as acute or chronic.
- Acute causes include infectious mononucleosis (glandular fever) and cytomegalovirus.
- Chronic causes include tuberculosis, sarcoidosis, HIV and secondary syphilis. These would normally cause bilateral cervical enlargement rather than unilateral. Tuberculosis invading lymph nodes can sometimes present as a cold abscess – the lymph node will be caseating and may have a point that can burst, leading to what is known as a collar-stud abscess. Tuberculosis usually affects the cervical lymph nodes (especially the deep cervical) but may also involve axillary and mesenteric nodes.

Hodgkin's lymphoma can also present with bilateral painless cervical lymphadenopathy. The affected lymph nodes often appear enlarged, swollen and rubbery, but remain smooth and of normal shape because the capsule is not usually invaded. Some patients may present with systemic symptoms, known as 'B' symptoms, which include fever, weight loss and night sweats. There may also be hepatosplenomegaly.

Axillary
When palpating for lymph nodes in the axillary area it is important to ask the patient if they would like a chaperone. Again, the patient should be seated, but this time you should sit in front of them. Begin by examining the right axilla. Do this by supporting their right elbow in your right hand whilst gently abducting the shoulder, opening up their axilla. With the fingertips of your left hand begin to palpate the axilla. Start by palpating the central nodes located deep in the underarm. Next move on to palpate the anterior (pectoral) chain on the anterior axillary fold and then the posterior (subscapular) chain on the posterior axillary fold. Finally, feel the lateral nodes with the palm of your hand facing the humeral head. Repeat your examination for the other side.

Local causes of axillary lymphadenopathy include infections or malignancies of the upper limb or the breast. In a breastfeeding patient with breast tenderness, axillary lymphadenopathy may be caused by mastitis whereas a painless breast lump with a lump in the axilla should raise the suspicion of breast cancer.

> **TOP TIP!**
>
> When considering your differential diagnosis, always attempt to classify your findings into (a) local or general, (b) infectious, neoplastic or other, and (c) acute or chronic.

Table 2.7 Causes of localized and generalized lymphadenopathy		
Lymph node groups	**Localized lymphadenopathy**	**Generalized lymphadenopathy**
Cervical	**Infectious** • Dental infections • Tonsillitis • Folliculitis of scalp • Ear infections • Infected skin lesions (sebaceous cyst) • TB • Toxoplasmosis and rubella **Neoplastic** • Nasopharyngeal cancer • Head and neck cancer metastasis (BCC, SCC) • Metastasis from abdomen, chest and breast	**Infectious** • Infectious mononucleosis • Syphilis • Cytomegalovirus • HIV • TB **Neoplastic** • Lymphoma • Leukaemia **Other** • Amyloidosis • Sarcoidosis
Axillary	**Infectious** • Upper limb infections • Mastitis **Neoplastic** • Metastasis from breast cancer	
Epitrochlear	**Infectious** • Forearm and hand infections • Secondary syphilis • Infectious mononucleosis **Neoplastic** • Metastasis from forearm cancers	
Inguinal	**Infectious** • STDs • Lower limb infections • Ulcers **Neoplastic** • SCC, BCC melanomas	
Popliteal	**Infectious** • Infections and ulcers of the lower leg and foot **Neoplastic** • SCC, BCC, melanomas	

Epitrochlear

Examine the epitrochlear region for enlarged lymph nodes. In order to do this, flex the patient's elbow at a 90 degree angle. For the right epitrochlear nodes, use your right hand to hold the patient's right wrist and approach the nodes with your left hand from behind their elbow. Place the palm of your left hand underneath the elbow and use your ring and index fingers to palpate superior to the medial epicondyle of the humerus. Repeat on the other side with your other hand. Epitrochlear lymphadenopathy usually occurs secondary to infections of the hand and forearm, but can sometimes be associated with a neoplastic process. Generalized causes include infectious mononucleosis and secondary syphilis as well as lymphomas and leukaemias. Infectious mononucleosis, also known as glandular fever, is caused by the Epstein–Barr virus (EBV). It usually affects young adults and is commonly known as the 'kissing disease' as it is spread by saliva. It often presents with generalized tender lymphadenopathy.

Inguinal

For this part of the examination the patient should be lying supine on a couch. The inguinal group of lymph nodes is divided into the horizontal (below the inguinal ligament) and vertical chains (along the path of the saphenous vein). The horizontal group drains the penis, vulva, scrotum and anus, whereas the vertical group drains the leg. It is quite common for adults to have shotty nodes in the inguinal regions, which are firm, discrete, mobile and less than 1 cm in size.

Localized unilateral inguinal lymphadenopathy is usually due to lower limb infections and ulcers, but you should always consider malignancies such as melanomas and squamous cell carcinomas as a possible cause. Tender and enlarged lymph nodes that occur in the inguinal region and nowhere else may also be due to sexually transmitted infections such as syphilis, herpes and chancroid.

Popliteal

Popliteal lymphadenopathy can be felt in the popliteal fossa when the knee is at a 45 degree angle. Place both hands around the knee to palpate for enlargement of lymph nodes in the popliteal fossa, which can occur secondary to infections below the knee.

Table 2.7 lists the causes of localized and generalized lymphadenopathy by lymph node group.

2.18.3 **Additional points**

The lymph node examination is not complete without examining the liver and spleen for enlargement, as the spleen is part of the lymphatic system. Hepatosplenomegaly associated with lymphadenopathy is found in lymphoma whereas splenomegaly can occur in infectious mononucleosis.

2.18.4 **Summing up**

Thank the patient for their co-operation and offer to cover them with a blanket to protect their dignity. Draw the curtain around them and give them appropriate time to gather themselves and get dressed. Make sure you acknowledge the patient's concerns. Remember to wash your hands again at the end of the examination.

2.18.5 **Common clinical scenarios**

The following are a list of common cases which you may encounter when undertaking an examination of the lymph nodes. For each one, consider:

- what the likely diagnosis is
- what key features you would look for
- what questions you would ask or further investigations you would order to refine or confirm your diagnosis

You could use role play with a friend, using the histories in the cases below as a framework.

CASE 1

A 16 year old girl presents with a headache, sore throat, fever and a transient rash after a school trip to France. She was seen by a local doctor while on the trip who had given her antibiotics for her sore throat. On examination there were generalized tender, enlarged, firm lymph nodes in the cervical, axillary and epitrochlear regions associated with palatal petechiae, a generalized macular rash and splenomegaly.

CASE 2

A 65 year old woman presented to her GP after she found a lump in her right armpit whilst shaving. On examination, a number of non-tender, hard, irregular, fixed lymph nodes were found in the central and pectoral axillary lymph node groups. On examination of the breasts a 2 by 2 cm firm, non-mobile lump was felt in the upper outer quadrant of the right breast. There were no significant findings in the left axilla and left breast.

CASE 3

A 55 year old man presents to A&E with painful 'lumps and bumps' in his left groin preventing him from sleeping comfortably. On examination, there were a number of soft, tender, warm, round, mobile and discrete lumps in the vertical chain of the left inguinal nodes. Similar lymphadenopathy was present in the left popliteal fossa. A large weeping ulcer with surrounding erythema was also noted above the medial malleolus of the same leg. His fasting glucose was 15.

CASE 4

A 20 year old man presented to his GP because of a 3 week history of severe night sweats and weight loss. He also explains that every time he drinks alcohol with his friends he notices pain in his neck. On examination, generalized non-tender, discrete, rubbery, enlarged cervical lymph nodes were present. Abdominal examination also reveals hepatosplenomegaly.

CASE 5

A 28 year old African man presents with night sweats, weight loss and haemoptysis. He recently arrived in the country from Kenya. On examination he has numerous cervical lymphadenopathy and a collar stud abscess.

Chapter 3.1
Hand washing

What to do . . .

- Introduce yourself to the examiner
- Enquire about the patient's *C. diff.* or MRSA status
- Remove rings, watches and bracelets and roll up sleeves
- Wet hands under running water and work soap into a lather
- Use six-step technique: palm to palm, palm over dorsum of hand, palm to palm with fingers interlaced, back of fingers to opposing palm with fingers interlaced, rotational rubbing of thumb with palm, rotational rubbing of palm with fingertips
- Rinse hands thoroughly under running water
- Dry hands with disposable paper towel and dispose in a pedal-operated bin
- Use paper towel or elbow to turn off the taps

Hand washing is perhaps one of the most neglected medical procedures to be performed, despite overwhelming evidence highlighting its vital role in preventing the transmission of infection. With the rise of hospital-acquired infections, in particular multi-drug resistant organisms such as MRSA and *C. difficile*, infection control procedures have come under much scrutiny. Doctors come into contact with a large number of unwell patients on a daily basis and each encounter exposes us to a wide variety of pathogens. Inadvertently, one may become a host for these microorganisms and help transmit them from patient to patient. By adopting good hand hygiene (see *Fig 3.1*) it should be possible to greatly minimize the risk of being contaminated and then spreading it to others.

Broadly speaking there are two classes of organisms that can be found on the body (see *Table 3.1*):

- resident flora which includes organisms such as *Staphylococcus* and diphtheroids; these colonize the hands and cause little harm to the host individual or to others
- transient microorganisms which are acquired through contact with patients, secretions and excreta, contaminated apparatus, foods and from the general environment; examples include *E. coli*, *Klebsiella* and *Campylobacter* and these are usually associated with the spread of infection and hence are the target of effective hand washing.

Hand washing is the process by which the hands are cleansed of visible dirt, transient microorganisms and organic contaminants. It involves the use of agents such as soap or antiseptic solutions which are rubbed into all areas of the hand before being washed off under flowing water and dried appropriately; see *Table 3.2* for details as to which type of hand washing to use when.

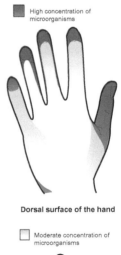

High concentration of microorganisms

Dorsal surface of the hand

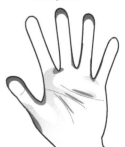

Moderate concentration of microorganisms

Palmar surface of the hand

Fig 3.1 Common areas that are missed by poor hand washing technique.

Table 3.1 Pathogenic transient microorganisms on the hands	
Bacteria	**Viruses**
Campylobacter jejuni	Avian influenza A
Candida albicans	Human coronavirus (common cold)
Clostridium difficile	Influenza A
Enterococcus faecalis	Norovirus
Escherichia coli	Swine flu (H1N1)
Klebsiella pneumoniae	
Listeria monocytogenes	
Pseudomonas aeruginosa	
Salmonella	
Shigella	
Staphylococcus aureus (including community-associated methicillin-resistant *S. aureus* [MRSA])	
Streptococcus pneumoniae	
Streptococcus pyogenes	
Vibrio cholerae	

TOP TIP!

It is important to know that alcohol gel is NOT effective against *Clostridium difficile*. If a patient is known to be infected with this organism, hands must be washed with soap and water!

TOP TIP!

Patients with MRSA should ideally be barrier nursed. If hands are not soiled, wash hands with alcohol gel.

TOP TIP!

When using alcohol gel to clean hands between patients, it should be allowed to dry naturally on the skin and not be dried with a paper towel.

Medical Guidelines
When to perform hand hygiene

- Before and after having direct contact with patients
- After removing gloves
- Before handling an invasive device for patient care, regardless of whether or not gloves are used
- After contact with body fluids or excretions, mucous membranes, non-intact skin or wound dressings
- If moving from a contaminated body site to a clean body site during patient care
- After contact with inanimate objects (including medical equipment) in the immediate vicinity of the patient

WHO Guidelines on Hand Hygiene in Healthcare, 2007

There are a number of different hand cleansing solutions available and each hospital trust may have different guidelines in relation to their use. It is generally accepted that bar soap should not be used for routine hand washing and liquid soap should always be used instead. Liquid soaps are effective in removing large contaminants on the hands such as dirt and excreta but provide little antimicrobial action.

If hands are not visibly soiled, for routine patient encounters doctors are recommended to use alcohol gel as a disinfectant. Although alcohol gel works rapidly to neutralize superficial pathogens, it does not act as a cleansing agent and hence has no role to play in cleaning soiled hands.

When undertaking any medical or invasive procedures, more potent antiseptic solutions such as chlorhexidine gluconate (Hibiscrub) or povidone iodine (Betadine) should be used. These agents are extremely effective in eradicating a wide spectrum of pathogens and are recommended for most sterile procedures.

Drying the hands appropriately is as important as cleaning them because adopting a poor drying technique may cause recontamination of the hands. The general consensus is that single use disposable paper towels are best for drying the hands rather than using cloth towels that may harbour organisms. Air dryers, by virtue of how they work, have been shown to spread microorganisms to the immediate environment.

3.1.1 Beginning the procedure

When preparing to wash your hands it is important to roll your sleeves up above your elbows and remove any jewellery, including watches, rings or bracelets. Such items, if worn, are known to shield bugs and organisms from the antiseptic solution and reduce its efficacy.

	Main purpose	Effect on microorganism	Cleansing agents
Routine hand wash	After patient contact and soiling	Partly removes transient flora	Non-antimicrobial liquid soap
Alcohol-based hand rubbing	After patient contact (do not use on soiled hands)	Removes transient flora and reduces resident organisms	Alcohol-based antiseptic solution
Procedural antiseptic hand wash	Hand antisepsis prior to invasive or surgical procedures	Removes transient and reduces resident organisms	Chlorhexidine gluconate (Hibiscrub); povidone iodine (Betadine)
			Alcohol-based waterless antiseptic

Table 3.2 **Hand washing options**

TOP TIP!

If you are in an exam situation, you should talk through each step of the hand washing procedure as you perform it to ensure that the examiner is aware of what you are doing and remove any potential for ambiguity or misinterpretation.

Establish the clinical context before washing your hands as this may affect the manner in which you perform this (*Table 3.2*). The type of antiseptic solution you use will be different if you are simply greeting a relative of a patient compared to undertaking an invasive procedure. If you are going to examine a patient with known *Clostridium difficile* infection in a side room it is imperative that you wash your hands using liquid soap and comply with barrier protocols.

Preparation

Before you start washing your hands, turn on both the hot and cold water taps and adjust to an optimal temperature. Make sure that you have a ready supply of paper towels available to dry your hands.

3.1.2 **The procedure**

There are many different techniques that have been suggested for effective hand washing, each of which tries to ensure that all areas of the hands are adequately washed and cleansed of microbes. The six-step technique (*Fig 3.2*), devised in 1978 and later updated by Ayliffe in 1992, has been widely adopted by most hospital trusts in the UK. It is characterized by a five stroke rubbing motion forwards and backwards for each step.

The six-step technique

Begin the procedure by wetting both hands under the running water and apply around 5 ml of cleansing solution or disinfectant from the dispenser onto the palm of one hand. Rub your hands together vigorously and thoroughly for at least 15 seconds until a soapy lather appears. This should generate sufficient friction to help dislodge any dirt or large particles that are present on the hands.

Proceed with the six-step technique as follows:

Step 1 – rub both of your palms against each other.

Step 2 – move your right palm over the dorsum of the left hand and rub over this area repeatedly, then repeat on the other hand.

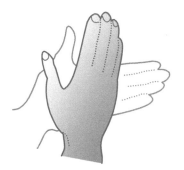

Rubbing palms together

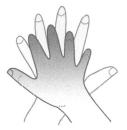

Rubbing one palm over the back of the other hand

Fig 3.2 The six-step technique for hand washing (continued overleaf).

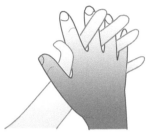

Rubbing the two palms together
with fingers interlaced

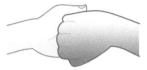

Bring together the opposing palms
with fingers interlocked

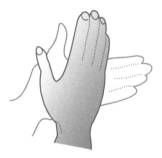

Rubbing palms together

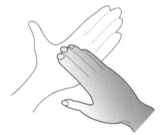

Rub your palm using the fingertips
of the other hand in rotatory motion

Fig 3.2 (Continued).

TOP TIP!

If you are washing your hands as part of a scrubbing up technique for theatre, you should use a sterile nail brush to clean under your fingernails. Ideally nails should be cut short and artificial nails and nail varnish should be avoided.

Step 3 – interlock the fingers of both hands together with the palmar surfaces opposing one another, then rub between the fingers carefully, ensuring that all areas between the fingers are cleaned.

Step 4 – lock the tip of the fingers of both hands together and place the back of the fingers into the palmar surface. Rub in circular motions ensuring that there is good contact between the palm and the interlocked fingers.

Step 5 – this is focused on washing the thumb; clasp the left thumb in the palm of your right hand. Using a rotatory movement, wash and rub the thumb from its base to the tip until it is thoroughly clean, then repeat the process for the left side.

Step 6 – rub your left palm using the fingertips of the right hand in a rotatory circular motion, then repeat the process for the other side.

Although not part of the six-step technique, some advocate the washing of the wrists by the opposing hands. This may be useful to remove any residual debris which was dislodged during the hand washing process.

Rinse

When you rinse your hands you should make sure that you keep them elevated above your elbows as this will help prevent contamination. Rinse both hands thoroughly under a stream of warm water from the fingertips downwards. Use your elbows to turn off the taps via the attached levers to prevent your hands being from being re-contaminated from the taps.

Dry

After washing your hands you must dry them thoroughly using single use disposable towels. When using the paper towels it is better to pat your hands dry rather than rubbing them across your skin. Dispose of the towels using a pedal-controlled bin so that you do not inadvertently contaminate your hands by touching the bin.

Hand protection

If you wash your hands frequently, your skin may become dry and begin to crack, which may increase the risk of infection and irritation. In order to prevent this ensure that you use a moisturizing hand cream after each wash. Such creams are often located within liquid dispensers adjacent to the antiseptic solutions.

3.1.3 **Finishing up**

In an examination situation, once you are happy that you have washed your hands effectively, you should thank the examiner and ask if they have any questions about your hand washing technique. You may be asked about the reasons why hand washing is important and when it is performed. You may also be required to explain the circumstances where alcohol gel or antiseptic solution use is preferred over liquid soap and vice versa.

3.1.4 **Common clinical scenarios**

The following are a list of common scenarios that you may encounter. For each one, determine the best course of action.

CASE 1

You are on your Consultant's ward round. You have just finished examining a patient's chest and have moved on to the next case. Should you choose to wash your hands with water, liquid soap, alcohol gel or Hibiscrub?

CASE 2

You have finished seeing a 40 year old lady in a side room. She is known to be barrier nursed because of *C. difficile* infection. Should you choose to wash your hands with water, liquid soap, alcohol gel or Hibiscrub?

CASE 3

You have visited the toilet and have washed your hands with liquid soap. You are due back on the ward round. There are a number of options to dry your hands – should you use a cloth towel, disposable paper towels, communal towel or electric dryer?

CASE 4

You have just finished examining a patient with MRSA in a side room. Should you choose to wash your hands with water, liquid soap, or alcohol gel?

Chapter 3.2
Surgical scrubbing

What to do ...
- Change into theatre attire, including a cap and clogs
- Remove all jewellery
- Introduce yourself to the theatre staff
- Prepare your gown pack and gloves and put on your mask
- Perform a simple pre-scrub wash using the antiseptic solution and the nail-pick
- Use the brush to clean the finger nails (thistle end)
- Use the sponge end to clean from fingertips to elbow
- Rinse with flowing water from hand to elbows
- Have hands held above elbows at all times
- Use elbow to turn off the taps
- Dry hands with sterile paper towel from distal to proximal
- Gown and glove using aseptic technique
- Tie the gown appropriately
- Maintain a sterile approach throughout

Surgical scrubbing describes the procedure of preparing oneself for theatre prior to an operation. During an operation, patients are in their most susceptible state for contracting infections, because any incision or insertion of surgical instrumentation that breaches the body's protective barrier, i.e. the skin, can lead to the introduction of harmful pathogens or microorganisms into the body. A thorough and methodical scrubbing technique must therefore be followed to reduce the risk of contamination and illness.

Scrubbing should take place in a designated scrub room; this is usually an area adjacent to, but separate from the operating theatre. Protective clothing such as a face mask, theatre hat and surgical gown must be worn. Surgical scrubbing entails the thorough cleaning of the hands, fingernails and forearms with a liquid antiseptic agent such as Betadine or chlorhexidine.

Whilst scrubbing may sound a relatively straightforward procedure, it can be quite a challenging skill to master. Maintaining a strict aseptic technique throughout the scrub, particularly when unpacking the surgical gown or when wearing sterile gloves, can be difficult even for the most dexterous amongst us. Although it is important to read the principles and steps involved, scrubbing is a skill that can only really be learnt through observation and practice.

3.2.1 Beginning the procedure

Preparation

It is important that you prepare yourself before you enter the scrub room by wearing surgical scrubs and clogs that fit comfortably. Without these you are likely to be refused entry. Do not forget to collect a face mask prior to entering the scrub room. Ensure that your nails are clean and cut short and with any nail varnish removed. You should remove any jewellery such as rings, bracelets or watches. Long hair must be tied and kept up in a bun whilst beards must be concealed behind the face mask.

Equipment

Collect the appropriate equipment that will be required for the procedure. You will need:

- Scrub brush
- Pair of sterile gloves
- Theatre shoes
- Theatre gown
- Mask and cap
- Scrubs

3.2.2 **The procedure**

Sterile field

You will need to set up a sterile field on the trolley before commencing – a sterile field is the area in which all materials are sterile and uncontaminated by foreign elements. This is essential to maintain an aseptic technique to reduce the risk of any contamination.

First, peel off the outer plastic covering of the theatre gown pack and slide it onto the trolley. Hold the inverted corners and open up the packet, as you would a sterile dressing pack, to create your sterile field. It is extremely important to maintain the sterility of this area throughout the procedure to reduce or eliminate the spread of infection or contamination.

Select the appropriate size of sterile gloves and peel off the plastic outer covering. Place this aseptically into one corner of your sterile field. Make sure that you do not touch the gloves directly until you have nearly completed the procedure.

Handwashing

Much of this procedure focuses on your ability to perform hand washing competently. For surgical scrubbing there are three stages for hand washing, as follows.

Pre-scrub wash

Remove the back packaging of the brush packet and leave it facing open-side up on the shelf above the washing area. Turn on the taps, ensuring that you have a steady stream to prevent splashing. The water should be set to an even temperature; be aware that too much hot water may lead to excessive drying of the skin; cold water, on the other hand, may inhibit lather formation when soaping and so there may be insufficient to eradicate contaminants and germs.

Wet your hands with running water before applying any antiseptic solution. Use your elbows to depress 5 ml from the chlorhexidine or Betadine dispensers. Work the lather onto your hands, forearms and then elbows, remembering to employ the six-step technique when washing the hands (see *Chapter 3.1*).

Once you have completed this phase, remember to keep your hands held above your elbows throughout the remainder of the procedure.

> **TOP TIP!**
>
> The manufacturers recommend that the antiseptic solution should be in contact with the skin for at least 3 minutes for maximal effect.

Scrub (brush and file) wash

Remove the nail pick from the brush pack and clean the areas under your fingernails. Discard the file into the waste bin. Collect the brush and dispense 5 ml of solution onto the sponge side. Now scrub, using this side down, from the fingertips to 2 cm beyond the elbows. Move on to complete the other arm and spend 1 minute in total washing both.

Position your arms under the running water to rinse down from the hands to the elbows. Ensure that the water flows away from your hands so that the hands do not become re-contaminated.

Once you have rinsed your arms, use the thistle end of the brush to perform a deeper clean of the fingernails. Spend 30 seconds doing this on each hand. Do not use the thistle side on the arms as this has been shown to cause abrasions and extracts deeper organisms from the hair follicles out on to the surface.

Move on to wash the digits and interdigit spaces with the sponge side of the brush, spending 30 seconds per hand. Progress down to include the dorsum of the hand and palm, also washing here for 30 seconds. Proceed down to the forearm and elbow and wash again for 30 seconds. Do not forget to do this for both arms. Finally, using flowing water from the taps, rinse off from the hands down to the elbows. Make sure that you turn off the taps using only your elbows.

Drying

Proceed to the gown pack. There should be two sterile towels contained within this which can be found lying on top of the surgical gown. Pick one up and use it to dry your hands. Ensure that you dry downwards from your fingertips to the elbows in a circular motion. Do not scrub the arms up and down with the towel nor return to an area that has already been dried. Make sure that when drying you use one surface of the towel for drying purposes and the other simply to hold it. Make sure that you do not cross-contaminate between the two surfaces. Once completed, dispose of the towel and pick up the remaining one to clean the other hand.

Gown

The gown will be prefolded with the inner surface facing you. It is important that you do not touch the outer surface of the gown directly nor allow any objects to break the sterility. Pick up the inner surface of the gown, ensuring that you have ample space around you. Gently shake the gown out so that it unfolds correctly before you. Locate the two sleeves and pass your arms through them. Do not push your hands through the cuffs but rather have the ends of your fingertips poking through. At this point request a member of the theatre staff to secure your gown from the back.

Gloves

Next move your attention to putting on the sterile gloves. Unfold the packet containing the gloves and, using the left cuff, pick up the right glove. Place it on your supinated right hand with the glove fingers pointing proximally towards your elbow. The thumb of the glove should be correctly aligned with your thumb to permit easy insertion into it. Tuck the fingers of your right hand into the opening of the glove and using the left cuff, grab the folded glove edge and pull it distally over the cuff and fingers to cover the rest of your hand. Slip your fingers into place by pulling back on the gown. Repeat the procedure for the

TOP TIP!

If the hands are still wet despite drying, putting on the gloves will become a more difficult task.

TOP TIP!

Always keep your hands above your waist at all times. If you are not engaged actively in surgery, stand with your hands held at chest height and with your palms together with fingers interlocked.

other hand. Since one hand is now gloved, this step should be markedly easier to complete.

3.2.3 **Finishing up**

The difficult part is over and you are almost ready to enter the operating theatre. Seek the assistance of a colleague to secure your gown properly. At the front of your gown you will find two ties with a piece of cardboard attached. Take hold of the cardboard and offer it to a colleague. Turn anticlockwise to allow the tie to go round you. Pull the tie held by your colleague and use it to make a knot with the remaining tie on the gown.

Be aware that if you ever accidentally break sterility yourself for whatever reason, you must remove yourself immediately from the theatre and re-glove and gown as appropriate. Failure to comply with this will put the patient at unnecessary risk.

> **TOP TIP!**
>
> You should only consider your anterior surface, between your chest and waist, to be sterile. Don't scratch your nose!

Chapter 3.3
Wound swabbing

What to do . . .

- Introduce yourself to the patient – establish rapport
- Confirm the patient's name, date of birth and hospital number
- Elicit the patient's symptoms and consider analgesia if the wound is painful
- Explain the procedure to the patient and obtain their consent
- Collect all the equipment
- Wash your hands and don a pair of non-sterile gloves
- Swab the wound using the zigzag method in a rotatory manner
- Re-dress the wound if appropriate
- Label the sample and correctly complete a Microbiology request form
- Document the procedure in the patient's notes
- Thank the patient and answer any questions

The skin is the largest organ of the human body and acts as the primary barrier preventing hostile foreign organisms from entering the body. Trauma or injury to the skin may create a wound that is susceptible to local infections that have the potential to spread systemically. Signs of local infection may include redness, warmth, swelling and tenderness around the site of injury. Systemic signs include a temperature, chills and rigors, tachycardia and low blood pressure.

Unfortunately, wound infections are commonplace within both the hospital and community settings. They can cause high morbidity, reduce the patient's quality of life, and may even extend inpatient hospital stays unnecessarily. The potential to develop a wound infection depends on a number of factors including the patient's age, nutritional state (malnourished or obese), presence of chronic illness (e.g. diabetes), and immunosuppression. If the wound was secondary to a surgical procedure then other variables come into play, including the surgical technique employed, length of operation and adequacy of wound drainage.

Most wounds become contaminated with the patient's own normal flora that can be found on the skin, mucous membranes, or hollow viscera. The types of pathogens found (see *Box 3.1*) differ depending on location. For example, Gram-positive cocci (staphylococci) are found on skin and mucosal surfaces, whereas Gram-negative aerobes and anaerobic bacteria are found predominantly in the groin and perineal areas.

A wound swab should be requested if a wound is suspected to be infected. It may occasionally be performed when a patient has been treated for a wound infection to evaluate the treatment's effectiveness. It is important that the procedure is performed correctly in order to reduce false positive results by

BOX 3.1 **Examples of potential wound pathogens**

Gram-positive cocci
- B-haemolytic streptococci (*Streptococcus pyogenes*)
- Enterococci (*Enterococcus faecalis*)
- Staphylococci (*Staphylococcus aureus*/MRSA)

Gram-negative aerobic rods
- *Pseudomonas aeruginosa*

Gram-negative facultative rods
- *Enterobacter* species
- *Escherichia coli*
- *Klebsiella* species
- *Proteus* species

Anaerobes
- Bacteroides
- Clostridium

Fungi
- Yeasts (*Candida*)
- *Aspergillus*

Medical Guidelines
Treating post-operation surgical wounds

Dressing and cleansing the wound
- Use an aseptic non-touch technique for changing or removing dressings
- Use sterile saline for wound cleansing up to 48 hours after surgery
- Advise patients that they may shower safely 48 hours after surgery
- Use tap water for wound cleansing after 48 hours if the wound has separated or has been surgically opened to drain pus
- Use an interactive dressing for surgical wounds that are healing by secondary intention
- Refer to a tissue viability nurse (or another healthcare professional with tissue viability expertise) for advice on appropriate dressings for surgical wounds that are healing by secondary intention

Do not use the following to reduce the risk of surgical site infections
- Topical antimicrobial agents for surgical wounds that are healing by primary intention
- Eusol and gauze, or moist cotton gauze

Antibiotic treatment
- If a surgical site infection is suspected (i.e. cellulitis), either *de novo* or because of treatment failure, give the patient an antibiotic
- Choose an antibiotic that covers the most likely causative organisms. Consider local resistance patterns and the results of microbiological tests

Specialist wound care services
To improve the management of surgical wounds:
- use a structured approach to care (including preoperative assessment to identify patients with potential wound healing problems)
- provide enhanced education to healthcare professionals, patients and carers, and share clinical expertise
NICE Guidelines: Surgical site infection (2008)

inadvertently swabbing pre-existing normal flora. Once the swab has been taken it should be sent to the laboratory for sensitivity and microscopy testing.

In the presence of an infected wound it may be appropriate to initially treat with broad spectrum antibiotics, even before the Microbiology results have come back, such as in cellulitis. Once the report has been made available and the wound infection has been confirmed, the choice of antibiotic can be altered depending on the pathogen isolated. A further wound swab may be indicated if signs of infection persist despite treatment.

3.3.1 **Beginning the examination**

Start by introducing yourself to the patient, stating your name and job title. Ask the patient for their name and date of birth and check against the patient's wrist band. Try to elicit from the patient any relevant clinical history such as whether they are suffering from pyrexia, sweating, chills or rigors. Also try to establish what antibiotics, if any, they are currently taking, as well as any drug allergies they may have. This information will be useful for the Microbiologist when completing the wound swab request form.

Check that the patient is comfortable and not in any obvious pain before proceeding. If the patient is experiencing any pain then consider offering them analgesia before undertaking the procedure.

Explain the procedure

Explain to the patient why you wish to take a wound swab, using simple language they would understand. Inform the patient that the procedure is unlikely to be painful but they should inform you immediately if they do suffer from significant discomfort. You may wish to say: '*Because of the pain, redness and swelling around your wound site, we will be taking a swab to check if it is infected. This is a simple and common procedure that will give us information about what bug is causing the problem and how to treat it. Although the swabbing may cause some discomfort, it should not be painful.'*

After explaining the procedure, check that the patient understands and is happy to proceed. At this point you may wish to offer them the opportunity to ask any questions.

Preparation

Ensure that the patient is comfortable and the wound site is adequately exposed. If the wound is dressed you should wash your hands and wear a pair of non-sterile gloves to remove it. Confirm with the patient that the correct wound site is being swabbed as they may have multiple sites.

Equipment

Wash your hands thoroughly and collect the appropriate equipment; it is sensible to try to collect the equipment on a trolley that can be positioned close to the patient.

- Non-sterile gloves
- Sterile swabs in culture tube
- Clinical waste bin
- Sterile dressing pack
- Gauze to re-dress wound
- Microbiology form

3.3.2 **The procedure**

If you have not already done so, wash your hands and put on a pair of non-sterile gloves. Remove the culture swab from its tube by rotating the cap end and breaking the seal. Hold the cap end carefully, ensuring you do not accidentally contaminate the tip of the swab. Insert the swab into the wound, rotating the tip whilst moving it in a zigzag motion (see *Fig 3.3*). This will help ensure that the swab collects a sample from all areas of the wound site and that the bacteria are evenly spread around its surface.

If the wound is particularly large, it is acceptable to take samples from a number of smaller sites within it, concentrating on swabbing those areas of the wound that show signs of infection. Viable tissue should be swabbed instead of scabs or slough as they are more likely to contain higher concentrations of bacteria than dead tissue.

Once you have collected sufficient material, place the swab back into the tube, ensuring that it is fully immersed within the culture medium. Apply moderate pressure to the top to make sure it seals well. Dispose of all clinical waste appropriately into the clinical waste bag, re-dress the wound if indicated and thank the patient.

Labelling

The swab tubes must be clearly labelled with the patient's name, date of birth and hospital number in addition to the date and time the sample was taken. Complete the Microbiology form using the same details and ensure that you sign it, leaving your bleep number for future contact. Tick the MC&S (microscopy, culture and sensitivity) box, documenting the site from which the swab was taken. Fill in the clinical details section with as much relevant information as possible. Record clearly on the form whether the patient is currently taking any antibiotic agents and what they are.

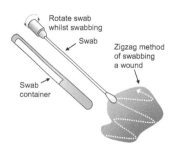

Rotate swab whilst swabbing

Swab

Zigzag method of swabbing a wound

Swab container

Fig 3.3 Swabbing a wound.

Once you have done this, place the swab tube into the pouch attached to the back of the request form and send to the Microbiology laboratory for analysis.

3.3.3 Finishing up

Once you have taken the patient's swab samples, do not forget to record this in the notes. It may be an idea to inform the patient that the results may take up to 2–3 days before they are ready. Thank the patient and answer any questions they may have.

TOP TIP!

Swabs should be sent to the laboratory within 24 hours of being taken. If they cannot be sent within this time, they should be stored in a refrigerator to reduce the likelihood of replication of bacteria as might occur at room temperature.

Chapter 3.4
Taking a blood pressure

What to do . . .

- Introduce yourself to the patient – establish rapport
- Ask the patient's name, age and occupation
- Explain the procedure to the patient
- Ensure that the patient has rested for at least 5 minutes
- Choose an appropriately sized cuff and palpate for the brachial artery
- Estimate the systolic pressure by feeling the radial pulse when the cuff is inflated
- Take an accurate (to the nearest 2 mmHg) blood pressure reading
- Take two subsequent readings
- Interpret the results appropriately and document the reading
- Thank the patient and conclude the consultation

TOP TIP!

In the ITU setting it is often the pulse pressure that is recorded and this is simply the difference between the systolic and diastolic pressure.

Medical Guidelines
Classification of blood pressure levels

Blood pressure category	Systolic BP (mmHg)	Diastolic BP (mmHg)
Stage 1 hypertension	140–159	90–99
Stage 2 hypertension	160–179	100–109
Severe hypertension	≥ 180	≥ 110

NICE Hypertension Guidelines (2011)

TOP TIP!

Although in an OSCE you are likely to be presented with a manikin arm in lieu of a real patient, you should still act courteously towards it as if you were talking to and treating a human being.

Taking a patient's blood pressure is perhaps one of the commonest procedures that you will be performing for the rest of your working life. Although electronic sphygmomanometers are becoming more readily available, you will always be expected to be competent in taking a blood pressure reading manually.

The blood pressure represents the force exerted by the circulating blood upon the surrounding vessel walls as it moves away from the heart. When you take a patient's blood pressure you will obtain two readings:

- the first reading represents the systolic pressure – this is the larger of the two and is defined as the peak pressure that is found in the artery following ventricular systole
- the second reading represents the diastolic pressure – this is the smaller of the two and represents the level to which the arterial blood pressure drops during ventricular diastole.

Although large variations exist in the definition of what constitutes normal and high blood pressure, the British Hypertension Society defines normal blood pressure as being less than 130/85 mmHg and hypertension being anything above 140/90 mmHg.

3.4.1 Beginning the procedure

Start by introducing yourself to the patient, stating your name and job title. Ask the patient for their name and age. Ask the patient if they are feeling well and not in any discomfort before proceeding with your check-up.

Explain the procedure

Explain to the patient what you intend to do next, using language that the patient would understand. Try to avoid using any medical jargon which may unnecessarily confuse the patient, whilst trying not to be patronizing. You could say, for example, *'I understand that you have attended today so that I may check your blood pressure. In order to do this I will need you to expose your upper arm. I will be placing a blood pressure cuff around your arm and slowly inflating it whilst listening with my stethoscope. This procedure should not cause undue discomfort. However, if you do experience any pain please do let me know.'*

After you have explained the procedure to the patient, it is important to check that they have understood and given you verbal consent to proceed. At this point you may wish to offer them the opportunity to ask any questions.

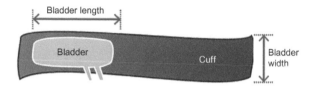

Fig 3.4 Selecting the correct bladder size.

The bladder length should encircle at least 80% of the circumference of the patient's arm for accurate blood pressure readings (BHS Guidelines).

Resting period

Blood pressure measurements may be affected by anxiety, emotional states, exercise or sleep. A common mistake which contributes to an artificially high reading is when the physician takes the blood pressure of a patient who has rushed into the treatment room, quickly taken off their jacket and then immediately presented their arm for examination. To prevent this from happening, it is important to ask the patient to remove their upper garments and expose the examining arm before remaining seated in a chair for at least 5 minutes.

3.4.2 **Taking the blood pressure**

Ideally the blood pressure should be measured in both arms to look for any significant pressure difference between the two sides. A systolic pressure difference of greater than 20 mmHg may suggest coarctation or dissection of the aorta and requires further investigation.

> **TOP TIP!**
>
> In the exam situation, simply inform the examiner that you would have asked the patient to wait for 5 minutes before taking their blood pressure.

Cuff

Bladder cuffs come in four different sizes: small, standard, large and thigh-sized. It is important to choose the correct size bladder cuff for the patient (see *Fig 3.4*). In order to do this you should measure the bladder length against the circumference of the patient's arm. A cuff size with a bladder length that encircles at least 80% of the patient's arm should give you the most accurate blood pressure reading. Using a smaller cuff may cause an inaccurately high reading whereas a larger cuff may give you a lower reading.

Fully deflate the cuff and attach it to the blood pressure manometer. Position the patient with the arm to be examined extended at the elbow and the antecubital fossa facing you. Have the manometer placed at approximately the same level as the patient's heart; this is easily achieved by having the patient sit on a chair with the manometer located beside them on an adjacent table.

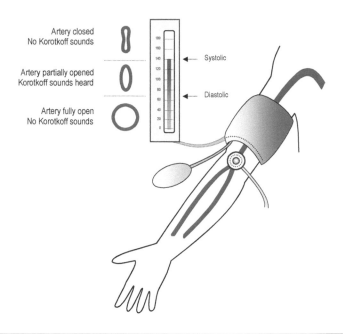

Fig 3.5 Taking blood pressure at the brachial artery.

Palpate within the antecubital fossa with the pulp of your fingers to locate the brachial artery; it is found one-third of the distance from the medial epicondyle to the lateral epicondyle. Neatly place the blood pressure cuff around the arm with the arterial point aligned with the brachial artery. Wrap the rest of the cuff around the arm securely, ensuring the patient is not in any discomfort.

Radial pulse

Before inflating the bladder cuff and measuring the blood pressure, palpate the patient's ipsilateral pulse over the radial artery. Whilst keeping two fingers on the radial pulse, slowly inflate the cuff until the pulse becomes faint and disappears. Slowly deflate the cuff by 3–4 mmHg per second until the pulse returns. This gives an approximate value for the systolic blood pressure; it is important to obtain an estimate of the systolic blood pressure first because this gives an indication as to how much to inflate the cuff when auscultating for a reading, whilst preventing undue discomfort due to over-inflation.

Auscultation

TOP TIP!

In the examination, you may be offered an adapted dual stethoscope whereby the examiner can listen to the sounds that you are hearing. Do not attempt to make up a false reading if you cannot hear the Korotkoff sounds clearly.

Place the diaphragm of your stethoscope over the brachial artery under the distal end of the cuff (*Fig 3.5*). Whilst listening with your stethoscope, inflate the cuff to the estimated systolic reading measured previously until the Korotkoff sounds disappear. At this point slowly deflate the cuff at a rate of 2–3 mmHg per second, watching the blood pressure level closely whilst listening out carefully for any sounds (*Fig 3.6*).

Korotkoff sounds

The first audible sound heard is defined as the first Korotkoff sound and represents the systolic blood pressure. It is often described as a loud thud. Continue

mmHg

.... Silence: No pulse

Systolic BP

〰〰〰 〰〰 〰〰 **Phase 1:** A sharp 'thud'

〰〰 〰〰 〰〰 **Phase 2:** Blowing sound

〰〰 〰〰 〰〰 **Phase 3:** Softer thud

Muffling Sounds

〰〰 〰〰 ▬ **Phase 4:** Disappearing
blowing sound

.... **Phase 5:** Silence

Diastolic BP

Blood pressure   Artery under the cuff   Korotkoff sounds

Fig 3.6 Korotkoff sounds and artery size.

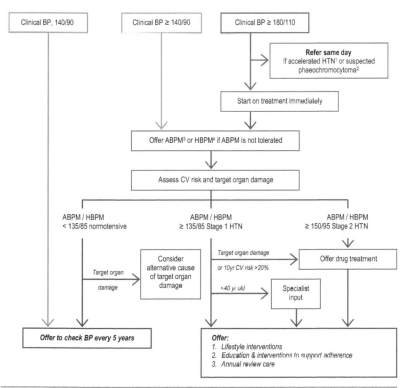

| Clinical BP, 140/90 | Clinical BP ≥ 140/90 | Clinical BP ≥ 180/110 |

Refer same day
If accelerated HTN[1] or suspected
phaeochromocytoma[2]

Start on treatment immediately

Offer ABPM[3] or HBPM[4] if ABPM is not tolerated

Assess CV risk and target organ damage

ABPM / HBPM
< 135/85 normotensive

ABPM / HBPM
≥ 135/85 Stage 1 HTN

ABPM / HBPM
≥ 150/95 Stage 2 HTN

Target organ
damage

Consider
alternative cause
of target organ
damage

Target organ damage
or 10yr CV risk >20%

Offer drug treatment

<40 yr old

Specialist
input

Offer to check BP every 5 years

Offer:
1. *Lifestyle interventions*
2. *Education & interventions to support adherence*
3. *Annual review care*

Notes to flow chart

[1]Signs of papilloedema or retinal haemorrhage.
[2]Labile or postural hypotension, headache, palpitations, pallor and diaphoresis.
[3]Ambulatory blood pressure monitoring.
[4]Home blood pressure monitoring.

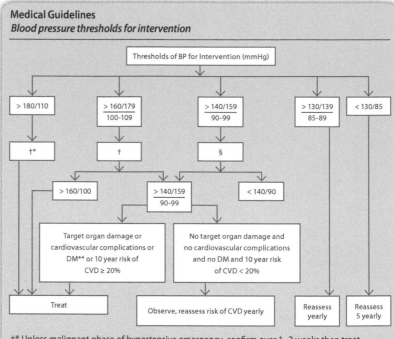

Medical Guidelines
Blood pressure thresholds for intervention

†* Unless malignant phase of hypertensive emergency, confirm over 1–2 weeks then treat.

† If cardiovascular complications, target organ damage, or diabetes are present, confirm over 3–4 weeks then treat; if absent, measure again weekly and treat if blood pressure persists at these levels over 4–12 weeks.

§ If cardiovascular complications, target organ damage or diabetes, confirm over 12 weeks then treat; if absent, measure again monthly and treat if these levels are maintained and if estimated 10 year cardiovascular disease risk is ≥20%.

British Hypertension Society Guidelines for Hypertension Management (BHS-IV) (2004)

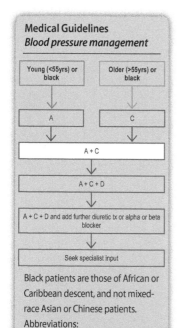

Medical Guidelines
Blood pressure management

Black patients are those of African or Caribbean descent, and not mixed-race Asian or Chinese patients.

Abbreviations:

A – ACE inhibitor (consider angiotensin-II receptor antagonist if ACE intolerant),

C – calcium-channel blocker,

D – diuretic.

NICE Hypertension Guidelines (2011)

to release the pressure slowly within the cuff until this sound muffles and then eventually disappears.

When the Korotkoff sounds disappear completely this represents the diastolic pressure reading. Under certain circumstances, such as pregnancy, the Korotkoff sounds may never disappear. In such situations, the fourth Korotkoff sound (the muffled blowing sound) should be used to indicate the diastolic pressure.

Measure the patient's blood pressure to 2 mmHg, but do not be tempted to round the reading up or down to the nearest 10 mmHg; this is inaccurate, may distort a patient's serial measurements, and may lead to an incorrect diagnosis.

Repeat blood pressure

You should ensure that you take two blood pressure readings a few minutes apart to get the most accurate measurement. The initial reading obtained should be disregarded and subsequent measurements taken if there are large differences between them. A common cause for an artificially raised blood pressure is a patient who is anxious when seeing a doctor. This is known as the 'white coat effect' and is believed to affect up to one in three readings.

Ensure that you deflate the bladder completely before removing the cuff from the patient's arm.

3.4.3 **Summing up**

Once you have taken the patient's blood pressure, ensure that you document it onto a blood pressure chart or in the patient's notes. You will need to interpret the blood pressure as to whether it is high or low (hypertensive or hypotensive) and make a clinical judgment as to what should happen next. If it is normal, reassure the patient and offer an appointment in an appropriate time to have a repeat check-up if necessary.

In cases of high blood pressure, you should follow the British Hypertension Society Guidelines for when to reassess. Deliver an appropriate explanation to the patient as to what the blood pressure is and what it indicates. You may say for example, 'I have taken your blood pressure today and it is 158/98. This result is slightly high. Normally we take the reading on two or three separate occasions because simple things like exercise and anxiety may falsely increase the reading. I suggest we repeat your blood pressure in 1 month's time to confirm whether it is in fact still high.'

Often the patient will be concerned about their blood pressure reading and it is important not to be dismissive of their worries. Reassure the patient that their reading is not life-threatening and that repeating it in a month's time is appropriate. Advise the patient that if they are worried about their blood pressure or develop symptoms such as headaches, blurred vision and vomiting, they should attend earlier for review. Thank the patient and confirm that they have understood what you have told them.

3.4.4 **Common clinical scenarios**

The following are a list of scenarios with different blood pressure readings. Read the cases carefully and determine whether it is necessary to recall or treat the patient.

CASE 1
A 54 year old carpenter who is newly diagnosed with type 2 diabetes. He is asymptomatic and was found to have a resting blood pressure of 154/90 by the practice nurse at his annual diabetic check.

CASE 2
A 27 year old semi-professional football player presents for his medical check-up before transfer to his new club. He is well and is found to have a blood pressure of 110/70.

CASE 3
A 55 year old widow presents complaining of a 2 week history of headaches and now feeling sick. She is a known hypertensive and was recently diagnosed with breast cancer. Her neurological examination is normal. Her blood pressure was found to be 185/122.

CASE 4
A 37 year old Afro-Caribbean lady with type 2 diabetes and stage 3 chronic kidney disease is referred to a local diabetologist due to poor glycaemic control. Her last HbA1C was 11.1. A dipstick urine showed 2 + protein. Her blood pressure was found to be 150/90.

CASE 5

A 62 year old retired banker newly registered with his local general practice. His blood pressure is found to be 132/86 on his health promotion check. He has no known chronic illnesses.

CASE 6

A 35 year old unemployed man has applied for life insurance and attends a medical check-up. He is noted to be very tall with long spindly fingers and a high arched palate. His blood pressure is noted to be 139/86 in the left arm and 110/72 in the right arm.

Chapter 3.5
Body mass index

What to do . . .

- Introduce yourself to the patient – establish rapport
- Ask the patient's name and age and confirm the reason for their appointment
- Establish the patient's understanding of BMI
- Explain and demonstrate to the patient how BMI will be measured
- Ask the patient to remove their shoes and stand straight against the stadiometer, lower the reading arm to the scalp and measure the height in metres
- Ask the patient to remove any heavy clothing, set the weighing scale to zero, and measure the weight of the patient in kilograms
- Calculate the BMI by dividing the weight in kilograms by the square of their height in metres (kg/m^2)
- Interpret the patient's BMI against the WHO scale and document the value
- Thank the patient and conclude the consultation – offer a follow-up appointment if required

The body mass index (BMI) is a simple measurement of weight-for-height that is commonly used to classify adult patients as underweight, overweight or obese. It is used to determine whether someone is at a 'healthy weight' for their height. Due to its simplicity it is in widespread use across a range of healthcare professions and it plays an important role in all areas of clinical practice ranging from primary care to operative surgery.

BMI is defined as the patient's weight in kilograms divided by the square of their height in metres (kg/m^2). The value produced from this calculation is then interpreted against a standardized BMI range that defines the patient's status (see *Table 3.3*).

The patient's BMI can also be determined using a BMI chart which displays the weight on the horizontal axis and height on the vertical axis. When plotting the patient's BMI, the chart has a useful colour scheme (matched in *Table 3.3*) that defines the category of weight to which they belong (see *Fig 3.7*).

In the adult population, the BMI values are age-independent and are the same for both men and women. In children and teenagers, the situation is more complex with age and gender-specific charts required for interpretation; this chapter focuses on how to undertake BMI measurement in adults.

Despite its apparent benefits, the BMI does have limitations. The BMI only measures the crude body weight and hence cannot differentiate between the weight contributed by fat or that of muscle. Because muscle is denser than fat, an athlete's BMI may be incorrectly interpreted as overweight or obese when in reality they may be perfectly healthy. The same can be said of a pregnant woman whose body weight increase is because of her pregnancy rather than accumulation of body fat. Hence, the BMI should not be looked at in isolation but rather interpreted within the clinical context.

Classification	BMI (kg/m²)	
	Principal cut-off points	**Additional cut-off points**
Underweight	<18.50	<18.50
Severe thinness	<16.00	<16.00
Moderate thinness	16.00–16.99	16.00–16.99
Mild thinness	17.00–18.49	17.00–18.49
Normal range	18.50–24.99	18.50–22.99
		23.00–24.99
Overweight	≥25.00	≥25.00
Pre-obese	25.00–29.99	25.00–27.49
		27.50–29.99
Obese	≥30.00	≥30.00
Obese class I	30.00–34.99	30.00–32.49
		32.50–34.99
Obese class II	35.00–39.99	35.00–37.49
		37.50–39.99
Obese class III	≥40.00	≥40.00

Table 3.3 **The International Classification of adult underweight, overweight and obesity according to BMI**

Data from the World Health Organization (2004).

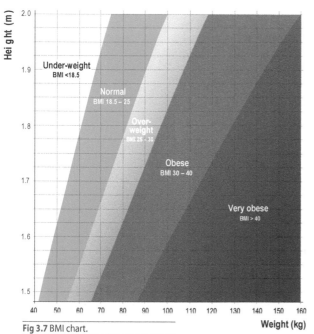

Fig 3.7 BMI chart.

Another shortcoming is that BMI results do not take into account fat distribution. There is increasing evidence (see Medical Guidelines box below) to suggest that distribution of fat plays a more significant role than the body weight of the patient as a risk factor for cardiovascular disease. A patient who has fat deposited around their waist area (so-called 'apple shaped') is at higher risk than a patient whose fat is located around the buttocks and thighs (so-called 'pear shaped'). As a result clinicians are including the waist circumference in conjunction with BMI measurements in their cardiovascular risk assessment.

BMI and health

Due to a media focus on the growing obesity epidemic, measuring BMI has become synonymous with checking for obesity. Although BMI plays a key role in diagnosing obesity it is equally useful in diagnosing patients who are underweight and at risk of malnourishment. Both extremes of BMI have associated severe health implications:

- obesity is associated with ischaemic heart disease, hypertension, diabetes, cancers and osteoarthritis
- a malnourished patient is at risk of osteoporosis, fractures, decreased immunity and electrolyte imbalances as well as heart failure and anaemia.

3.5.1 **Beginning the procedure**

Start by introducing yourself to the patient, stating your name and job title. Ask the patient for their name and age before proceeding. It may be relevant to try to establish risk factors for cardiovascular disease such as diabetes, hypertension, hypercholesterolaemia, and past medical and family history of ischaemic heart disease and smoking.

Check if the patient is well and not in any discomfort before carrying on. It may be useful before you begin to confirm the reason why the patient needs to have their BMI measured; it could be that they are attending a pre-assessment clinic and that a future operation hinges on their BMI being below a certain cut-off point.

Before starting to measure the BMI, make yourself familiar with the equipment so that you do not appear hesitant in front of the patient. You should have access to a stadiometer to measure the height, a weighing scale for the weight, and a calculator to work out the BMI. If a calculator is not present, you may be offered a standardized BMI chart which you should use instead.

Explain the procedure

Explain to the patient what you intend to do using language that the patient will understand. Explain to the patient what BMI is and why you intend to measure it; note that some people can be very conscious about their weight and will be uncomfortable being weighed. It is important that you do not appear to judge the patient based upon their weight or BMI status. You may wish to say to the patient: *'I have been asked to measure your BMI or Body Mass Index. This is a simple procedure that compares your weight against your height and allows us to determine whether your weight is healthy for your height. It involves us weighing you and then measuring your height.'*

After you have explained everything to the patient, it is important to check that they have understood what you have said so far and given you verbal consent to proceed.

3.5.2 **The procedure**

Height measurement

A stadiometer is a device for measuring a patient's height. It consists of a vertical ruler with a sliding horizontal arm which is moved up or down to rest on the top of the patient's head (*Fig 3.8*). Before asking the patient to stand by the stadiometer, you must first ensure that nothing is going to affect their height measurement. They should remove their footwear before continuing. People who have their hair tied up on top of their head may have to unfasten it if necessary.

Once they are ready ask them to stand straight against the stadiometer with their heels pressed back against the wall while facing towards you. The patient's chin should be lifted so that the external auditory meatus is in line with the lateral canthus (corner of the eye). Move the horizontal arm of the stadiometer down to touch the patient's head. If the patient's hair is thick, make sure to lower the arm until it rests against the patient's scalp. Patients who have difficulty standing with their back straight against the wall, such as those with kyphosis

Medical Guidelines
Waist circumferences and risk to health in overweight individuals

For men, a waist circumference of less than 94 cm indicates a low risk to health, 94–102 cm is a high risk, and more than 102 cm is a very high risk.

For women, a waist circumference of less than 80 cm is low, 80–88 cm is high and more than 88 cm is very high.
Adapted from NICE Guideline: Obesity guidance (2006)

TOP TIP!

Whilst measuring waist circumference is important in assessing cardiovascular risk it is not normally included in the BMI exam station.

TOP TIP!

If you just remember kg/m², you will never forget that weight needs to be divided by height.

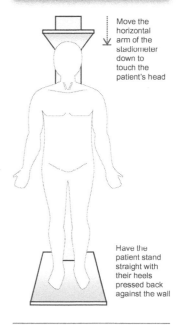

Move the horizontal arm of the stadiometer down to touch the patient's head

Have the patient stand straight with their heels pressed back against the wall

Fig 3.8 Patient standing against a stadiometer.

Medical Guidelines
Health benefits of losing weight

The health benefits of a modest 10% weight loss are described below; the precise benefits will vary between individuals and will depend on the initial body weight, health and degree of weight loss.

Mortality
• 20–25% reduction in premature death
• 30% reduction in the risk of dying from diabetes-related complications
• 40% reduction in the risk of dying from cancer

Blood pressure
• 10 mmHg decrease in systolic blood pressure
• 20 mmHg decrease in diastolic blood pressure

Diabetes
• 50% fall in fasting blood glucose levels

Lipids
• 10% fall in total cholesterol (15% fall in LDL cholesterol)
• 8% increase in HDL cholesterol

SIGN Guidelines: Obesity in Scotland: Integrating prevention with weight management (1996)

or scoliosis, may need an alternative method for measuring height, such as the Demispan.

Record the patient's height by taking the reading from the stadiometer or from the ruler adjacent to it. Make sure that you record the height in metres because this is the value you need to use for the BMI calculation.

Weight measurement

Ideally the patient should remove all of their outer clothing and have their weight measured whilst wearing only their undergarments. However, in a busy clinical situation this is not practical. Instead ask the patient to remove as much of their heavier outer clothes as they are comfortable to do, particularly any thick coats and knitwear. You should try to ensure that they wear similar amounts of clothing for any subsequent measurements and this will allow you to accurately monitor whether the patient's BMI has changed. Ideally the same scales or weighing machine should also be used on each occasion.

Set the scales to zero before continuing. Ask the patient to stand up straight on the scales with their feet together in the centre of the platform. Allow the needle to rest at the given weight before recording the value. The weight should be recorded in kilograms and not in stones or pounds.

Once you have obtained the height and weight, it is courteous to tell the patient that they can get dressed before you begin the calculation.

Calculation

With the aid of a calculator, use the patient's height and weight to work out the BMI. Use the formula below and ensure that you are using the correct units:
$$BMI = \text{Weight in kg} / (\text{Height in m})^2$$

3.5.3 Interpreting the BMI

Once you have calculated the BMI, ensure that you document it in the patient's notes. You will then need to interpret the result to determine whether the patient is a healthy weight for their height, and then structure your clinical advice accordingly.

It is important to be aware of the BMI ranges and understand what they mean. In an exam situation you may be requested to plot the patient's BMI on a chart.

The World Health Organization (WHO) considers an adult with a BMI of less than 18.5 to be underweight and this may indicate malnutrition, an eating disorder or other health problems. Some consider a BMI of less than 17.5 as part of the criteria in the diagnosis of anorexia nervosa. An adult with a BMI of over 25 is regarded as overweight and those with a BMI above 30 are considered clinically obese. BMI values do not predict health, but the higher the BMI, the more likely a patient is to suffer with cardiovascular disease and diabetes.

If the BMI is normal, reassure the patient and encourage them to continue as they are. In cases where the BMI is above 25, you should advise the patient on how to lose weight through diet and exercise as per the NICE guidelines. Deliver an appropriate explanation to the patient as to what the BMI is and what it

TOP TIP!

In the examination you may be presented with a sliding weight beam scale to measure a patient's weight. Ensure that you are familiar with it and how to prime the scale for first time use.

indicates. You may say, for example, *'I have calculated your BMI today and it is 28. This result is slightly high and indicates that you are not at a healthy weight for your height. This can put you at an increased risk of developing diabetes or heart disease. It is good that you have come to see us early so that we can offer you advice on how to reach a healthy weight.'*

Medical Guidelines
A guide to determine the initial level of intervention to discuss

BMI classification	Waist circumference			Co-morbidities
	Low	High	Very high	
Overweight				
Obese class I				
Obese class II				
Obese class III				

General advice on weight and lifestyle
Diet and physical activity
Diet and physical activity, consider drugs
Diet and physical activity, consider drugs, consider surgery
NICE Guideline: Obesity guidance (2006)

Medical Guidelines
Advice and management of obesity

Information given to the patient should be structured around advice about eating a low calorie diet and increasing their regular exercise. Depending on their BMI it may be necessary to consider medication or even surgery if the patient fulfils the criteria.

Diet
- Eat starchy foods such as potatoes, bread, and brown rice; choose wholegrain where possible
- Eat fibre-rich foods such as oats, beans, peas, lentils, grains, seeds, wholegrain bread
- Eat at least five portions of fruit and vegetables each day
- Eat a low-fat diet and avoid high calorie foods (fried foods, drinks high in added sugars)
- Watch the portion size of meals and snacks, and how often you are eating
- Minimize the calories you take in from alcohol

Activity
- Make enjoyable activities such as walking, cycling and swimming part of everyday life
- Minimize sedentary activities, such as sitting watching TV, playing computer games
- Build activity into the working day, e.g. take the stairs instead of lift, have regular walks

Drugs (Orlistat)
- Prescribe as part of an overall plan for managing obesity in those who have a BMI of 28 kg/m² or more with associated risk factors, or a BMI of 30 kg/m² or more
- Continue treatment for longer than 3 months only if they have lost at least 5% of their initial body weight since starting the medication (less strict goals for type 2 diabetics)
- Continue for longer than 12 months (for weight maintenance) after discussing potential benefits and limitations with the patient

Medical Guidelines
Advice and management of obesity (Continued)

Surgery

Bariatric surgery can be considered as a first-line option in patients with a BMI of more than 50 kg/m². It can be recommended at lower BMIs if all of the following criteria are fulfilled:

- they have a BMI of ≥40 kg/m², or between 35 kg/m² and 40 kg/m² and other significant disease (e.g. type 2 DM or HTN) that could be improved if they lost weight
- all appropriate non-surgical measures have been tried but failed to achieve adequate beneficial weight loss for at least 6 months
- the person will receive management in a specialist obesity service, is generally fit for anaesthesia and surgery, and commits to the need for long-term follow-up

Adapted from NICE Guidelines: Obesity guidance (2006)

3.5.4 Summing up

Often the patient will be concerned about their BMI and it is important not to be dismissive of their worries. Reassure the patient that their BMI may not be life-threatening and that simple things like a healthy diet and exercise can help to reduce their weight. Offer the patient an appointment with the dietician who can give detailed guidance regarding their diet. Thank the patient and confirm that they have understood what you have told them.

3.5.5 Common clinical scenarios

The following are a list of common clinical scenarios which you may encounter. For each one, consider:

- what the BMI is
- whether they are underweight, normal overweight or obese as according the WHO BMI classification

CASE 1
A 41 year old Afro-Caribbean lady presents for a new patient registration. She has no medical problems. Her height is 1.63 metres and her weight is 70 kg.

CASE 2
A 35 year old Bengali restaurant waiter has been recently diagnosed with diabetes. He attends his yearly diabetic check. His height is 1.7 metres and his weight is 95 kg.

CASE 3
A 16 year old college student attends complaining of reduced appetite and lack of interest in food. She demands that her weight be checked as she strongly believes she is overweight. Her height is 1.75 metres and her weight is 50 kg.

CASE 4
A 62 year old retired builder suffers from ischaemic heart disease, raised blood pressure and hypercholesterolaemia. He attended his pre-assessment clinic for bariatric surgery and is found to weigh 120 kg with a height of 1.5 metres.

Chapter 3.6
Recording an ECG

What to do . . .

- Introduce yourself to the patient – establish rapport
- Ask the patient's name and age and confirm the reason why the patient needs an ECG; establish any symptoms as relevant
- Explain the procedure to the patient and gain consent
- Expose the patient's chest, arms and ankles
- Gather and prepare equipment, wash hands
- Attach the sticky pads, limb leads and chest leads in the correct positions
- Calibrate the ECG machine, filter and print the ECG
- Document the patient's details, time and date on the ECG as well as the indication for the test
- Remove leads and sticky pads and dispose of waste
- Interpret the results and document in the notes
- Explain findings to patient and answer any questions they may have
- Thank the patient and conclude the examination

The ECG (electrocardiogram) tracing is a non-invasive, trans-thoracic recording of the electrical activity of the heart using electrodes placed on the patient's skin. The machine picks up electrical activity of the heart through these electrodes and generates a number of interpretable ECG tracings which analyse the heart from different angles. Although different types of ECG machines exist (such as the three lead or five lead), the most commonly used is the 12 lead ECG: this gathers electrical activity from limb and chest electrodes to form a 12 lead trace (see *Box 3.2*).

ECGs are performed for a number of different reasons; the most important is in the diagnosis of cardiac chest pain. They also have a role in detecting abnormalities of the cardiac rate and rhythm. The ECG is an extremely useful diagnostic tool and should be used in conjunction with a detailed history and thorough examination. Although in the hospital setting nurses are normally responsible for performing an ECG on a patient, you should be fully competent in carrying it out and interpreting the results.

TOP TIP!

Although the typical ECG is referred as the '12 lead ECG', it actually contains only 10 physical leads that connect to the patient (six chest leads and four limb leads including one neutral). The six leads, i.e. I, II, III, aVL, aVF and aVR, are electronically extrapolated from the four physical limb leads (RA, LA, RL and LL).

BOX 3.2 **Leads representing areas of the heart**

V1, V2, V3, V4	Anterior surface (right ventricle and septum)
V5, V6, aVL and I	Lateral surface (left ventricle)
II, III, and aVF	Inferior surface
aVR	Right atrium

Electrical activity of the heart

When the heart muscle contracts, an electrical change known as depolarization takes place. This activity can be detected by electrodes. In a healthy patient depolarization (see *Fig 3.9*) occurs in an orderly fashion starting at the sino-atrial node (SAN), spreading through the atria (atrial systole) and then on to the atrio-ventricular node (AVN). From here it is transmitted down through the His–Purkinje system within the septum before spreading to the right and left ventricles causing ventricular systole.

When a depolarization wave spreads towards a lead the needle on the ECG trace will move upwards, known as a positive deflection. Conversely, when the wave moves away from the lead, the needle will move downwards, producing a negative deflection. The extent of the electrical activity recorded is proportional to the muscle mass though which it passes. For example, as the atria have smaller muscle bulk than the ventricles the ECG records a smaller deflection. Appreciating this fact will make interpreting ECG traces much easier.

> **TOP TIP!**
>
> Patients should remain still and relaxed during an ECG recording as skeletal muscle activity may cause a distortion to the ECG trace.

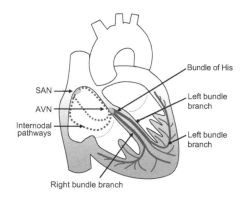

Fig 3.9 Cardiac depolarization.

3.6.1 **Beginning the procedure**

Introduce yourself to the patient by stating your name and job title. Confirm the patient's name and date of birth and check this against their ID wrist band. It is important to record these details on the ECG tracing once it is performed because an anonymous ECG will be routinely discarded.

Ensure that the patient is well and not in any discomfort. In an OSCE you may be faced with either a real patient or a manikin that can generate cardiac rhythms; when faced with a manikin you should follow the same procedure as you would do with a real patient.

Before you begin it is useful to confirm the reason why the patient is having an ECG. This may give you valuable insight as to possible changes you may expect to see on the tracing. Briefly note any cardiac symptoms and whether the patient has had a pacemaker fitted in the past.

Explain the procedure

Explain to the patient what you wish to do, using language that the patient will understand. Inform them why you wish to do an ECG and remind them that it is a painless procedure. You could say: '*I understand that you have been having some chest pain recently and I would like to carry out an ECG trace of your heart. This procedure is quick, simple and painless and only involves attaching a number of stickers to your body at various places. I will then connect up the ECG machine by attaching a number of leads to these points. The machine will then record a trace of your heart, monitoring its electrical activity. At no point should it be painful and I would like to reassure you that you will not be receiving an electrical shock.*'

Preparation

Before beginning it is essential that you ask if the patient would like a chaperone to be present and then seek consent to proceed.

Make sure the patient is lying comfortably on the couch and resting against a pillow at 45 degrees with their arms by their side. An anxious patient may create enough interference on the ECG to make it difficult to interpret. Ask the patient to expose their chest, upper arms and ankles so that you can place the electrodes correctly. In order to get a clear trace you will need to ensure good electrical contact between the electrodes and the skin; it may be necessary, particularly over the chest, to shave any excess hair to improve contact.

Ask the patient to remove any jewellery, watches or metallic objects because they may interfere with or distort the reading.

Equipment

Before you start make sure that you have washed your hands and collected all of the equipment that you will require. You will need the following:
- ECG machine
- 6 chest electrodes (V1–V6) and 4 limb electrodes (red, yellow, green, black) Electrode stickers and leads

> **TOP TIP!**
>
> Spend a little time untangling the leads before starting as this will simplify the procedure and also prevent any cross-lead electrical interference.

3.6.2 **The procedure**

Warn the patient that you will start by placing small stickers on their arms, legs and chest wall. Remind them of the need to remain relaxed and still for the duration of the procedure.

Limb leads

The limb leads look at the heart in the vertical plane and are colour co-ordinated. They consist of both unipolar (aVR, aVL and aVF) and bipolar leads (I, II and III). In the active unipolar leads, the aV stands for 'augmented vector' and the last letter denotes the position of the lead (Right, Left and Foot respectively). Each lead independently monitors electrical activity from that point. Together they form the three corners that make up Einthoven's triangle (*Fig 3.10*).

The bipolar leads measure electrical activity between two points. The machine extrapolates a lead from the information gathered between two electrodes such that lead I is generated from aVR and aVL, lead II from aVR and aVF and finally lead III from aVL and aVF.

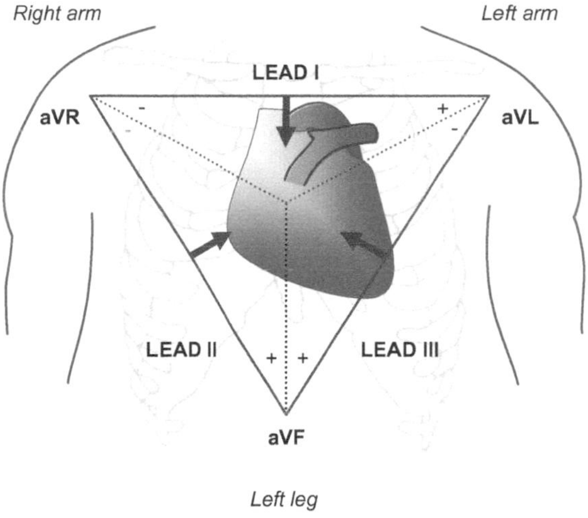

Fig 3.10 Einthoven's triangle and limb leads.

Place four sticky pads in the correct position (see *Fig 3.11*) on the patient's limbs to form the attachment points for the limb leads. Place one pad on the distal aspect of the forearms just above the wrist. Next place a pad just above each ankle. Ensure that the flap end of the pads are facing downwards so that you can attach the leads with minimal inconvenience.

The four limb leads are noticeably longer in length than the chest leads. Attach the red limb lead (corresponds to aVR) to the right forearm and then connect the yellow lead to the left forearm (corresponds to aVL). Move down to the left leg and attach the green lead to it (corresponds to aVF). Finally, connect the black lead to the right leg. This is the neutral lead and its presence helps complete the electrical circuit.

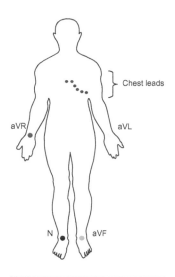

Fig 3.11 Position of chest and limb leads.

Chest leads

The chest leads look at the heart in a horizontal plane and are labelled from V1 to V6:

- V1 and V2 look at the right ventricle
- V3 and V4 look at the interventricular septum
- V5 and V6 look at the left ventricle

Start by attaching the sticky electrode pads to the chest. A good knowledge of the anatomical landmarks will ensure that you place them in the correct position (*Fig 3.12*).

Locate the angle of Louis (sternal angle) which corresponds to the second intercostal space. Count down two further spaces until you locate the fourth intercostal space. Stick the V1 pad just right of the sternum in this area. The V2 pad should also be aligned along the fourth intercostal space but placed to the left of the sternum. Next attach the V4 pad in the fifth intercostal space bisecting the mid-clavicular line. Approximate a midway point between the V2 and V4 stickers and place the V3 pad there; this should normally be on the fifth thoracic rib. Locate the fifth intercostal space and find the point where it bisects the anterior-axillary line: place the V5 pad at this location. Finally, move along this plane until you reach the mid-axillary line and place the V6 pad there.

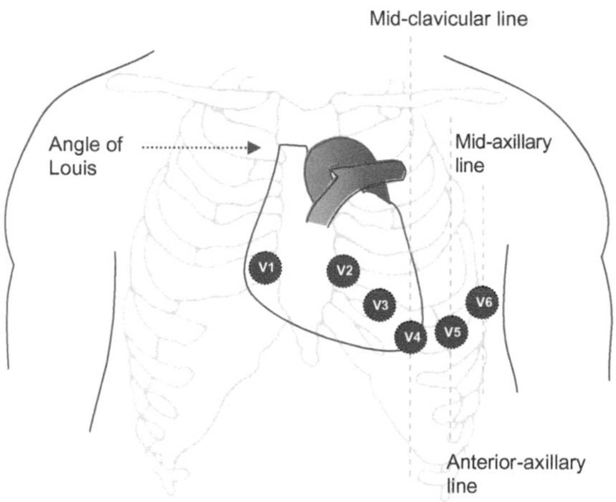

Mid-clavicular line

Angle of
Louis

Mid-axillary
line

V1 V2 V3 V4 V5 V6

Anterior-axillary
line

Fig 3.12 Location of the chest leads.

Calibration

Before recording the trace, it is important that you check that the ECG machine is calibrated. The standard setting should be where 1 mV is equivalent to 1 cm (2 large squares on the paper) vertical deflection on the ECG. The printing speed of the paper should be set at 25 mm per second. You should remember that 1 large square on the ECG is equal to 0.2 seconds and each small square represents 0.04 seconds. Altering the standard setting may change the tracing and make it difficult to interpret.

Print

Now you are ready to print the ECG. Before you press the print button, make sure that the patient is lying still, relaxed and breathing normally. Check that all pads have good contact with the skin. If the machine requires it, enter the patient's name, date of birth and hospital number as appropriate. If not, remember to complete these details on the ECG itself after it has been printed.

Press the print button and allow the machine a few seconds to generate the ECG printout. Immediately check that the trace has all the leads recorded clearly and that a readable ECG has been obtained. If you feel that an inadequate ECG has been obtained you should not hesitate to repeat it. Also check that the machine has printed the correct date and time onto the trace.

Once you are satisfied with the recording, disconnect the patient from the ECG machine and remove all of the stickers. It may be an idea to ask the patient to remove the pads over their chest area as doing so may cause some discomfort.

TOP TIP!

Modern ECG machines often display the trace on an LCD screen before printing. It may be an idea to briefly look at it prior to printing your ECG. You can use it to check that you have a good trace or whether any leads are incorrectly connected.

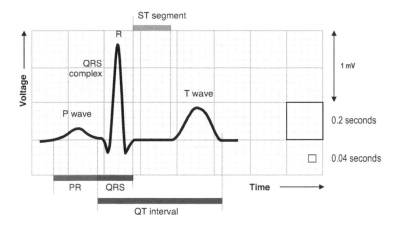

Fig 3.13 Basic ECG complex.

If the patient requires serial ECGs you may wish to leave the electrode stickers in place until they are no longer required.

Dispose of any waste and place the leads back on the ECG trolley without twisting them. Check that the patient is comfortable and give them the opportunity to get dressed. Let the patient know that you are going to interpret the ECG and inform them of the results.

3.6.3 Interpreting the ECG tracing

An ECG trace reveals detailed information about the function and health of the heart. It is easy to miss or overlook subtle changes that may indicate significant underlying pathology and so, irrespective of how experienced you are, it is always best to interpret the tracing in a systematic manner. A simple framework would be to examine the rate, rhythm and cardiac axis first before proceeding to the waveforms and their intervals.

A typical ECG (see *Fig 3.13*) comprises:
- a P wave – represents atrial systole
- a QRS complex – represents ventricular systole
- a T wave – represents ventricular repolarization

Rate

The heart rate, if the rhythm is regular, can be calculated by dividing the number of large squares between two consecutive R waves into 300. For example, if there are three large squares between adjacent R waves, this would mean a heart rate of 100 beats per minute (300/3). If there were four large squares, then the rate would be 75 beats per minute (300/4). A rate less than 60 beats per minute is known as bradycardia, whilst a rate greater than 100 is known as tachycardia. A heart rate between 60 and 100 beats per minute is considered normal in a healthy adult.

Sinus bradycardia
Sinus bradycardia can be normal (e.g. during sleep and in athletes) or abnormal (e.g. in hypothermia, hypothyroidism and raised intracranial pressure (Cushing's response)).

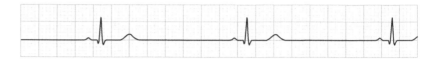

Sinus tachycardia

Sinus tachycardia can be a normal physiological response to exercise and excitement or can occur with fever and anaemia.

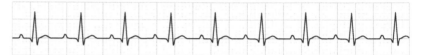

Rhythm

When assessing rhythm you should note whether it is regular or irregular and if it is a sinus rhythm or not. Check for the presence of P waves and their relationship to the QRS complex. Look at the morphology of the QRS complex and note if it is broad or narrow.

Sinus rhythm

Sinus rhythm typically has a normal upright P wave followed by a single QRS complex that repeats in a regular pattern. Regardless of how 'regular' the pattern may appear, you should try to determine it objectively using a piece of paper placed horizontally over lead II (rhythm strip) of the ECG trace. Mark out four consecutive R waves on to the paper and slide this across onto the subsequent four R waves. Note whether the current set of R waves match up with the markings on the paper from the first set of four R waves. If they do, then the rhythm strip can be considered to be in sinus rhythm.

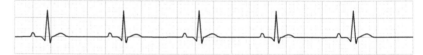

Atrial fibrillation

In atrial fibrillation there is disorganized activity which originates in the atria resulting in the absence of P waves, a wandering baseline and irregularly irregular QRS complexes. Atrial fibrillation is a common arrhythmia occurring in 5–10% of patients over 65 years of age. It has a number of causes including ischaemic heart disease, infection and thyrotoxicosis.

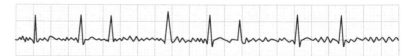

Atrial flutter

Atrial flutter is usually associated with organic heart disease and presents with a sawtooth pattern of the baseline known as flutter waves. Although the atria contract at a rate of 300 beats per minute only a portion of the impulses are transmitted to the ventricle (usually 150 bpm) due to AV note blockade. The QRS complexes are narrow and regular and are preceded by two P waves.

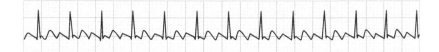

Junctional (nodal) rhythms

Sinus rhythm occurs when the sino–atrial node (SAN) depolarizes. If the depolarization originates elsewhere, then the rhythm is named after the site in which it originated. An AV nodal rhythm presents with P waves that are closer to the QRS complex or they may not be seen at all, but the QRS will always be narrow.

Ventricular tachycardia

A ventricular rhythm will have wide QRS complexes and lack P waves. Ventricular tachycardia is likely when there are three or more consecutive broad QRS complexes occurring at a rate of over 120 bpm. Sustained ventricular tachycardia can transform into ventricular fibrillation resulting in death.

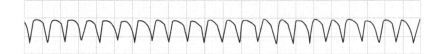

Ventricular fibrillation

Ventricular fibrillation is a medical emergency which occurs when there is chaotic ventricular electrical activity that is not compatible with life (i.e. the patient will be unconscious with no pulse). As the muscle fibres in the ventricles contract independently and not as a collective unit a bizarre, disorganized trace with no QRS complexes results. This rhythm requires immediate DC cardioversion.

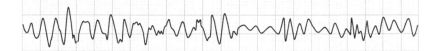

Cardiac axis

The cardiac axis describes the direction of electrical activity through the heart (see *Fig 3.14*). In a healthy adult, this should pass from the right atrium down towards the apex and range between –30 degrees and + 90 degrees. It is determined by looking at the direction of QRS wave forms in limb leads I, II and III. A normal axis should have positive QRS complexes in leads I, II and III with lead II having the greatest positive deflection.

Axis deviation

If the heart's electrical activity shifts from the normal range it is known as axis deviation and may indicate an underlying pathology. An easy way to interpret cardiac axes is by looking to leads I and III and noting the direction of their deflections.

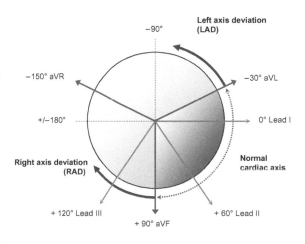

Fig 3.14 The cardiac axis.

- If there is a positive deflection in lead I with a simultaneous negative deflection in lead III (i.e. lead I and III are leaving each other), this may indicate left axis deviation (LAD). Common causes of this include an inferior MI, Wolff–Parkinson–White syndrome or left anterior hemiblock.
- If there is a negative deflection in lead I along with a positive deflection in lead III (i.e. leads I and III are reaching out to one another), then this may suggest the presence of right axis deviation (RAD). Causes include dextrocardia, pulmonary embolism (or any cause of right ventricular overload) and left posterior hemiblock.
- A negative QRS in leads I and II could either indicate that the leads have been placed incorrectly or may be due to dextrocardia.

Waveform

Having assessed the rate, rhythm and cardiac axis of the overall ECG you should now focus on the individual waves that make up the tracing. Look to the P wave, QRS complex and T wave for their shape and size. Check the ST segment for depression or elevation and finally measure the interval between different waveforms.

P waves

Check for the presence of P waves. If they are absent it may mean that the patient is suffering from atrial fibrillation. If P waves are present, check their morphology and length; normal P waves should be less than 0.12 seconds (3 small squares) wide and less than 2.5 mm tall. Broad and bifid P waves (> 0.12 sec) are known as 'P mitrale' and occur with left atrial hypertrophy, e.g. due to mitral stenosis. Tall peaked P waves (> 2.5 mm) are known as 'P pulmonale' and occur in right atrial hypertrophy, e.g. in tricuspid stenosis or pulmonary hypertension.

QRS complex

Next move to the QRS complex. The Q wave is an initial downward deflection of the QRS complex that is caused by septum depolarization away from the left ventricle. Normal Q waves may be found in the lateral (V5, V6) and ventricular leads (I, aVL). The wave should be less than 1 mm wide and less than 2 mm deep. Large, deep Q waves are pathological and usually indicate the presence of scar tissue in the heart post-MI.

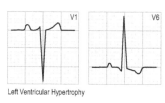

Left Ventricular Hypertrophy

The height of the R and S waves may provide extra information about the muscle bulk of the ventricles. In left ventricular hypertrophy (LVH), the muscle mass is increased and leads to tall R waves (> 25 mm) in the left ventricular leads (V5 and V6) and deep S waves in the right ventricular leads V1 and V2. This may be confirmed by adding the height of the S wave in V1 with that of the R wave in V6 with a result in excess of 35 mm confirming LVH. The most common cause of this is systemic hypertension.

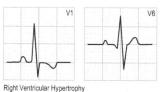

Right Ventricular Hypertrophy

In right ventricular hypertrophy (RVH) the opposite changes are seen, with deep S waves in V6 and the height of the R wave becoming greater than the S wave depth in V1. This can be caused by pulmonary hypertension.

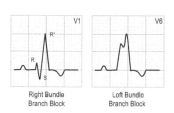

Right Bundle
Branch Block

Left Bundle
Branch Block

A normal QRS complex (narrow) should be no longer than 0.12 seconds (3 small squares). A widening of the QRS complex may indicate a conduction defect within the Bundle of His and its accompanying branches, resulting in a slowing down of electrical impulses through the ventricles.

In right bundle branch block (RBBB), there is a lack of electrical impulse being transmitted through the right conducting pathway. As a result the left ventricle depolarizes before the right creating two upward deflections (two R waves). This creates a unique arrangement known as the RSR pattern, otherwise known as the M sign, best seen in V1. You may also find a deep S wave in V6.

In left bundle branch block (LBBB), due to a lack of conduction down the left pathway, the ventricle depolarization from right to left creates an 'M' arrangement best seen in V6 and a 'W' shape in V1.

T wave

T waves are normally inverted in aVR and V1, and in V2 in young people and in V3 in some Afro-Caribbean people. The most common abnormality seen is T wave inversion which usually occurs in ischaemia or infarction.

Drug toxicity and electrolyte abnormalities can also cause T wave abnormalities. Hyperkalaemia causes tall tented T waves whereas hypokalaemia causes flat T waves and a subsequent U wave (see *Box 3.3*).

ST segment

This is the segment between the end of the QRS and the start of the T wave and should appear as an isoelectric straight line across the baseline of the ECG. Abnormalities of the ST segment include elevation and depression.

ST elevation of over 1 mm in two or more contiguous leads in a concave upward fashion indicates the early stages of an MI. Later stages may reveal a 'tombstone' appearance in this segment. The leads in which changes occur indicate the part of the heart that has been affected (see *Box 3.4*). ST elevation in a convex up (saddle-shaped) fashion occurring in most leads (except aVR and V1) is seen in pericarditis. ST depression of over 0.5 mm occurs in ischaemia, angina and a posterior infarct (seen in V1 and V2 as reciprocal changes). It may also occur with digoxin toxicity whereas the ST changes are seen as a 'reverse tick'.

Intervals

PR interval

The PR interval is the distance from the start of the P wave to the beginning of the QRS complex. It represents the time it takes for a wave of depolarization to

> **TOP TIP!**
>
> LBBB can be easily remembered with the mnemonic WiLLiaM indicating that a 'W' shape to the QRS complex can be seen in V1 and an M shape arrangement in V6. RBBB can be remembered using the mnemonic MaRRoW with the opposite being true.

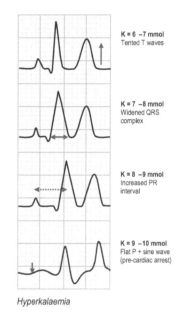

K = 6 –7 mmol
Tented T waves

K = 7 –8 mmol
Widened QRS complex

K = 8 –9 mmol
Increased PR interval

K = 9 –10 mmol
Flat P + sine wave (pre-cardiac arrest)

Hyperkalaemia

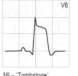

MI – 'Tombstone'   Pericarditis – 'Saddle shape'

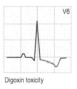

Digoxin toxicity

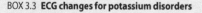

> BOX 3.3 **ECG changes for potassium disorders**
>
> Hypokalaemia
>
> ST depression
> Flat and depressed T wave
> U waves
> Long QT interval
> Ventricular dysrhythmia
>
> Hyperkalaemia (see traces)
>
> Tall tented T waves (K = 6–7 mmol)
> Widened QRS complex (K = 7–8 mmol)
> Increased PR interval (K = 8–9 mmol)
> Flat P wave and sine wave (K = 9–10 mmol)
> Cardiac arrest rhythms

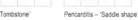

BOX 3.4 **MI location, involved leads and affected artery**

Anterior
ST elevation and Q waves in V2–V4
Anterior descending coronary artery

Posterior
ST depression and tall R in V1 and V2 (reciprocal changes).
Right coronary artery

Inferior
ST elevation and Q waves in II, III and aVF
Right or left coronary artery

Lateral
ST elevation and Q waves in I, II, aVL, V5 and V6
Circumflex coronary artery

Septal
ST elevation and Q waves in V1–V2

leave the SAN and travel through the AVN to reach the ventricles. A normal PR interval is expected to lie between 0.12 and 0.2 seconds and any abnormality in this conduction may prolong or shorten the PR interval. A prolonged PR interval of greater than 0.2 seconds is termed a heart block, of which there are three degrees:

- First degree heart block – this describes a delay along the conduction pathway between the atria and ventricles such that the PR interval is prolonged with a fixed distance of greater than one large square. Every P wave is accompanied by a QRS complex.

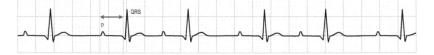

- Second degree heart block – if the impulses intermittently fail to pass from the atria to the ventricles such that some P waves are not followed by QRS complexes, this is known as second degree heart block, of which there are three types:
  - Mobitz type 1 (Wenkebach) – the PR interval gets progressively longer with each QRS until eventually a P wave fails to conduct and no QRS follows. The PR interval then returns to normal and the cycle repeats itself.

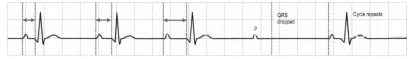

o Mobitz type 2 – this occurs when the PR interval stays constant but occasionally a QRS complex is dropped. This can occur in the absence of a particular pattern.

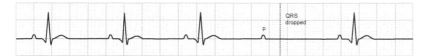

o Fixed degrees of atrioventricular block (2:1/3:1) – for every two or three P waves there is a single QRS complex. This means that the atria may have to contract up to three times before the ventricle contracts.

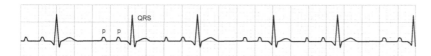

- Third degree heart block (complete) – this is where there is a complete dissociation between atrial activity and ventricular contractions. There is no direct link between P waves and the QRS complexes. With careful inspection P waves can sometimes be seen anywhere along the trace and sometimes be seen even within the QRS complex. The QRS complexes will be wide and abnormal as they originate from the ventricles and the rate will be around 40 bpm.

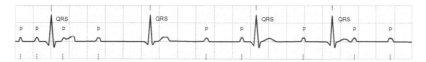

> **TOP TIP!**
>
> To confirm a third degree heart block rhythm, mark the P waves on a piece of paper held beneath the rhythm strip. Once you have done this move the paper across until you line up the marks with the first QRS complex. Note if the markings on the paper correlate with the QRS complexes. In complete heart block there will be no association.

Wolff–Parkinson–White

Short PR intervals occur in the presence of a faster conducting aberrant pathway between the atria and ventricles such as in Wolff–Parkinson–White (WPW) syndrome. In such conditions one may notice a slurred upstroke of the QRS complex known as a delta-wave. This is often accompanied by a widened QRS.

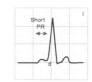

Wolff–Parkinson–White syndrome

QT interval

This interval is measured from the start of the QRS to the end of the T wave. It represents the time taken for the ventricles to depolarize and repolarize. The QT interval is usually corrected for heart rate (QTc) and should not generally exceed two large squares. Causes of long QT syndrome can be congenital or acquired, such as electrolyte imbalances (low potassium, magnesium and calcium), ischaemia and drugs (sotalol, chlorpromazine and macrolide antibiotics).

3.6.4 **Summing up**

Once you have taken and interpreted the ECG, ensure that the patient's name, date of birth and the date and time the ECG was performed are recorded clearly and legibly. Next document in the patient's notes your interpretation of the ECG and compare it if possible with old ones. The patient may have developed changes, such as a new LBBB, that may have to be acted upon.

If the ECG is normal, reassure the patient and offer an appointment to have a repeat check-up if necessary. In cases of abnormal results you should interpret them according to the clinical context and know what symptoms the patient has presented with. Deliver an appropriate explanation to the patient about what the ECG results indicate and what should happen next. Often the patient will be concerned and it is important not to be dismissive of their worries.

Conclude the scenario by thanking the patient, confirming their understanding and checking if they have any further questions to ask.

3.6.5 Common clinical scenarios

The following are a list of common ECG traces which you may encounter. For each one, consider:
- what the possible diagnosis of each could be
- what key features you noticed

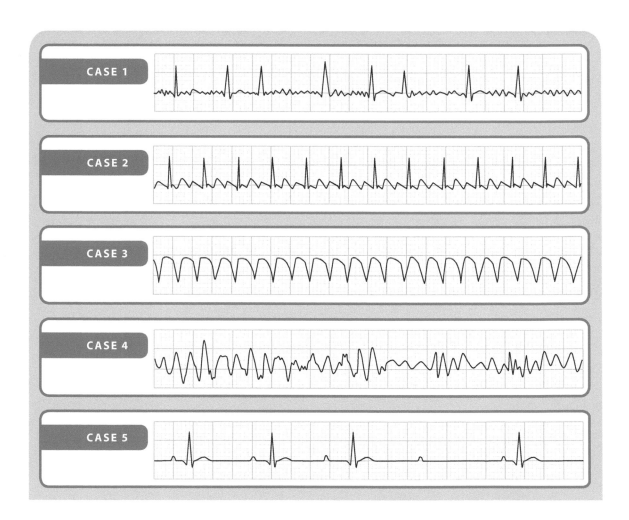

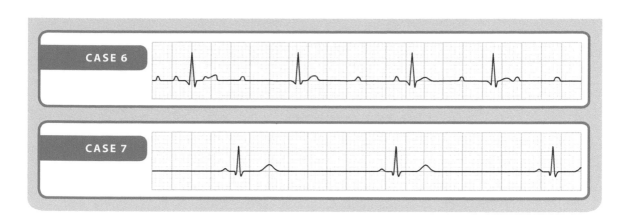

Chapter 3.7
Measuring blood glucose

What to do . . .

- Introduce yourself to the patient – establish rapport
- Ask the patient's name, age and occupation and confirm the reason why they need to have their sugar levels monitored
- Explain the procedure to the patient
- Wash your hands and ask the patient to wash their hands too
- Gather and prepare the equipment, put on gloves
- Switch on the machine and insert the corresponding test strip correctly
- Select a finger and place the lancet firmly against the skin then release the needle
- Place the drop of blood on the assembled BM test strip and glucose monitor
- Discard lancet needle into a sharps bin
- Offer patient a cotton wool ball or plaster to stop any bleeding
- Interpret the results correctly and document the reading in the log book
- Thank the patient and conclude the consultation

Glucose is an important carbohydrate that is used by the body as a vital source of energy. In healthy individuals blood glucose levels are tightly controlled and should range between 3.5 and 8 mmol/l, despite varying amounts of food and exercise, or fasting. There are a number of conditions (see *Box 3.5*) whereby this control is lost and this may result in either high sugar levels (hyperglycaemia) or low sugar levels (hypoglycaemia).

BOX 3.5 **Causes of hyperglycaemia and hypoglycaemia**

Hyperglycaemia	**Hypoglycaemia**
Diabetes	Dietary intake
Cushing's syndrome	Alcohol-induced
Pancreatitis	Drugs (sulphonylureas, insulin injection)
Pancreatic carcinoma	Insulinoma
Hyperthyroidism	
Drugs (β-blockers, thiazide diuretics, steroids, antipsychotic agents such as olanzapine)	

Table 3.4 **Reference ranges for plasma glucose levels**	
	Plasma glucose (mmol/l)
Normal	
Random	<7.8(*)
Fasting	<6.1
Diabetes mellitus	
Random	>11.1
Fasting	>7.0
Borderline ranges	
Random	7.8–11.0
Fasting (impaired fasting glycaemia**)	6.1–6.9
An **oral glucose tolerance test** (OGTT) is performed if a patient has impaired fasting glycaemia or borderline random glucose level. The patient fasts overnight and is then given 75 g of glucose. Plasma glucose levels are checked 2 hours later:	
Not diabetic	<7.8
Impaired glucose tolerance	7.8–11.0
Diabetic	>11.1

*2 hours after taking 75 g of glucose.
**Impaired glucose tolerance and impaired fasting glycaemia are risk factors for developing diabetes and cardiovascular disease in the future.

The presence of raised glucose levels (see *Table 3.4*) can be detected and monitored in a number of different ways and it is important to understand the roles each of these have to play:

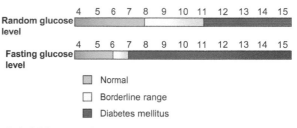

Fig 3.15 Interpreting plasma glucose levels.

- Urine dipstick provides a non-invasive screening tool to detect raised glucose levels; it is particularly useful for the diagnosis of gestational diabetes.
- Measurement of HbA1C (glycosylated haemoglobin) is helpful in assessing the average plasma glucose concentration over a prolonged period of time; it is commonly used in the monitoring of a patient's diabetic control.
- Venous plasma glucose provides the most accurate measurements for glucose levels, with fasting tests being the gold standard method of diagnosing diabetes.
- Capillary BM test (or finger prick test) offers a rapid, near-patient test that gives an accurate estimate of the patient's sugar levels.

Because of the increasing prevalence of conditions such as diabetes, the BM test is becoming more common in primary care. Patients are now given BM machines to monitor their own sugar levels and are then trusted to make simple adjustments to their own insulin doses. As a result they should be able to achieve tighter glucose control and so prevent future complications. The BM test is also useful in the acute setting and is routinely used in emergency departments. Conditions such as hyperglycaemia may mimic neurological diseases causing confusion, loss of consciousness or even fits. The BM test provides a rapid diagnostic tool (see *Fig 3.15*) to help exclude this differential in an unwell patient.

TOP TIP!

The 'BM' test refers to 'Boehringer Mannheim' which is the pharmaceutical company that manufactured the most commonly used brand of test strips for measuring blood glucose. When measuring blood glucose with a finger prick method (the 'BM' test) you are actually testing the capillary blood glucose as opposed to venous blood. Capillary blood glucose is about 7% higher than venous values.

Diabetes

Diabetes is characterized by a syndrome of disordered metabolism resulting in hyperglycaemia. Glucose levels are normally tightly controlled in the body through a complex interaction of chemicals and hormones such as insulin. Persistently raised blood glucose levels can cause a person to suffer acutely with symptoms of thirst, tiredness, polyuria and weight loss. Complications can be macrovascular in nature, such as myocardial infarctions and stroke, or microvascular in nature, such as retinopathy, neuropathy and nephropathy. These complications can be reduced with tight glucose control.

Diabetes is usually classified into three different types; type 1, type 2 and gestational.

Type 1 is associated with early onset in life due to islet cell dysfunction.

Type 2 usually occurs later in life and is largely linked to obesity and has a strong genetic component.

Medical Guidelines
Diagnosing type 2 diabetes

Type 2 diabetes should be diagnosed using the following criteria:

1. Diabetes symptoms (i.e. polyuria, polydipsia and unexplained weight loss) PLUS
   • a random venous plasma glucose concentration >11.1 mmol/l OR
   • a fasting plasma glucose concentration >7.0 mmol/l OR
   • after a positive OGTT (checked at 2 hours) >11.1 mmol/l OR

2. With no symptoms diagnosis should not be based on a single glucose determination but rather two separate measurements on different days. Raised venous plasma glucose should be shown via fasting (>7.0 mmol), from a random sample (>11.1 mmol), or from the OGTT (>11.1 mmol after 2 hours).

WHO: Definition and diagnosis of diabetes mellitus and intermediate hyperglycemia (1999)

Medical Guidelines
Self-monitoring of type 2 diabetes

- Offer self-monitoring of plasma glucose to a person newly diagnosed with type 2 diabetes only as an integral part of his or her self-management education
- Discuss the purpose of self-monitoring and agree how it should be interpreted and acted upon
- Self-monitoring of plasma glucose should be available:
  - to those on insulin treatment
  - to those on oral glucose-lowering medications to provide information on hypoglycaemia
  - to assess changes in glucose control resulting from medication and lifestyle changes
  - to monitor changes during intercurrent illness
  - to ensure safety during activities, including driving
- Assess at least annually and in a structured way:
  - self-monitoring skills
  - the quality and appropriate frequency of testing
  - the use made of the results obtained
  - the impact on quality of life
  - the continued benefit
  - the equipment used
- If self-monitoring is appropriate but blood glucose monitoring is unacceptable to the individual, discuss the use of urine glucose monitoring.

NICE Guideline: Type 2 diabetes: the management of type 2 diabetes (update) (2008)

Gestational diabetes is discovered during pregnancy and may subsequently lead to early onset type 2 diabetes.

Patients with any of the three types of diabetes may need varying levels of insulin to control their symptoms.

In insulin-dependent diabetics, regular blood monitoring is essential to prevent hypoglycaemia and permit titration of insulin doses. However, in non-insulin dependent diabetes, the role of regular BM testing is more controversial; for this reason NICE (see *Medical Guidelines* box) have offered a number of recommendations on the testing of blood glucose in diabetic patients.

3.7.1 Beginning the procedure

Start by introducing yourself to the patient, stating your name and job title. Ask the patient for their name, age and occupational status if relevant. Patients who are insulin-dependent diabetics have to inform the DVLA of their diagnosis and will be prevented from holding an LGV (large goods vehicle) or PCV (passenger carrying vehicle) licence.

Before you begin, confirm the reason why the patient needs to have their sugar levels checked. Try to establish any symptoms of hypoglycaemia such as sweating, tremor, anxiety, palpitations or symptoms of hyperglycaemia, such as polydipsia, polyuria, nausea and abdominal pain. It is also useful to ask if the patient is using insulin or any oral hypoglycaemic agents.

Explain the procedure

Explain to the patient why they need to have their glucose levels checked regularly and what the monitoring entails. You could say, for example, '*I understand that you have recently been diagnosed with diabetes and you have been given a blood glucose monitor to help keep a record of your blood sugar levels. We need to monitor your sugar levels to ensure you are responding well to your medication and that your blood glucose levels are not going too high or too low. In order to do this we need to use a handheld glucose meter. This is a simple device with an LCD screen with a port where the test strips are inserted. We will need to take a drop of blood from your finger for it to be analysed. To do this we will use a lancet to prick the side of your finger. You may feel a small scratch when the needle goes in, but it should not be too painful.*'

After you have explained the procedure to the patient, it is important to check that they have understood what you have said and given you verbal consent to proceed. At this point you may wish to offer them the opportunity to ask any questions.

Preparing the patient

Have the patient wash their hands in warm soapy water. Apart from reducing the risk of introducing an infection and inaccurate results due to contaminants, the warm water will also help dilate the capillaries and hopefully make it easier to gain a sample.

Ask the patient to sit down and relax. Take the blood sample from their non-dominant hand. Avoid using the thumb or index finger because these are used regularly for day-to-day activities. If you have to repeat the test, make sure that you choose another site or preferably another finger.

> **TOP TIP!**
>
> You are likely to be faced with a scenario in the exams in which the patient is diabetic and you are going to teach them how to use a BM monitor and explain why they need to check their blood glucose regularly.

TOP TIP!

Make sure that you have set up the machine before drawing the drop of blood from the patient's finger otherwise the sample may clot and be unreadable.

The equipment

Before you start make sure that you have washed your hands and collected all of the equipment that you will require:

- pair of gloves (non-sterile)
- sharps box (make sure it isn't full)
- cotton wool balls
- lancet device with needle
- glucometer and calibrated BM test strips
- log book

The lancet is designed to penetrate the skin only as far as needed to draw a drop of blood. Each patient will be given their own lancet with disposable sharps and a sharps bin to take home with them. Remember, there are many different types of blood glucose monitors, so ensure you have the correct BM test strip for the monitor.

3.7.2 **The procedure**

After washing your hands, put on a pair of non-sterile gloves because this procedure involves sharps as well as contact with blood. The gloves should provide an additional barrier in helping prevent a needle stick injury.

Switch the monitor on and check that it is in good working order and calibrated ready for measurement of blood glucose levels. Make sure that you select a test strip that is compatible with the glucose meter; this can be confirmed by cross-referencing the code on the test strip bottle with that on the meter.

The test strips have enzyme-impregnated reagent contained within them that must be kept in a cool, dry environment away from sunlight or excessive heat. Ensure that the strips are within date by checking the expiry date before use. Insert the strip into the machine and check that it has been accepted. Once you have inserted the strip into the meter, you should next assemble the lancet.

Assemble the lancet by inserting the needle at one end. Prime the mechanism by applying gentle pressure on the lever. Once it has been primed place it firmly against the side of the chosen finger. Make sure that you do not apply it against the pulp of the finger as this will be extremely painful for the patient. Warn the patient to expect a sharp scratch before releasing the lancet device. Gently squeeze the finger medial to the puncture site to collect a drop of blood that can be placed on the surface of the strip. Immediately dispose of the sharp within a sharps container and apply cotton wool to the finger to help stop the bleeding.

Allow time for the meter to process the sample and display the glucose level (*Fig 3.16*). If the meter displays an error it may be that the blood sample collected was too small and another one must be taken. Dispose of the strip accordingly and repeat the test using a fresh test strip and lancet needle.

Record the glucose reading in the patient's notes and log book if indicated. Interpret the measurement according to the clinical scenario.

After the patient has seen you go through the procedure, offer them the chance to demonstrate it back to you. This will help you check that they have understood everything and are competent to take a blood glucose reading on their own.

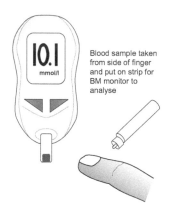

Blood sample taken from side of finger and put on strip for BM monitor to analyse

Fig 3.16 Technique for taking blood glucose reading.

Interpretation of glucose level

The glucometer provides a quick and relatively accurate estimate of the patient's glucose level. The results should not be acted on in isolation, but rather in light of the clinical context:

- in a patient presenting for the first time with symptoms suggestive of diabetes, such as polyuria, polydipsia, nocturia and weight loss, a random BM of greater than 11.1 may indicate diabetes but the patient will require a plasma glucose sample to confirm
- in a patient with established diabetes who is on treatment, BM levels of less than 3.5 with symptoms of dizziness, confusion, hunger, sweating and personality change may indicate hypoglycaemia and should warrant review of their medication and dietary practices.

3.7.3 **Summing up**

It is important that the patient knows what blood glucose level they should be aiming for and what range is abnormal. Education and patient understanding is a crucial part of successful management of diabetes. The glucometer empowers the patient by giving them control of the management of their illness. It provides near instantaneous quantitative measurement of their sugar levels and allows it to be compared with previous readings.

When summarizing back to the patient you should remind them of the importance of keeping tight glucose control. The patient should also be told when to take the blood glucose measurements and how often to record them. You may wish to say to the patient:

- *'In general the target blood glucose value we aim for in diabetic patients is 4–7 mmol/l before meals and 4–10 mmol/l after meals. Keeping a tight control of your blood sugar will reduce the risk of complications associated with diabetes. Poorly controlled diabetes can affect the large blood vessels causing increased risk of heart attacks and stroke; it can also affect the small blood vessels in the eyes, kidneys and nerves. If this happens it can affect your vision, and may eventually lead to blindness and can also affect the sense of feeling, especially of the feet, leading to you potentially being unaware of injuries to your feet.'*
- *'We usually advise newly diagnosed diabetics to start by checking their blood glucose about three times a day, before breakfast, two hours after lunch and just before bed. The results of these measurements will guide how we dose your medication so that we can effectively manage your diabetes and prevent low sugar levels occurring.'*
- *'Make sure that you record all your readings in a log book so that you can show it to your doctor or diabetic nurse who can then adjust your medications accordingly. Once your blood sugars are stable you may be able to reduce the frequency of monitoring.'*

It is important to warn the patient of the symptoms of hypoglycaemia and hyperglycaemia. 'If you begin to feel sweaty, anxious, hungry or shaky, it may be that your blood sugar is very low and you need to eat something. If you feel that you are very thirsty and passing a lot of urine, it is again important to check your blood sugar as it may be high.'

Confirm with the patient that they have understood everything they have been told and offer them the opportunity to ask any questions. Thank the patient and give them other sources of information, such as Diabetes UK (www.diabetes.org.uk), or an appointment with the diabetes specialist nurse.

3.7.4 **Common clinical scenarios**

The following are a list of common blood glucose-related scenarios which you may encounter. For each one, consider:

- what the possible differential diagnosis could be
- what key features you would look for
- what further investigations you would request to refine or confirm your diagnosis
- what the best method of treatment is

You could use role play with a friend, using the histories in the cases below as a framework.

CASE 1

You are called to the ward by a nurse because a 40 year old insulin-dependent diabetic man has become unresponsive. He has not had much to eat today because he claims that he does not like the hospital food, but you note from the drug chart that he has still received all his usual medications, including insulin. On testing the BM was found to be 1.5 mmol/l and the patient is making groaning noises; he is not able to respond to your questions or open his eyes to command.

CASE 2

A 70 year old type 2 diabetic man has been sitting in A&E for the last 3 hours waiting to be seen by a doctor about his painful, swollen ankle after a fall. He takes metformin and rosiglitazone for his diabetes. He has started to feel anxious and sweaty. When you see him he tells you he can feel his heart beating very fast and cannot stop his hands from shaking. His BM is 2.4 mmol/l and the patient is alert and communicating with you.

CASE 3

A 60 year old woman presents to her GP complaining of a 3 day history of a productive cough with green sputum and some shortness of breath. She is known to have insulin-dependent type 2 diabetes and COPD. As she has been feeling unwell she has not taken her medications as regularly as she usually does. Examination of her chest reveals inspiratory wheezes and some fine crackles in the left base. On checking her BM it is 15 mmol/l.

CASE 4

A 30 year old obese Pakistani man presents with increased frequency of nocturia and tiredness for the past few months. His BM was noted to be 16 mmol/l.

CASE 5

A known type 1 diabetic man has recently returned from holiday complaining of heavy respiration, sickness and abdominal pain. His glucometer failed to provide a reading but notes it was high.

Chapter 3.8
Urine dip testing

What to do . . .

- Introduce yourself to the patient – establish rapport
- Ask the patient's name, date of birth and occupation
- Establish the patient's symptoms and relevant medical history
- Explain the procedure to the patient including how to collect a mid-stream sample
- Collect all the equipment and check the dipstick container's expiry date
- Remove one urine dipstick and immediately reseal the container
- Fully immerse the dipstick in the urine sample for 1 second and tap off excess
- Read the urine dipstick after 60 seconds against the standardized charts
- Interpret the results in the context of the clinical situation
- Complete a Microbiology request form
- Thank the patient and answer any questions they may have

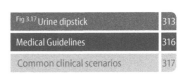

A urine dipstick is a long, thin plastic strip that is layered with several squares of chemical reagents. These reagents react to different molecules in a urine sample and change colour (see *Fig 3.17*) depending on the presence and concentration of, for example: protein, glucose, ketones, blood, leukocytes, nitrites, bilirubin and urobilinogen; they also indicate pH and specific gravity. However, not all dipsticks are the same. Some may test for all the molecules described above, and these are known as multistix, whilst others only test for single substances such as glucose, ketones or albumin.

The urine dipstick test can be performed while the patient waits as it provides nearly instantaneous results. It is useful in the detection of a number of diseases including renal stones, urinary infections, diabetes and ketoacidosis. For this reason it is a useful screening tool that plays a vital role in the initial assessment of a patient presenting to primary or secondary care.

In order to obtain accurate results it is important to follow a stringent procedure both when collecting and testing the sample. A fresh mid-stream urine specimen should be collected in a sterile container. This is because the first phase of micturition may contain bacterial contaminants that can be found on the skin which confound the culture and sensitivity.

Do not forget that urine dipsticks should only be used as an investigatory tool and should not be relied upon when making a diagnosis. An abnormal result should always be accompanied by a relevant detailed history and appropriate further investigations as necessary.

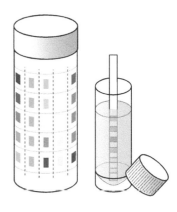

Fig 3.17 Urine dipstick.

3.8.1 **Beginning the procedure**

Ask the patient for their name and date of birth. Take a focused history from the patient to establish whether they have urinary symptoms such as dysuria (a burning sensation on passing urine), frequency, haematuria or urethral discharge. It may be useful to elicit whether the patient suffers from any chronic illness such as diabetes, renal failure or recurrent renal stones.

Ask if they are taking any prescribed medications including antibiotics; drugs such as rifampicin, metronidazole and amitriptyline are known to alter the colour of the urine sample, whilst antibiotics may affect the bacterial yield if the sample is later sent for a microbiology, culture and sensitivity (MC&S) check.

Explain the procedure

You must emphasize to the patient the importance of obtaining a sample which is as free from contamination as possible. This can be achieved by requesting the patient to firstly clean their external genitalia before micturition prior to collecting a mid-stream sample. You may wish to advise them: *'Because of the problems you are having I would like to perform a urine dipstick test. In order to prevent contamination of the sample that may give us inaccurate results, it is important that you collect the urine in a certain way. Before providing the sample, clean your genitalia thoroughly and make sure nothing touches the neck of the collection pot. Initially pass urine into the toilet and then slide the bottle into the stream and catch a mid-stream sample. Once you have finished, secure the bottle with a cap and return it to me.'*

Equipment

Before you test the urine sample, ensure that you have washed your hands thoroughly and have all the following equipment ready:
- equipment tray/kidney dish
- pair of gloves (non-sterile)
- urine sample
- paper towels
- urine dipsticks

3.8.2 **The procedure**

Put on a pair on non-sterile gloves and take the urine sample from the patient. Observe the urine for its colour and turbidity. Check the expiry date of the dipstick container and remove a single reagent strip; immediately close the container. Insert the stick into the urine sample for 1 second, ensuring that all the reagent squares are covered. Tap away the excess urine and lay it on the paper towel. Wait for 60 seconds before comparing the coloured squares against the standardized chart found on the side of the container; note that some containers may recommend different times depending on the assay concerned. Record the result(s) in the notes and dispose of the dipstick and gloves appropriately.

3.8.3 **Interpretation**

Once you have noted down the results of the dipstick and your observations, it is important that you interpret them in the context of the patient's presenting symptoms. Urine dipstick results in isolation are rarely used to make a clinical

> **TOP TIP!**
>
> Ask male patients to retract their foreskin and female patients to separate the labia before collecting a mid-stream urine sample.

> **TOP TIP!**
>
> Be aware that in an exam you may be offered a dipstick container that is past its expiry date!

> **TOP TIP!**
>
> When testing, it is vital that the strips have been kept in a cool and dry environment away from sunlight. Dipsticks that are exposed to air for prolonged periods of time may alter the reagent properties of the nitrite assay in particular, leading to false positives.

Table 3.5 **Causes of urine coloration**	
Colour	**Causes**
Orange / brown	Liver failure (bilirubinuria), metronidazole, nitrofurantoin, carrots, fava beans
Red	Frank haematuria, myoglobinuria, lead or mercury poisoning, rifampicin (pink), beetroot, rhubarb
Green or blue	Urinary tract infection (*Pseudomonas*), hypercalcaemia, biliverdin, amitriptyline
Colourless	Excessive fluid intake, diabetes insipidus, diuretics

diagnosis. If any abnormal results are found the patient should be offered further investigations such as a blood test, urine microscopy and culture, ultrasound scan or cystoscopy.

General appearance

A fresh sample of urine should be straw-coloured, transparent and free from any debris. A change in colour may indicate a disease process or may simply be due to drug or food ingestion (see *Table 3.5*).

Other features that may direct you towards a diagnosis include the smell of the urine as well as its turbidity. A change in urine consistency may be due to infection (pyuria) or hyperoxaluria (kidney stones). A foul smelling sample may indicate a urine infection or dehydration, whereas a sweet smell may suggest ketoacidosis.

Blood

One of the most important and common uses of a urine dipstick test is to detect microscopic haematuria. Haematuria is defined as the presence of more than three erythrocytes per high power field (when viewed at $400 \times$ magnification), whilst microscopic refers to the fact that the erythrocytes in haematuria cannot be seen by the naked eye. The concentration of blood in the urine is reflected by the degree of colour change in the dipstick test.

Blood in the urine can be caused by pathology anywhere along the urinary tract and can be classified as:
- renal – causes include glomerulonephritis, IgA nephropathy, interstitial nephritis, polycystic kidney disease and renal cancer
- extra-renal – causes include urinary tract infection, kidney stones, hypertension, and sickle cell disease.

Do not forget that trauma, severe dehydration, haemoglobinuria, myoglobinuria and menstruation can also produce a positive result.

Although startling to find, only around 5% of patients with microscopic haematuria are later found to have underlying pathology. It is important to take into account the patient's age, gender and symptoms before considering the need for further assessment (see also *Medical Guidelines* box).
- Painless haematuria in an elderly patient should warrant further investigation to exclude renal tract tumour.
- Microscopic haematuria with severe colicky pain may be suggestive of renal stones.

- Proteinuria in conjunction with haematuria may be caused by a urinary tract infection or glomerulonephritis.

Protein

The presence of protein in the urine is known as proteinuria – this is almost never detected in a fit and healthy individual. If proteinuria is suggested, it may indicate a urinary tract infection, pre-eclampsia or intrinsic kidney dysfunction such as renovascular, glomerular or tubulo-interstitial disease. A patient with persistent proteinuria should be investigated further with MC&S, serum urea and electrolytes as well as a 24-hour urinary protein collection.

Patients with chronic kidney disease and significant proteinuria may require specialist input. In patients with diabetes it is better to check for microalbuminuria.

Nitrites and leukocytes

The nitrites test, in conjunction with the leukocyte esterase test, are the most useful to identify urinary tract infections. Because of the test's high specificity, positive nitrites usually indicate the presence of significant amounts of bacteria in the urine, with Gram-negative rods such as *E. coli* being most commonly implicated. However, negative nitrites do not exclude a UTI due to its lower sensitivity levels.

The leukocyte esterase test detects bacterial pyuria usually produced by neutrophils. A positive test may suggest a UTI. However, contamination from vaginal discharge, such as with chlamydia, may give a false positive result. The leukocyte esterase test has a high sensitivity but a low specificity and so a negative result cannot exclude the presence of infection. However, a positive nitrite test in addition to a positive leukocyte esterase test is an excellent indicator for a UTI. If in doubt, a urine sample should be sent to the lab for MC&S.

Glucose and ketones

The glomeruli are very efficient in reabsorbing glucose and preventing it from entering the urine; thus in a normal healthy person, the urine dipstick test should be negative for glucose. However, glucose can enter the urine when the renal threshold has been exceeded (above 10 mmol/l), most notably due to diabetes. The urine dipstick test is specific for glucose only and does not test for other sugars such as galactose and fructose (these are tested for, particularly in neonates, using the modified Benedict's test).

The discovery of glucose in the urine can be useful in establishing diabetes in a symptomatic patient. However, a positive urine dipstick test for glucose should not be used in isolation to diagnose diabetes: a fasting blood glucose test should be offered to all patients with noticeable glycosuria. Other causes of glycosuria include pregnancy, Cushing's disease and pancreatitis as well as intrinsic kidney disease such as acute glomerulonephritis and nephrotic syndrome.

Ketones are also not usually present in the urine sample. Ketones are the by-product of fat metabolism and are seen in starvation, high protein diets (or crash dieting) or diabetes. It is a useful qualitative indicator for admitting vulnerable patients such as children, pregnant women and the elderly suffering with dehydration and vomiting.

pH

Urine is usually acidic (ranges from a pH of 4.5 to 7) due to the body's metabolism. It is regulated by the renal tubules that reabsorb sodium and secrete hydrogen and ammonium. The urine becomes more acidic due to diet (meat), dehydration and diabetic ketoacidosis (DKA). In patients with renal stones due to uric acid, cystine or calcium oxalate, more acidic urine is also likely to be found.

Alkaline urine can be caused by diet (vegan), chronic renal failure or renal tubular acidosis. Bacterial UTIs commonly cause alkaline urine due to the bacterial urease enzymes converting urea into ammonia. In addition, staghorn stones such as calcium phosphate and carbonate are readily precipitated in alkaline urine.

Specific gravity

Urine specific gravity measures the concentration of molecules in urine. It normally ranges between 1.003 and 1.030. Lower values indicate urinary dilution such as in diabetes insipidus, renal failure and excessive fluid intake. On the other hand, raised specific gravity suggests urinary concentration that may be due to shock, dehydration and SIADH. Patients with glycouria or ketouria usually have raised specific gravity.

3.8.4 Finishing up

Labelling the specimen

Ensure that you label the urine collection pot clearly and legibly with the patient's name, date of birth, hospital number, and the date the sample was taken. Cross-reference these details with the urine request form and check that the urine MC&S box has been ticked and relevant clinical details have been provided. Do not forget to mention on the form any antibiotics the patient is taking as this information will be useful to the Microbiologist.

Check that your name and contact details are left on the form. Place the urine sample in the pouch attached to the form, ensuring that you have sealed it before dispatching it to the lab.

3.8.5 Common clinical scenarios

The following are a list of common urine dipstick scenarios which you may encounter. For each one, consider:
- what the possible differential diagnosis could be
- what key features you would look for
- what further investigations you would request to refine or confirm your diagnosis.

CASE 1
A 30 year old man complains of sudden onset of colicky abdominal pain radiating to the groin. You find 4+ blood on the dipstick and urinary pH is 7.5.

CASE 2
An 18 year old woman with dysuria and frequency. The dipstick shows positive nitrites and 2+ leukocytes.

CASE 3
A 28 year old woman who is 32 weeks pregnant is noted to have raised blood pressure and 2+ proteinuria.

CASE 4
A 16 year old boy complains of generalized abdominal pain and nausea and vomiting with polydipsia and polyuria. Urine shows 3+ glucose and 3+ ketones.

CASE 5
A 25 year old man attends his GP on a hot day. His 'new patient check' urinary dipstick shows 1+ ketones.

CASE 6
A 35 year old Afro-Caribbean man attends A&E complaining of intermittent sweats and chronic cough. His urine colour is noted to be pink.

Chapter 3.9
Venepuncture

What to do . . .

- Introduce yourself to the patient – establish rapport
- Confirm the patient's name, date of birth and check why they are having their blood taken
- Explain the procedure to the patient and obtain verbal consent
- Identify the tests required from the blood form and any associated requirements, e.g. fasting status
- Gather and prepare the equipment and put on gloves
- Select a vein in the antecubital fossa by palpation after applying tourniquet
- Clean selected site with alcohol wipe and leave to air dry
- Steady vein with left hand and insert needle keeping an angle of 30 degrees with bevelled edge upwards
- Observe for flashback and release tourniquet – withdraw sufficient volume of blood into the syringe
- Withdraw needle and dispose of in sharps box
- Place a gauze or cotton wool ball over puncture site and apply gentle pressure
- Attach new needle on syringe and fill the test bottles in correct order
- Dispose of needle and syringe in sharps container
- Dispose of gloves and waste material appropriately

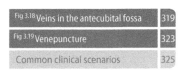
Venepuncture is the process by which a needle is inserted into a vein in order to draw blood; it is one of the most common medical procedures performed. The blood that is taken is sent to haematology and biochemistry laboratories for processing and the results provide information on: blood count, infection and inflammatory response, and kidney and liver function. The results can be compared against standardized values, allowing any organ dysfunction to be noted.

You must become fully competent in venepuncture, but as a junior doctor you will be given plenty of chance to practise! Venepuncture on a manikin may give you an idea of how to perform it successfully, but the key to mastering this skill is continuous practice on real life patients.

Anatomy

The most common site for taking blood is the antecubital fossa in the forearm. This is because the veins located there are large, have wide lumina and thick walls and are less sensitive to pain. There are three

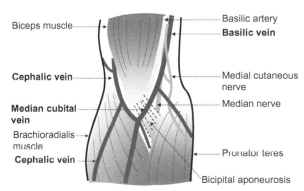

Fig 3.18 Veins in the antecubital fossa.

veins in the antecubital fossa that are most appropriate for venepuncture. They include the median cubital vein, cephalic vein, and the basilic vein (*Fig 3.18*). The first choice vein for venepuncture is the median cubital vein. It arises from the cephalic vein and runs obliquely to drain into the basilic vein. It is the most prominent vein in the forearm and is well anchored, preventing displacement upon needle insertion. In addition, the vein is surrounded by fewer nerve endings, offering the chance of a less painful puncture.

If the median cubital vein is unavailable, then the second choice for venepuncture is the cephalic vein. This runs superficially across the outer aspect of the arm and lies lateral to the biceps muscle.

In the event that your preferred choices of veins are inaccessible, you should move on to the basilic vein. This vein ascends from the hand along the medial surface of the forearm. It passes along the medial margin of the biceps muscle before crossing the brachial artery as well as branches of the median nerve. Because of its anatomy, there may be an increased risk of puncturing the brachial artery in addition to causing damage to the median nerve.

If you are unable to locate any of these veins or have failed to draw blood, then you may wish to consider the metacarpal veins located on the dorsal surface of the hands.

Sites to avoid in venepuncture

There are certain cases where you should avoid performing venepuncture on a specific arm.

- If a patient has an IV cannula *in situ*, taking blood from the same arm may lead to inaccurate results, because the blood sample will be affected by the fluid composition contained within the drip.
- Avoid taking blood from the same limb as an arterio-venous fistula in a dialysis patient. The fistula is an artificial communication between an artery and vein reserved for quick access for dialysis and any damage to this may affect the patient's ability to be dialysed.
- In stroke patients, do not take blood from the affected limb. This is because they may lack sensation in that area and as a result you may inadvertently cause damage to the surrounding structures.

Other situations where you should avoid taking blood from a specific site include an oedematous post-mastectomy arm, areas of inflammation or infection (phlebitis, severe eczema), or a haematoma.

3.9.1 **Beginning the examination**

Start by introducing yourself to the patient, stating your name and job title. Confirm the patient's name and date of birth to ensure that you draw blood from the correct person. This will also help you complete the patient's identifier details on the blood form before sending off the sample.

Check if the patient is well and not in any discomfort before proceeding with the procedure. In the exam situation, you are more likely to be presented with a simulated manikin arm in lieu of a real patient. In such circumstances, treat the manikin as if it were a patient, maintaining your standards of professional courtesy and rapport building.

It may be useful before you begin to confirm the reason why the patient is having the blood test so that you can correctly identify the appropriate blood bottles as well as determine the right time the sample should be taken:

- a fasting glucose or cholesterol requires the patient to fast from midnight with blood taken first thing in the morning
- blood tests for an early morning cortisol measurement should only be performed at 9 am.

Explain the procedure

Explain to the patient what you intend to do using simple language that the patient will understand. Venepuncture is a procedure that may cause pain to the patient and, although most patients may have had an injection in the past, not all have had blood taken from them. It is therefore important that you explain the procedure clearly and gain verbal consent to proceed. You may wish to say: *'I understand that you have come today to have some blood taken. It is a short and simple procedure. I will be using a syringe and needle to take blood from your forearm. You may feel a sharp scratch when the needle enters the vein, but this shouldn't be too painful.'*

Preparation

Ask the patient to remove any clothes that may obstruct access to the antecubital fossa. If the patient is wearing a shirt, it may be sufficient simply to ask them to roll up their sleeve. It is usually sensible to select the non-dominant arm to take blood from because there may be some residual discomfort after the procedure.

Ensure that the patient is either sitting or lying comfortably. Some patients may faint when blood is taken and, if they think this is possible, it is recommended that they lie down for the procedure. Rest the arm either on a table or pillow for the patient's comfort. Have them fully extend the arm and lower it below the level of the heart to help the veins fill and improve venous access.

Equipment

Before you start, make sure that you have washed your hands and collected all of the equipment that you will require. Check the request form to see what tests have been ordered and select the corresponding blood bottles. You will need the following equipment:

- tray/kidney dish
- pair of gloves (non-sterile)
- 21G needle (green)
- tourniquet
- syringe (20 ml) or Vacutainer needle holder (see *Box 3.6*)
- Vacutainer blood bottles (purple/yellow top, etc.)
- sharps box (make sure it is not full)
- cotton wool balls
- tape/ plaster
- alcohol swab

> **TOP TIP!**
>
> Make sure you position the sharps box no more than an arm's length away from you and in a position which means that you do not have to lean across the patient with the used needle.

Selecting the vein

Place a tourniquet around the patient's upper arm around the lower border of the biceps muscle. Use a suitable tourniquet with a quick release mechanism so that the arm can be freed instantly when needed. It is becoming more common to have disposable tourniquets on the ward as it is believed to reduce cross-contamination

---

BOX 3.6 **Vacutainer system**

Vacutainers are becoming a common sight on wards and are slowly replacing the standard barrel syringe and needle as a way to take blood samples. The system employs a vacuum to automatically draw blood from the vein and fill the blood bottles directly. The Vacutainer is a container that has an internal needle with a rubber sleeve in which the blood tubes are inserted as well as an external mouthpiece to which a needle can be attached.

They help to reduce the chance of a needle stick injury and they take less time than conventional methods because blood bottles can be filled directly from the system. Once the technique has been mastered it is often found to be more efficient and less fiddly than the classic syringe. However, it does have some disadvantages that include the lack of flashback, which makes it difficult for the physician to know if they have successfully entered the vein or not, as well as reports that the vacuum system causes haemolysis.

Using the Vacutainer
Attach a 21G sheathed needle to the mouth end of the Vacutainer. Rest a blood sample bottle in the container without puncturing it with the internal needle. Unsheath the needle and insert it into the vein with the bevel pointing upwards. Sense for a change in resistance as you pass the needle through the skin and into the lumen of the vessel. Once in place, use your thumb to push in the blood bottle into the internal needle. Allow it to fill automatically and remove once sufficient blood has been collected. Keep the Vacutainer system stable as you continue to replace the bottle with another one. Once finished, remove the final bottle before withdrawing the needle and disposing of the container and the needle into the sharps box.

---

rates between patients. Make sure you tighten it sufficiently to allow the veins to fill but not to compromise arterial supply. Check with the patient that they are comfortable with the tourniquet in place and that it is not on too tight.

Glance over at the patient's antecubital fossa looking for a vein to bleed. As discussed before, your preference should begin with the median cubital vein, followed by the cephalic and then the basilic vein. Palpate the vein using your index finger and identify the position and direction in which the vein runs. The vein should feel firm and bouncy. Make sure it does not have a pulse, in which case it is an artery and this should be avoided.

If you are finding it difficult to find a vein there are a number of techniques that you may wish to employ to help improve venous access. Gently tap over the area to release local histamines that cause vasodilation and make the veins more prominent. It may also be helpful to ask the patient to clench and release their fist a few times in the ipsilateral hand. This process will cause muscles to contract and relax, acting as a pump to force blood into the veins. If, despite your efforts, the veins remain elusive, you may try immersing the area in hot water or applying a warm compress. The heat generated induces vasodilation and should bring the veins to the fore. If all else fails, the application of a local GTN patch or cream should generate a similar effect.

3.9.2 **The procedure**

Wear a pair of non-sterile gloves. It is important to remember that all blood, like bodily fluids, should be considered potentially infectious and handled accordingly.

TOP TIP!

The tourniquet should not be left on for more than a minute, as blood will become static. Also if the tourniquet is too tight and the arterial circulation is obstructed, then the flow of blood into the sample tube will be impaired. Release the tourniquet immediately if you notice the patient's arm going blue!

TOP TIP!

You should be aware that fist clenching with venous occlusion can cause pseudohyperkalaemia (a falsely raised potassium measurement) and could potentially mask hypokalaemia in the patient.

Take an alcohol swab and wipe over the vein with a single stroke. Allow the area to air dry before proceeding. There has been much discussion about the role of alcohol swabs in venepuncture. Although evidence indicates that swabbing reduces bacteria on the surface of the skin, there is little evidence to suggest that it reduces subsequent phlebitis or infection. However, most people still advocate its use.

Attach a green hypodermic needle to the syringe and carefully unsheathe the cap. Once unsheathed, ensure that you keep the needle sterile and prevent contamination from the local environment. You are now ready to draw blood.

Inserting the needle

Try to anchor the chosen vein with the thumb of your non-dominant hand, a few centimetres below the site of the needle entry. This will help tether the vein and prevent it from rolling away.

Remind the patient that they may feel a sharp scratch and then insert the needle (bevel pointed up) into the vein at an angle of 30 degrees to the patient's arm (*Fig 3.19*). Try to perform this task with a swift and smooth motion to prevent prolonged discomfort.

Insert the needle steadily until you see a flashback in the neck of the needle. This will indicate that you are correctly located in the vein. If you do not see flashback, continue to advance or retract it until it is achieved. Avoid moving the needle sideways as this will cause undue pain and may induce a haematoma.

Once the needle is in the vein, stabilize the syringe between your index finger and thumb. Release the tourniquet before using your non-dominant hand to slowly draw back on the plunger. Pull back with an adequate force such that blood fills the barrel of the syringe at a moderate speed. Excessive force may cause the blood to haemolyse within the needle.

Removing the needle

Once you have collected enough blood to adequately fill the sample bottles, withdraw the needle whilst applying a cotton wool ball or gauze over the puncture site. Immediately dispose of the needle in the sharps box. Never re-sheath a used needle as this may lead to a needle stick injury.

Apply digital pressure over the wound site for 30 seconds to ensure haemostasis. Check that bleeding has stopped and that no haematoma has formed. Warn the patient to watch out for other complications such as bruising, phlebitis or superficial cellulitis. Stick a plaster over the puncture site before completing the procedure.

Filling the blood bottles

Connect a fresh needle to the syringe and proceed to fill the appropriate blood bottles as requested on the blood form. When doing so, it is important that you fill the blood collection bottles in a particular order to prevent the cross-contamination of additives between the tubes (see *Table 3.6*). It is recommended that tubes be drawn in the following order if all such tests are required:
- blood culture bottles
- light blue (coagulation)
- yellow or red (if available)
- green, purple and grey top (glucose).

> **TOP TIP!**
>
> Once you have cleaned the area you must not palpate the vein again, so make sure you know where it is!

> **TOP TIP!**
>
> Try using a green needle when taking blood as larger gauges may cause sample haemolysis.

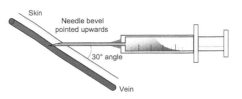

Fig 3.19 Venepuncture.

> **TOP TIP!**
>
> If you feel you punctured at the wrong site, remove the needle completely and start again; never re-introduce the needle once it has been partially withdrawn.

Table 3.6 Blood bottles and their indications

Tube colour	Tube type	Use	Instructions
	Sodium citrate	Coagulation screen, APTT, D-dimer, INR, thrombophilia screen, anticardiolipins	Must be completely filled (often 1.8 ml required); invert 3–4 times
	Sodium citrate ESR	ESR	Full bottle
	Serum separator tube (SST)	Endocrine tests (TFT, FSH , LH), LFTs, urea and electrolytes, lipid serology, immunology and virology, maternal screening, Paul–Bunnell test, tumour markers	Invert 5–6 times
	Heparin and plasma separating tube (PST)	Carboxyhaemoglobin, methaemoglobin, cytogenetics	Invert 8–10 times
	EDTA	Full blood count, plasma, B_{12} and RBC, folate, sickle cell screen, PCR, HbA1c, electrophoresis	Should be at least half full; invert 8–10 times
	EDTA / cross match	Blood group / cross-match	Must be labelled correctly with patient's details; invert 8–10 times
	Fluoride oxalate	Glucose	Invert 8–10 times

APTT – activated partial thromboplastin time; EDTA - ethylenediaminetetraacetic acid; ESR – erythrocyte sedimentation rate; FSH – follicle-stimulating hormone; INR – International Normalized Ratio; LFTs – liver function test; LH – luteinizing hormone; PCR – polymerase chain reaction; RBC – red blood cells; TFT – thyroid function test.

Make sure the blood sample is mixed sufficiently with the additive in the tube by inverting it 8–10 times (except for the sodium citrate bottle which should only be inverted 3–4 times). Do not vigorously shake because this can cause haemolysis and affect the sample.

Dispose of the needle and syringe in the sharps box and remove your gloves. Dispose of any waste in the appropriate disposal bin.

Label the bottles

Ensure that you label the bottles clearly and legibly with the patient's name, date of birth, hospital number, and the date and time the sample was taken, and sign it. Cross-reference these details with the blood form and check that all parts of the form have been completed. It is important to include relevant clinical details on the form otherwise some more expensive tests may not be performed by the lab, for example troponin, D-dimers, HbA1c, and some specific antibody tests.

Check that your name and bleep number are left on the blood form so that you can be contacted urgently by the laboratory for any grossly abnormal results. Place all the blood bottles into the pouch attached to the back of the form, ensuring that you have sealed it before dispatching it to the lab.

3.9.3 **Finishing up**

It is the duty of the physician who requested the blood tests to check if they are abnormal and to act accordingly. If they are all normal, inform and reassure the patient of the results.

In cases of abnormal results you should interpret them according to the clinical context of the patient. Often the patient will be concerned about their blood results and it is important not to be dismissive of their worries.

3.9.4 **Common clinical scenarios**

The following are a list of scenarios of patients presenting with different medical symptoms. Read the cases carefully and determine which coloured bottle would be most helpful in aiding the diagnosis.

CASE 1
A 48 year old obese man presents to his GP complaining of a 3 month history of nocturia, excessive thirst and tiredness.

CASE 2
A 70 year old woman presents with poor vision in her left eye. She has also been experiencing headaches, pain in her jaw on chewing food for a long time, central muscle tiredness and trigger points on her shoulder. On examination she has tenderness on palpation of the scalp and a pulseless temporal artery.

CASE 3
A 35 year old woman has been complaining of generalized lethargy. She used to be very fit and now gets breathless going up a flight of stairs. For the last 6 months she has been experiencing very heavy periods. On examination her conjunctiva and mucous membranes are very pale.

CASE 4
A 50 year old man presents to his GP complaining of abdominal distension. During the consultation the GP notices that he can smell alcohol on his breath and the patient appears unkempt. Examination reveals yellow sclera, spider naevi, a distended abdomen consistent with ascites and caput medusa. He is also tender in the right upper quadrant.

CASE 5
A 62 year old woman who had a mechanical heart valve fitted years ago, has noticed that recently she has been bruising very easily and now has very large bruises all over her body. She cannot recall any trauma which could have caused these and she is worried.

CASE 6
A 40 year old woman arrives in your clinic complaining of fatigue and hair loss over the last few months. She has recently felt depressed and wishes to be started on medication. On examination, she is hypotensive, and bradycardic with hypo-reflexia.

Chapter 3.10
Blood cultures

What to do . . .

- Introduce yourself to the patient – establish rapport
- Confirm the patient's name, date of birth and relevant history
- Explain the procedure to the patient
- Gather and prepare equipment including the correct blood culture bottles (pair)
- Wash hands and put on gloves
- Select a vein in the antecubital fossa by palpation after applying tourniquet
- Clean selected site with alcohol wipe and leave to air dry
- Remove cap from anaerobic culture bottle and clean with alcohol wipe and allow to air dry; repeat process with a fresh alcohol swab for the aerobic bottle
- Take blood from the patient, drawing up between 15 and 20 ml of blood
- Apply fresh needle and fill anaerobic bottle with 5–10 ml, then replace the needle and fill the aerobic bottle with a similar volume
- Discard clinical waste appropriately
- Label bottles and complete forms
- Thank the patient and answer any questions they may have

The culturing of blood is a useful investigatory test employed when patients show signs of sepsis. It involves taking a sample of blood from the patient and culturing it in either an aerobic or anaerobic environment. It is later analysed under a microscope by a Microbiologist looking for the presence of microbes and sensitivities to common antibiotics.

Blood cultures are not routinely performed unless there is some clinical indication to do so; usually a patient's clinical condition, presenting complaint and past medical history should be taken into account. Patients with a focal infection which later presents with systemic signs that include a raised temperature, sweating, chills and rigors, tachycardia, tachypnoea, hypotension, in addition to a raised white cell count, should have a blood culture because these signs may indicate a spread of infection into the bloodstream (septicaemia).

It is often assumed that blood cultures can only detect bacteria in the blood. However, a wide variety of microorganisms including mycobacteria, viruses, mould and yeast can be detected, depending on the type of medium used.

The most commonly used bottles test for aerobic and anaerobic bacteria. Aerobes are those bacteria that require oxygen to grow, whereas anaerobes grow without it. For this reason blood culture bottles come as a pair with blood samples needing to be added to both.

Maximizing the yield of blood cultures

When taking blood for culturing, there are a number of factors that may improve the yield of microorganisms produced from the sample.

- *Timing* – when blood cultures are taken is important. They should be taken as soon as bacteraemia (bacteria in the blood) is suspected, with some recommending that they should be taken when the patient first develops a temperature.
- *Antibiotics* – samples for culture should be taken before antibiotics have been initiated. This improves the likelihood of identifying and isolating the offending organism. If antibiotics have already been started, this does not preclude the need for blood cultures, but the Microbiologist should be informed of the antibiotic agent used.
- *Site* – one set of blood cultures taken from a single site at one time may not be adequate. It is often recommended that two or more samples from different sites at different times should be obtained in order to improve the chances of isolating the causative organism. Certain conditions necessitate the need to take more blood cultures; for example, in endocarditis it is advisable to take at least three blood cultures from different sites within 24 hours of admission.

Interpreting results

Once blood samples have been taken and sent to the lab for culturing, a preliminary report is provided within two days. This provides brief information on the type of organism found, detailing whether it is Gram-positive or Gram-negative, as well its type, e.g. rods or cocci. A more comprehensive report normally follows within 3–5 days stating the specific organism found as well as its sensitivities to various antibiotics.

Due to the relatively long time it takes for the final results to be available, patients who are unwell are usually started on broad spectrum antibiotics by the admitting physician. Once the blood culture results are provided, the antibiotic would be reassessed and usually changed to a more specific one.

If blood culture results come back positive for an organism, this may not necessarily mean that the patient's symptoms are caused by it. There are numerous microbes that exist on the surface of people's skin, known as commensal organisms (or normal flora), that may contaminate the blood culture sample if an aseptic technique was not strictly observed.

> **TOP TIP!**
>
> The key to avoiding contaminants in blood culture bottles is an aseptic technique.

3.10.1 Beginning the procedure

Start by introducing yourself to the patient, stating your name and job title. Confirm the patient's name and date of birth and check against the blood culture form. Try to establish any relevant clinical information from the patient such as pyrexia, sweating, chills and rigors as well as noting their vital signs. Also ask about any antibiotics they are currently taking as well as any drug allergies. This information will be useful for the Microbiologist when completing the blood culture request form.

Check that the patient is comfortable and not in any obvious pain before proceeding. You are likely to have a manikin's arm in the examination, but remember to treat it as if you were dealing with a real patient.

Explain the procedure

Explain to the patient the reasons why you would like to take blood from them using language they will understand. As for venepuncture, let the patient know that the procedure maybe a little painful. You may wish to say: *'As you know, you have been suffering from a fever and this may mean that you have an infection. We would like to take a sample of blood which would be sent to the lab to be analysed for any microorganisms. The procedure is the same as taking blood for a blood test and may be a little painful when we insert the needle into your vein.'*

Preparation

Ensure that the patient is comfortable and that you have good access to the arms.

Equipment

Wash your hands thoroughly and collect the appropriate equipment. Make sure that you choose the correct blood culture bottles for the procedure. Bear in mind that separate blood culture bottles exist for virology as well as for paediatric cases. You should collect:
- tray/kidney dish
- pair of gloves (non-sterile)
- 21G needle (green) × 3
- tourniquet
- syringe (20 ml)
- pair of blood culture bottles (anaerobic and aerobic)
- alcohol swabs × 3
- sharps box (make sure it is not full)
- cotton wool balls and alcohol wipe
- tape/plaster

3.10.2 The procedure

Select and clean the site

After deciding which arm you will take the cultures from (opt for the non-dominant arm if possible), apply a disposable tourniquet 10 cm above the chosen vein. Select a vein in the antecubital fossa by palpation, as described in *Chapter 3.9*. You should not take blood from an existing central or peripheral cannula, unless it is the central line that is thought to be the source of bacteraemia. Blood should also not be taken from veins which lie very close to any cannulas because of the risk of contamination.

Once you have selected the vein you must disinfect the area thoroughly to prevent any flora from the patient's skin entering and contaminating the blood culture bottles. This is done by wiping the area with an alcohol wipe in a circular motion, starting from the centre and working outwards. Allow the area to air dry for around 30 seconds. Do not re-palpate the vein after swabbing.

Prepare the blood culture bottles

While you are waiting for the area to dry you should prepare the blood culture bottles. Check that the bottles have not expired or been tampered with. Remove the caps by flicking off the protective seal on the top of the bottle. To reduce the risk of contamination, use an alcohol swab to disinfect the top with a single swiping motion, then discard the swab and repeat the process for the other bottle.

Venepuncture

Having prepared the blood culture bottles you are now ready to take blood from the patient. Wash your hands and put on a pair of non-sterile gloves. Using the same technique as described in the venepuncture chapter (*Chapter 3.9*), draw between 15 and 20 ml of blood which will be divided equally between the two bottles.

> **TOP TIP!**
>
> Remember that blood culture bottles are the first to be collected so fill them before any other blood samples.

Filling the blood culture bottles

Once you have collected your blood sample, dispose of the needle safely in the sharps box. Attach a new sterile needle to the end of the syringe and inject between 5 and 10 ml of blood into the anaerobic bottle (coloured red) first. Make sure that you do not aspirate any air into this bottle.

Replace the green needle, again ensuring that you dispose of it correctly. Inject a further 5 to 10 ml of blood into the aerobic bottle (coloured blue) to complete the procedure. Inoculating more than 10 ml or less than 5 ml of blood can affect the ratio of blood to culture medium and give rise to false negative results.

> **TOP TIP!**
>
> Unlike in venepuncture where you invert the tubes, blood culture bottles should be rotated in the palms of your hands to thoroughly mix the blood with the culture medium.

It is important that the anaerobic bottle is always filled first to reduce the risk of oxygen being aspirated into it and affecting the sample.

Dispose of any blood-soiled material or any sharps into the relevant containers, then remove your gloves and wash your hands with soap and water.

Label the bottles and fill in the Microbiology request form

The blood culture bottles must be clearly labelled with the patient's name, date of birth and hospital number as well as the date and time the sample was taken. Complete the Microbiology form using the same details and ensure that you signed it and provided your bleep number for future contact. Tick the MC&S (microscopy, culture and sensitivity) box, documenting that it is a blood culture sample. Fill in the clinical details section with as much relevant information as possible. If the patient is currently taking any antibiotics, record clearly on the form what they are.

Once you have done this, place the culture bottles into the pouch attached to the request form and send to the Microbiology lab for analysis.

3.10.3 **Finishing up**

Once you have taken the patient's blood culture samples, do not forget to record this in the notes. It is also important to mention what site the culture was taken from so that when repeat samples are drawn they may be taken from another location.

Advise the patient that preliminary results will be available within 48 hours, but that definitive results may take up to 5 days. Answer any questions that the patient may have.

Chapter 3.11
Cannulation and IV infusion

What to do . . .

- Introduce yourself to the patient – establish rapport
- Confirm the patient's name and date of birth
- Explain the procedure to the patient
- Gather and prepare equipment, put on gloves
- Select a vein by palpation after applying tourniquet
- Clean selected site with alcohol wipe and leave to air dry
- Steady vein with left hand and insert cannula, keeping angle around 30 degrees with bevelled edge upwards
- Once there is flashback, advance the cannula and needle looking for a second flashback
- Release tourniquet and place gentle pressure over the vein near the cannula; remove the needle and discard into sharps bin; attach Luer lock cap to end of cannula
- Secure cannula with sticker and flush with 5 ml of normal saline
- Confirm IV fluids to be given by checking the drug chart
- Inspect bag for damage and also check its expiry date
- Close clamp on giving set and insert into fluid bag portal
- Squeeze fluid chamber until half full and open the clamp to expel any air bubbles; close clamp when complete
- Attach giving set to the end of the cannula and open the clamp; ensure there is no extravasation of fluid
- Date and sign the drug chart for fluid administration as well as the sticker over the cannula
- Thank the patient and check whether they have any questions

Inserting an IV cannula and setting up a drip is an important skill to master because it allows access to the veins for the administration of fluids, blood or medication. In the acute setting, securing venous access is crucial and follows on immediately after securing a patient's airway and breathing. This is because a patient brought in unconscious is unable to take anything orally and is therefore fully dependent on IV access to maintain hydration and electrolyte balance, and perhaps to receive life-saving treatment.

An IV cannula is a fine plastic tube; one end is covered with a small white cap that can be removed for a giving set to be attached, whilst at the other end is an exposed needle. The trunk of the cannula contains flexible wings which act as an aid when locating it in addition to being a raised injection

Table 3.7 Maximum flow rates through IV cannulas		
Cannula colour	**Gauge**	**Flow rate (ml/min)**
Yellow	24G	23
Blue	22G	36
Pink	20G	65
Green	18G	95
White	17G	142
Grey	16G	200
Orange	14G	305

port that allows for flushing and the administration of medication (see *Fig 3.20*).

Cannulas come in a range of different sizes and corresponding colours (*Table 3.7*). Their sizes are often described in 'gauges' whereby a lower gauge indicates a cannula with a wider diameter. They follow Poiseuille's law which states that the flow rate of a fluid through a tube is proportional to the fourth power of the luminar radius – effectively this means that the larger the cannula lumen, the faster fluid can pass through it. Hence larger cannulas (14–16G) are ideal in the resuscitation setting, whilst smaller cannulas (22–24G) are more suited for a paediatric and neonatal setting. Beware that the lower gauge cannulas use a larger bore needle and are therefore likely to cause more pain to the patient.

3.11.1 Beginning the procedure

Start by introducing yourself to the patient, stating your name and job title. Confirm the patient's name and date of birth. Try to establish why the patient needs a cannula as this may give you an idea as to what gauge should be used. If in doubt and the patient is well and stable, a pink 20G cannula should suffice.

In an OSCE you are likely to be presented with a simulated manikin arm in lieu of a real patient, but you should still act courteously towards it as if you were talking to and treating a human being. It is good practice to ask the patient whether they are right- or left-handed and whether they would prefer a specific arm to be used. Remember to avoid using an arm with an AV fistula, one that is paralysed or the ipsilateral arm post-mastectomy.

Explain the procedure

Explain to the patient the procedure you intend to perform and why it is necessary. Most patients can be quite apprehensive when seeing a cannula for the first time. Many assume that the full length of the needle will be left in their vein and the whole process will be extremely painful. It is important that you try to allay their fears by explaining that the needle simply acts as a guide to scratch the skin and gain access to the vein before being removed and disposed of. You may wish to say: *'I would like to insert a cannula into one of your veins so that we can treat your dehydration by giving you some fluids. A cannula is a small plastic tube that carries a needle. The needle is there simply to scratch the skin and find a vein. Once the tube is inserted the needle is removed and discarded. You may feel a small prick when the needle goes in but the whole process should not be too painful.'*

After you have explained the procedure to the patient, check that the patient is happy to give consent to proceed.

Preparation

Ensure that the patient is either sitting or lying down comfortably. It may be an idea to rest the patient's arm on a pillow to help them relax. Ensure that you have good lighting before starting and that you yourself are positioned comfortably.

Choose an appropriate site for the cannula to be inserted. This often depends on the clinical situation. In the resuscitation setting, large bore cannulas are usually located in both antecubital fossae (see *Fig 3.18* in *Chapter 3.9*). For routine fluids the cannula should ideally be placed in the dorsum of the hand as this is more comfortable for the patient and is less likely to catch on their clothing or to kink.

> **TOP TIP!**
>
> Except in a resuscitation setting, try to avoid the antecubital fossa when inserting a cannula as it will be uncomfortable for the patient and also obstruct the flow of fluid when the patient bends their elbow.

Equipment

Before you start, wash your hands and assemble together all the equipment that you require. Collect sufficient number of cannulas in case you are unsuccessful in your first attempts. Always prepare the equipment before you apply the tourniquet to prevent any discomfort for the patient. You need the following:

- equipment tray/kidney dish
- pair of gloves (non-sterile)
- cannula (pink or grey depending on the clinical scenario)
- tourniquet
- sharps box (make sure it is not full)
- cotton wool balls or gauze swab (in case the cannulation fails or blood spills)
- alcohol wipes
- adhesive cannula plaster
- correct fluid bag
- IV drip stand
- Giving set
- Flush: draw up 10 ml normal saline into a 10 ml syringe with a green needle; discard the needle in the sharps box once you have drawn it up.

> **TOP TIP!**
>
> Make sure you position the sharps box no more than an arm's length away from you and in a position which ensures that you do not have to cross over the patient with the used needle, i.e. if you are cannulating with your right hand, place the sharps box to the right of you.

3.11.2 **The procedure**

Vein selection

When choosing which vein to cannulate, always start distally at the hand and work your way up if unsuccessful. Place a disposable tourniquet about 10 cm above the site you wish to cannulate and encourage venous filling by lowering the arm below the level of the heart. Choose a large vein that is easily palpable, preferably on the non-dominant hand and on the contralateral side to any surgical procedures that the patient may have (AV fistula). The veins on the back of the hand are usually easily accessible for cannulation, particularly the dorsal metacarpal veins or the cephalic veins located radially and higher up the hand.

Preparation

Once you have identified a suitable vein, put on a pair of non-sterile gloves. Palpate the vein to orientate yourself before you begin and then clean the area over the vein with an alcohol swab, making sure that you allow it to air dry before proceeding.

Whilst you are waiting, remove the cannula from its packaging and loosen the white Luer lock cap (*Fig 3.20*). When the patient is positioned suitably and you are ready to begin, remove the protective cover from the needle.

With your non-dominant hand hold the patient's flexed hand in position and stabilize the vein distally with your thumb. With your dominant hand hold the cannula in a position that you feel comfortable with so that you have good control over it. Although there are different ways that you can hold the cannula, most people tend to grasp it using their index and ring finger across the wings, with their thumb firmly over the Luer lock.

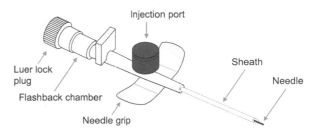

Fig 3.20 Elements of a cannula
This shows a pink 20G cannula.

Inserting the cannula

Make sure the needle is facing bevel side up at a shallow angle of about 30° to the skin. Warn the patient that they may feel a 'sharp scratch' as you pierce their skin with the needle. Advance the needle into the vein until you see a flashback of blood into the cannula chamber indicating that you are in the correct location.

Lower the angle of the cannula and advance a further 2 mm into the vein. This will ensure the plastic tube has entered the vein along with the needle. Hold the needle steady and advance the plastic tube further in. If you have been successful, you should see blood tracking back into the cannula. Once the cannula has been fully inserted into the vein, release the tourniquet and apply firm pressure over the vein slightly above the cannula site. This may help prevent any leakage of blood when removing the needle. Take the Luer lock cap off the end of the needle and immediately dispose of the needle in the sharps bin. Quickly re-secure the cap over the end of the cannula and release the pressure from the tip of the cannula.

Take the 10 ml syringe that has already been drawn up and flush the cannula with 5 ml of normal saline through the injection port. Ask the patient if they experience any pain or burning sensation and observe for any signs of extravasation around the cannula site; if you observe any of these signs or feel resistance whilst flushing then this may indicate that the cannula has not been sited correctly and it should be removed.

If the cannula flushes and the patient is in no discomfort, the cannula should be secured in place. Apply the adhesive plaster over the cannula, securing it firmly to the skin. Document on the back of the sticker, or within the medical notes, the date and time the cannula was sited.

Reducing the risk of infection

The skin acts as a barrier to prevent any infection from entering the body. The insertion of the cannula breaks this barrier as it penetrates the skin and the vein and so it may inadvertently act as a portal for infection. The risk of this happening can be reduced by adherence to strict infection control procedures, including hand washing, using a sterile technique when inserting the cannula, cleaning the skin with an alcohol swab and monitoring the site for signs of phlebitis. All cannulas should be removed within 72 hours of insertion because this has been shown to reduce the risk of infection.

TOP TIP!

You may be asked about the complications associated with cannulation; these include phlebitis, embolus, haematoma formation and vein thrombosis.

Fluid	Na⁺ (mmol/l)	K⁺ (mmol/l)	Cl⁻ (mmol/l)	Ca²⁺ (mmol/l)	HCO₃⁻ (mmol/l)	Osmolarity (mOsmol/l)	pH
Normal saline (0.9%)	154	0	154	0	0	308	5.5
Dextrose (5%)	0	0	0	0	0	252	4.1
Hartmann's	131	5	112	4	29	279	6.5
Gelofusine	154	0.4	123	0.4	0	308	7.4

Table 3.8 **Composition of common IV fluids**

Types of IV fluids

The IV drip is used to infuse fluid into a patient's vein through a cannula. It is usually used to fluid resuscitate (i.e. to correct dehydration), maintain daily fluid balance, to correct electrolyte imbalance or to deliver blood products.

Broadly speaking, IV fluids (see *Table 3.8*) fall into two categories:
- crystalloid – crystalloid fluids contain essential body minerals and electrolytes, e.g. normal saline, Hartmann's solution and dextrose fluids
- colloid – colloid fluids are plasma expanders, e.g. blood, Gelofusine and albumin.

There is much discussion about what type of fluids one should use in a critically unwell patient, but it is generally agreed that there is little to distinguish between colloids and crystalloids for fluid resuscitation. However, common practice is to use normal saline or Hartmann's solution in such cases. Dextrose (5%) is used as maintenance fluid or when a patient is suffering from hypoglycaemia or hypernatraemia.

Preparing the fluid bag

Having prepared the cannula, the IV drip should now be set up. First, compare the patient's details against those found on the drug chart to ensure that the correct patient is receiving the right fluid. Check the type and amount of fluid prescribed and note the duration over which it should be administered.

Collect the fluid bag and check that it has not passed its expiry date. Remove the bag from its protective cover and check its integrity, looking for any holes or contaminants. Hang the top end on a drip stand. Now prepare the giving set which is essentially a long tube that connects the IV fluid bag to the cannula. It has two ends, one with a sharp plastic stake that punctures the fluid bag and the other with a threaded cap that screws onto the cannula. Just below the sharp end is a filling chamber that allows you to see water dripping through; this permits you to calculate the rate at which fluid is passing into the cannula. Midway down is a regulating gauge with a roller that controls the flow rate into the cannula.

Be careful when removing the giving set from the packaging to ensure there is no contact with the sterile ends. Push the roller down fully in order to place the giving set in the 'off' position, so that when you insert it into the fluid bag there will be no leakage. Remove the blue wing of the IV fluid bag port and insert the sharp plastic end of the giving set. Squeeze the filling chamber until it is half full with fluid. Now open the regulating gauge by pushing the roller upwards fully

TOP TIP!

To avoid spillages, it may be easier to run the fluid through by holding the Luer lock end of the giving set at the level of the fluid bag.

to allow the fluid to run through and to remove any excess air from the set; this will reduce the risk of introducing an air embolus into the patient's vein. Once the set has been primed, close the clamp and move the stand, bag and giving set close to the patient.

Setting up the infusion

Now that both pieces of equipment are ready, they can be attached together. Remove the Luer lock cap from the end of the cannula and screw on the giving set. Unclamp the roller and set it to an appropriate rate as described on the drug chart: one drop per second is equivalent to giving 1 litre of fluid over 6 hours.

3.11.3 Finishing up

Check again whether there is any extravasation of fluid around the cannula site. If not, tape the distal end of the tube to the patient's arm in a way that will prevent accidental dislodgement of the cannula. Make sure you throw away any clinical waste in the appropriate waste bin.

Document on the drug chart the time and date when the fluid was started and sign next to it. Encourage the patient to report any signs of pain or swelling to a staff member. Finally, thank the patient for their co-operation and ask them if they would like to ask any questions or if they have any concerns.

Chapter 3.12
Blood transfusion

What to do . . .

- Introduce yourself to the patient – establish rapport
- Ask the patient's name and date of birth
- Establish the reason the patient is having a blood transfusion and any history of adverse reactions
- Explain the procedure to the patient and obtain informed consent
- Ensure that a patent large bore cannula is *in situ*
- Check that the patient's details are consistent across the drug chart, wrist band, compatibility form, and on the blood bag
- Check that the expiry date, blood group and serial number match the compatibility form and the blood bag
- Inspect the blood bag for any leaks, contamination, clots or signs of haemolysis
- Attach the blood bag to the stand and connect to the cannula
- Begin transfusion and check observations at regular intervals (every 15 minutes)
- Document the time and date the transfusion was commenced in the drug chart and place compatibility tag in the patient's notes
- Thank the patient and dispose of any waste appropriately

Blood transfusion is a common procedure that can be life-saving, particularly after acute blood loss from trauma or surgery. Other indications for having a blood transfusion include correction of severe symptomatic anaemia, haemophilia and in end-stage renal disease.

Although a common procedure, having a blood transfusion carries significant risks, some of which may be potentially life-threatening. It is therefore important to have a number of stringent checks and safeguards in place when undertaking this procedure.

Blood constituents

Blood consists of red blood cells (RBC), white blood cells (WBC), platelets and plasma. Each of these individually can be transfused from a donor to a recipient if necessary. The most common transfusion performed is that of red blood cells which is indicated in heavy blood loss such as from trauma, surgery or childbirth. It is also undertaken to correct severe symptomatic anaemia when a patient has a haemoglobin concentration of less than 8 g/dl and is suffering from shortness of breath, tachycardia, fatigue and dizziness.

Platelets can be transfused if a patient is found to be dangerously depleted and significantly thrombocytopaenic, such as in leukaemia, blood disorders or perhaps as a side effect of chemotherapy. In such situations a patient can be transfused with platelets to prevent the risk of bleeding.

Fresh frozen plasma contains plasma proteins in addition to a number of clotting factors. It is usually used to replace clotting factor deficiencies and to correct plasma depletion. It is indicated in acute disseminated intravascular coagulation, thrombotic thrombocytopaenic purpura, emergency reversal of warfarin anticoagulation, and plasma loss due to severe burns.

Albumin is useful in the acute setting when treating a patient who has been severely shocked or burnt. It is also used for replacement therapy in patients with advanced liver disease and ascites, who usually suffer from hypoalbuminaemia.

Although all the components above can be transfused, in clinical practice the one you would be expected to be competent in undertaking is red blood cell transfusion.

Red blood cell transfusion

Blood groups

Before transfusing a patient it is important to be aware that a number of blood group systems (including the ABO and Rhesus blood groupings) exist and a mismatch can cause incompatibility reactions.

The ABO blood group system

Broadly speaking, people are categorized as having blood from the A, B, AB or O blood groups. These groups are defined by the antigen found on the surface of their red cells. Patients with group A blood have an A antigen along with circulating anti-B antibodies. Patients with group B blood have B antigens on their surface with anti-A antibodies in the serum. Patients with group AB blood have both the A and B antigens, but no circulating antibodies. Finally, patients with group O blood have neither A nor B surface antigens, but have anti-A and anti-B antibodies in the bloodstream.

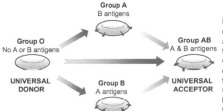

Each blood group can be donated to another person in their own group. Group O blood can be donated to all groups. Group A and B blood can donate to group AB.

Fig 3.21 Blood group compatibility.

In relation to blood transfusions, patients with blood group A can receive blood types A or O but not type B; the existence of anti-B antibodies in the group A recipient's blood would induce a haemolytic reaction with a group B donor's blood. For the same reason, group B patients can receive blood from individuals with the same group or group O but not from group A (see *Fig 3.21* and *Table 3.9*).

Blood group O has neither A nor B surface antigens and so this blood can safely be given to any group in an emergency – people with group O blood are known as 'universal donors'. However, because they have both anti-A and anti-B

Blood group	Surface antigen	Serum antibody	Can donate blood to:	Can receive blood from:	Frequency in UK population
O	None	Anti-A and anti-B	Any groups	Only O	44%
A	B antigen	Anti-B	A and AB	A and O	45%
B	A antigen	Anti-A	B and AB	B and O	8%
AB	A and B antigen	None	Only AB	Any group	3%

Table 3.9 **Characteristics of the different blood groups**

antibodies circulating, they cannot receive blood from any of the other blood groups.

Patients with group AB blood are known as 'universal acceptors' because they lack any antibodies in their blood serum and consequently can receive blood of any group. However, since both A and B antigens are present on their red blood cells, group AB donor blood can only be used in an AB recipient.

The Rhesus system

The Rhesus system is another blood group system that can cause incompatibility issues between a donor and recipient. The majority (85%) of people in the UK are Rhesus-positive (RhD positive) and have the D antigen present on the surface of their red blood cells. They are able to accept blood from both RhD positive and RhD negative people.

The remaining 15% of people are RhD negative and they lack the D antigen. However, unlike in the ABO system, they do not have any circulating antibodies to the antigen. This means that it is theoretically safe for them to receive a single blood transfusion from a RhD-positive individual without any immediate side effects. However, in doing so, the recipient's blood will become sensitized and develop anti-D antibodies that will lead to a haemolytic reaction if exposed again to Rhesus-positive blood. This is particularly significant for RhD-negative women of child-bearing age because they are at risk of developing anti-D antibodies and causing haemolytic disease of the newborn in any subsequent pregnancy.

Risks of a blood transfusion

Receiving donor blood can cause significant risk to the recipient if it has not been screened properly. More significantly, giving blood that is incompatible may induce a life-threatening haemolytic transfusion reaction. Following strict guidelines and protocols will reduce the risk of any adverse event occurring.

Haemolytic transfusion reactions

These are normally a result of blood group incompatibility. The most common cause is an ABO incompatibility due to a clerical error, leading to a rapid intravascular haemolysis, which can be life-threatening. Symptoms include a persistent fever, lumbar pain, sweating and dyspnoea which can develop fairly rapidly. If the transfusion is not immediately ceased then disseminated intravascular coagulation (DIC), haemoglobinuria, renal failure and cardiovascular collapse can follow.

Allergic reactions

Some people can have allergic reactions to the blood given during transfusions. Although relatively rare it is most often found in those who suffer from immunoglobulin A (IgA) deficiency. Allergic reactions can be mild or severe, with symptoms ranging from anxiety and nausea to anaphylactic shock (hypotension, tachycardia, fever and stridor).

Infectious diseases / blood-borne viruses

Some infectious agents, such as HIV, hepatitis B and hepatitis C, can survive in donor blood products and infect the recipient during blood transfusions. However, to minimize the risk, since the early 1990s blood banks in the UK have been carefully screening donated blood for these infections. As a result the risk of developing an infection post-transfusion is now:

- about 1 in 2 million for HIV infection

- 1 in 205 000 for hepatitis B
- 1 in 2 million for hepatitis C.

Iron overload

Repeated blood transfusions can cause a build-up of iron in the blood which is known as iron overload. People with blood disorders such as thalassaemia may require multiple transfusions over a period of time. As a result they are at more risk of developing iron overload than others. Iron overloading can cause damage to the liver, heart, pancreas and joints of the body.

3.12.2 Beginning the procedure

Start by introducing yourself to the patient, stating your name and job title. Ask the patient for their name and date of birth. Given the high risks involved with any blood transfusion, you should always check that the patient's identification band correlates correctly with these details and also get another member of staff to check all details again. Check that the patient is well and not in any discomfort before proceeding. Before you begin, it may be useful to confirm the reason why the patient needs a blood transfusion. Try to establish any symptoms they may be having, such as bleeding, shortness of breath, lethargy or weight loss. Ascertain if they have received blood before and whether they had any reactions or allergies. Establish if the patient has any religious or personal objection to having the transfusion; Jehovah's Witnesses, for example, are not allowed to receive a blood transfusion.

Explain the procedure

Explain to the patient about blood transfusions and the procedure you intend to follow. The patient may be apprehensive about having a blood transfusion and may raise concerns about receiving 'foreign' blood from a donor. It is important to deal with the patient's concerns and reassure them about the thorough screening checks now undertaken on the donor blood. You may wish to say: *'Your blood results show that the level of blood in your body is low. This is known as anaemia and explains why you have the symptoms you have described. In order to correct this we would recommend having a blood transfusion. This involves giving you blood through a small plastic tube (cannula) located in your arm. Some people can be apprehensive of having a blood transfusion. However, I can reassure you that the blood sample taken from any donor has undergone a number of tests to ensure that it is safe to use and is compatible with you.'*

After you have explained the procedure to the patient, inform the patient about the possible side effects and risk of having a blood transfusion. It is important that they have understood what you have said so that they can make an informed choice as to whether they should proceed or not. At this point you may wish to offer them the opportunity to ask any questions, before asking them to give you verbal consent to proceed.

Preparation

Ensure that the patient is lying down comfortably on the bed. Insert a large bore cannula, preferably 16G, into the antecubital fossa as described in *Chapter 3.11*, and flush it with normal saline.

Equipment

The equipment required is similar to that used for inserting a cannula and setting an IV drip, with the exception that a blood bag is required rather than

> **TOP TIP!**
>
> All blood transfusion giving sets must be replaced after 12 hours or after 2 units of blood have been given in order to limit bacterial growth.

a fluid bag, and a dedicated transfusion giving set is needed that has a double-barrel chamber with a micron filter.

- equipment tray/ kidney dish
- pair of gloves (non-sterile)
- cannula (large bore – 16G)
- tourniquet
- sharps box
- cotton wool balls or gauze swab
- alcohol wipes
- adhesive cannula plaster
- 1 unit of blood
- IV drip stand
- double-barrel giving set

3.12.3 **The blood transfusion procedure**

Checks

When obtaining a unit of blood, you must carry out a series of thorough checks before connecting it up to the patient's cannula; these checks will reduce the risk of any serious incompatibility reactions. Often these checks require two people, one of whom must be either a doctor, registered general nurse, registered sick children's nurse or a registered midwife.

Patient's details
Look at the patient's prescription and confirm that the patient has been prescribed a blood transfusion. Note the specific blood components to be administered, the number of units to be transfused, the date and time of the transfusion and its duration. Look out for any special instructions mentioned on the chart such as a request for CMV seronegative or irradiated blood components. Determine if any medications, such as furosemide, have also been prescribed before, during or after the transfusion.

Check that the patient's name, date of birth and hospital number on the drug chart match with what they have told you as well as with the information found on their wrist band. Do not transfuse if they are not wearing an identification wrist band or if there is any mismatch in any of these details.

Blood bag and compatibility form
Cross-check that the blood bag and compatibility form match the details of the patient (*Fig 3.22*). If these match, confirm whether the compatibility sheet has the same expiry date, serial number and blood group as that found on the blood bag. If there any inconsistencies, abort the procedure and contact the blood transfusion centre immediately, reporting your findings.

Inspect the blood product
Observe the blood bag for any leaks, contaminants, haemolysis, unusual discoloration or the presence of any clots. Return the bag to the laboratory if any suspicions are raised.

Setting up the transfusion

Once you are satisfied with all the checks and are confident that it is safe to proceed, place the unit of blood on a drip stand and insert the sharp end of the double-barrel giving set into it. Squeeze the double chamber to half fill it with

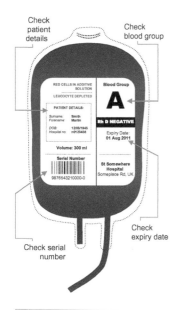

Check patient details

Check blood group

RED CELLS IN ADDITIVE SOLUTION

LEUCOCYTE DEPLETED

Blood Group

A

PATIENT DETAILS:

Surname: Smith
Forename: Martin

DOB: 12/03/1945
Hospital no: n0123456

Rh D NEGATIVE

Expiry Date:
01 Aug 2011

Volume: 300 ml

Serial Number

9876543210000-0

St Somewhere Hospital
Someplace Rd, UK

Check serial number

Check expiry date

Fig 3.22 Checking the blood transfusion bag's details.

blood and then prime the giving set by allowing the blood to flow through to expel any air. Connect the end of the giving set to the patient's cannula and then set the transfusion to run at an appropriate rate as directed by the drug chart.

Transfusion observations

Patients should be closely observed at regular intervals for signs of acute adverse reactions. Most reactions occur within 15 minutes of starting the transfusion. Observations should include checking their temperature, blood pressure, heart rate, respiratory rate and O_2 saturation. You should also inspect for any new rashes or sites of bleeding (DIC).

3.12.4 Finishing up

Ask the patient to inform a staff member if they develop any features of an adverse reaction such as itching, shivering, shortness of breath, flushing or rashes.

Sign and document the drug chart with the time and date the transfusion was commenced. Place the detachable sticker from the compatibility tag in the patient's notes. Dispose of any waste in the appropriate waste containers and thank the patient.

3.12.5 Common clinical scenarios

The following are a list of scenarios of patients who require a blood component transfusion. Read the cases carefully and determine which component or transfusion is most appropriate.

CASE 1 A 32 year woman presents complaining of weakness, dizziness and shortness of breath post-partum.

CASE 2 A 55 year old man post-chemotherapy presents with petechiae and easy bruising.

CASE 3 A 63 year old man with AF on warfarin is found to have frank haematuria and haematemesis.

CASE 4 A 35 year old cachectic man with gynaecomastia, spider naevi and caput medusa with new onset abdominal swelling and peripheral leg oedema.

CASE 5 A 28 year old male motorcyclist is brought into A&E. He is found to have a pelvic fracture and a haemoglobin level of 7 g/dl.

CASE 6 A 21 year old haemophiliac woman presents suffering from severe anaemia requiring a blood transfusion. Her blood group is O RhD-negative.

Chapter 3.13
Peak flow meter explanation

What to do . . .

- Introduce yourself to the patient – establish rapport
- Ask the patient's name, age and occupation
- Explain the procedure to the patient
- Ensure that the patient is standing upright and check that the pointer on the peak flow meter is at zero
- Hold the peak flow meter horizontally and keep fingers away from pointer
- Take a deep breath and close lips around mouthpiece firmly, and then blow as hard and fast as possible
- Look at the pointer to check reading, reset pointer to zero and do this twice more
- Record the highest reading in the asthma diary
- Interpret the results appropriately by checking the patient's reading against predicted normal values for age, sex and height using a chart
- Thank the patient and conclude the consultation

The peak flow meter is a small hand-held device that measures the maximum speed of expiration or peak expiratory flow rate (PEFR). It is a simple and cheap tool that measures the airflow through the bronchi and estimates the degree of obstruction. It is therefore useful in patients who suffer from obstructive airway disease such as asthma or COPD.

The peak flow meter, if used appropriately, can be valuable in determining the level of lung function, assessing symptom severity and monitoring response to treatment.

Peak flow readings can range from 0 to 800 litres per minute, with higher readings signifying patent airways and lower readings suggestive of airway constriction. Values also vary depending on gender, age and height. A single peak flow reading provides little clinical information if taken out of context; for example, a reading of 450 litres per minute would be quite normal for a 30 year old woman whilst the same value in a man of the same age would be only 70% of that expected.

Peak flow readings are also useful in providing an objective test in diagnosing asthma. Measurements that are consistently below the expected flow rate for the patient and later increase by more than 15% after a trial of β-agonist or steroids would support this diagnosis. In addition, serial measurements that demonstrate variability over a day may also add weight to your diagnosis (*Fig 3.23*). The classical variability seen is one where there is diurnal variation, with the peak flow reading worse during the night and first thing in the morning.

The peak flow meter is extremely useful in determining whether a patient's exacerbation of asthma is moderate, severe or life-threatening. By comparing the patient's current peak flow value with the patient's best or predicted, one can adopt the most appropriate treatment or management algorithm.

Medical Guidelines
Levels of severity of acute asthma exacerbations

Near-fatal asthma	Raised $PaCO_2$ and/or requiring mechanical ventilation with raised inflation pressures
Life-threatening asthma	Any one of the following in a patient with severe asthma:
	– PEF <33% best or predicted – bradycardia
	– SpO_2 <92% – arrhythmia
	– PaO_2 <8 kPa – hypotension
	– normal $PaCO_2$ (4.6–6.0 kPa) – exhaustion
	– silent chest – confusion
	– cyanosis – coma
	– feeble respiratory effort
Acute severe asthma	Any one of:
	– PEF 33–50% best or predicted
	– respiratory rate ≥25/min
	– heart rate ≥110/min
	– inability to complete sentences in one breath
Moderate asthma exacerbation	– Increasing symptoms: PEF >50–75% best or predicted
	– no features of acute severe asthma
Brittle asthma	Type 1: wide PEF variability (>40% diurnal variation for >50% of the time over a period >150 days), despite intense therapy
	Type 2: sudden severe attacks on a background of apparently well-controlled asthma

British Thoracic Society: British Guideline on the Management of Asthma (2008)

3.13.1 **Beginning the procedure**

Start by introducing yourself to the patient, stating your name and job title. Ask the patient for their name and age and occupational status; workplace exposure to animal products, dusts or chemicals is often associated with occupational asthma.

Check if the patient is well and not in any discomfort before proceeding. Before you begin it is useful to confirm the reason why the patient needs to have their peak expiratory flow rate measured. Try to establish any symptoms they may be having, such as cough, wheeze or shortness of breath and if they have any family history of asthma, eczema or atopy.

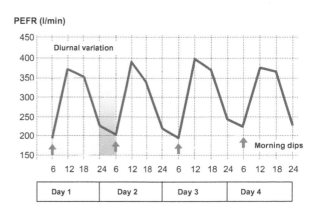

Fig 3.23 Diurnal variation in asthma.

Elicit understanding

Part of the success of patient compliance in taking peak flow measurements is to ensure that they understand why they are doing it. Many patients may already have an understanding as to what a peak flow meter is and how to use it, whilst others may never have seen one before. It is therefore important to gauge the patient's level of understanding before attempting to give your explanation. You may wish to say to the patient: *'I understand that you have been coughing and wheezing for some time. I would therefore like to take a peak flow reading to check if you have asthma or not. Have you ever used one of these devices before? Do you know how to use it?'*

Explain the procedure

> **TOP TIP!**
>
> Peak flow measurement is often combined with testing inhaler technique, so make sure you know both well.

Begin by explaining what a peak flow meter is and what it is used for. Try to keep your explanation simple and to the point and allow the patient time to digest what you are saying. You may wish to say: *'A peak flow meter is a small tube which you blow into that measures how fast you can push air out of your lungs. It will help us monitor how well your lungs are working and whether you suffer from asthma. In asthma, because the airways are narrowed, the peak flow readings are usually lower than normal. In order to use the peak flow meter correctly I will first demonstrate it to you and then you can show me what you have learnt.'*

After you have explained the procedure to the patient, it is important that they have understood what you have said and given you verbal consent to proceed.

3.13.2 Demonstrating how to use the peak flow meter

Firstly prepare the peak flow device by resetting the pointer to zero and placing a fresh mouthpiece onto the end of the device. Stand up and take in a few deep breaths, ensuring that you hold the device horizontally with your fingers either side of the pointer. Advise the patient that they should then take a single deep breath in order to inflate their lungs fully. Place your lips around the mouthpiece and make a tight seal. Now blow as hard and fast as possible as if you are trying to 'blow out candles'. Remember that it is the speed of the blow that is being measured and this should be made clear to the patient.

> **TOP TIP!**
>
> In the exam, the patient may often make a deliberate mistake such as pointing the device downwards or putting their fingers over the gauge. Correct the patient's mistake and demonstrate accordingly.

Show the patient how to read the peak flow meter by observing where the pointer lies against the graduations (see *Fig 3.24*). Record this reading on a piece of paper and repeat the process twice more. Do not forget to reset the pointer to zero each time.

Advise the patient that they should take the highest of the three readings and document it in their asthma diary. Once you have finished demonstrating the procedure, ensure the patient understood the process and ask them to demonstrate back to you. Remember to replace the mouthpiece with a fresh one.

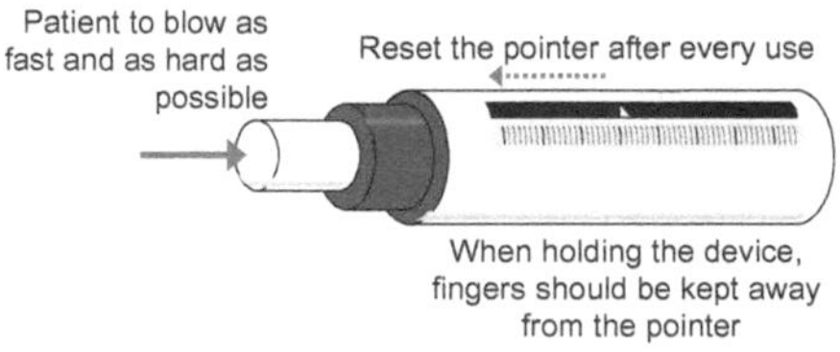

Patient to blow as fast and as hard as possible

Reset the pointer after every use

When holding the device, fingers should be kept away from the pointer

Fig 3.24 Peak flow device.

Interpreting the peak flow measurements

Compare actual PEFR to predicted value

Once you have obtained the patient's highest reading, compare this against the standardized peak flow chart of normal predicted values (*Fig 3.25*), taking into account their age, sex and height.

To use this chart, select the appropriate curved line which represents the patient's sex and height. Draw a vertical line from their age at the bottom of the chart and note where it intersects the chosen curved line. Read across to the y-axis and note the patient's predicted peak flow value. For example (see *Fig 3.26*), for a 50 year old woman who is 152 cm tall, the predicted peak flow will be about 450 litres per minute.

Peak flow diary

Although predicted PEFR charts are readily available, the patient's personal best peak flow result is the most useful in determining the severity of symptoms. Peak flow diaries are an effective way to demonstrate the variability of asthma as well as symptom control after medication use. In order to do this, the patient should take two readings a day, one in the morning and the other in the evening, over a two week period. They also should record in the diary when they experience symptoms such as coughing, wheezing or tightness of the chest. After a few days of monitoring they should then start using an inhaled steroid and continue taking readings as before.

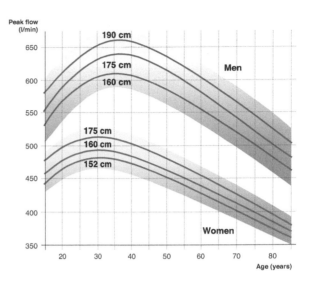

Fig 3.25 Predicted peak flow measurements.

Note the different measurements expected based on differences in height.

In asthma, the untreated chart would show a diurnal variation with consistently low values, whilst post-inhaler use the variation should be become less with higher peak flow readings (*Fig 3.27*).

3.13.3 **Finishing up**

Once you have obtained the patient's peak flow results and interpreted them using the chart provided, ensure that you document it in the peak flow diary and in the patient's notes. You will need to interpret the peak flow reading as to whether it is low or normal (asthmatic or not asthmatic) and make a clinical judgment as to what should happen next. If it is normal, reassure the patient and offer an appointment in an appropriate time to have a repeat check-up if necessary. In cases of peak flow readings lower than those predicted for the patient, you should give an appropriate explanation to the patient as to what the peak flow is and what it indicates. You may say, for example, '*I have taken your peak flow reading today and the value is 300 l/min. This result is slightly*

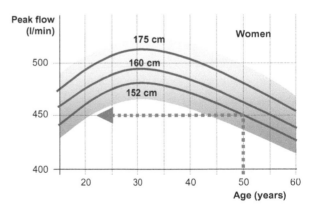

Fig 3.26 How to use the PEFR chart.

low for someone of your sex, age and height. Normally we take account of your symptoms as well as the readings and because you have been feeling breathless and wheezy, these findings suggest that you may have asthma. I recommend that we start you on a 'reliever' inhaler to reduce these symptoms and draw up an Asthma Action Plan for you. It would be very useful if you could record your peak flow readings for 2 weeks as explained above and I will see you in a fortnight to check whether the inhalers are helping.'

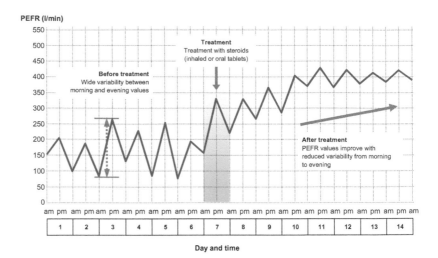

Fig 3.27 Improvement in peak flow measurement after using a steroid.

Often the patient will be concerned about their peak flow reading and it is important not to be dismissive of their worries. Advise the patient that if they are worried about their peak flow reading or develop symptoms such as severe breathlessness and wheeze, they should attend earlier for review or go to hospital. Thank the patient and confirm that they have understood what you have told them.

3.13.4 **Common clinical scenarios**

The following are a list of scenarios with different peak flow readings. Read the cases carefully and determine the best possible way to treat the patient.

CASE 1

A 20 year old student has been experiencing shortness of breath and intermittent wheeze. He was found to have a peak flow reading of 450 l/min which later increased to 600 l/min after being given a salbutamol inhaler.

CASE 2

A 27 year old teacher was seen as an emergency appointment by the GP. She felt so breathless that she couldn't complete her sentences. Her respiratory rate was 35, she was tachycardic and her peak flow was 270 l/min compared to her best of 550 l/min.

CASE 3

A 16 year school boy who was diagnosed with asthma 1 year ago presents complaining of worsening symptoms. He has been experiencing a dry cough every night and needs to use his inhaler almost every day. His peak flow was found to be 400 l/min. He is 1.75 m tall.

CASE 4

A 65 year old woman has poorly controlled asthma. She has poor respiratory effort, appears cyanotic and has a silent chest. Her peak flow after several unsuccessful attempts is 80 l/min.

Chapter 3.14
Inhaler explanation

What to do . . .

- Introduce yourself to the patient – establish rapport
- Ask the patient's name and age and confirm the reason for their appointment
- Establish the patient's understanding of asthma and inhalers
- Explain and demonstrate the procedure to the patient:
  - remove cap and shake inhaler vigorously
  - breathe out slowly and completely
  - hold inhaler in upright position and insert mouthpiece into mouth between closed lips
  - press the canister once whilst simultaneously taking a slow and deep breath in
  - remove the inhaler and hold breath for 10 seconds
  - wait for 30 seconds before starting second puff
- Explain side effects of medication, when to use it and when to seek help
- Thank the patient and conclude the consultation

Inhalers are small pocket-sized devices that are commonly used in respiratory conditions such as asthma and COPD. They are able to deliver medication in an aerosol form that can be inhaled through the oropharynx and into the lungs. As inhalers allow drugs to be delivered directly to the airways, much smaller doses are required compared to orally ingested medication. This reduces the likelihood of side effects and accidental overdose.

Many different shapes and sizes of inhalers (*Fig 3.28*) are available on the market, each of which have their own unique qualities and uses. It is important to familiarize yourself with the more common ones and to be aware of the groups of patients who could benefit most from their usage.

Metered dose inhaler

Perhaps the most commonly used inhaler available is the metered dose inhaler (MDI). These use a chemical propellant mechanism to deliver a measured dose of medication to the lungs. The inhaler is made up of a pressurized canister containing the medication, a metering valve that ensures the correct dose is dispensed and a mouthpiece.

The standard MDIs rely upon good hand co-ordination as well as a degree of dexterity. It requires an individual to apply sufficient pressure to the top of the canister to trigger the release mechanism, whilst simultaneously taking a deep breath in (*Fig 3.29*). Although the inhalers are suitable for the vast majority of adults, they may pose difficulty for elderly patients and those who have rheumatological conditions that particularly affect the hands. In such patients it may be more useful to use breath-actuated MDIs which reduce the need for hand co-ordination and instead release medication upon inspiration.

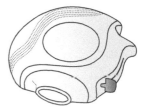

Accuhaler

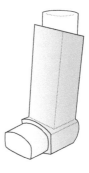

MDI

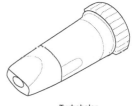

Turbohaler

Fig 3.28 Different types of inhaler.

TOP TIP!

Traditionally, the propellant used was CFC-based, but most inhalers are now CFC-free, containing a hydrofluoroalkane (HFA) propellant instead.

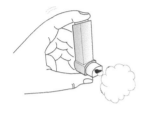

Fig 3.29 Use of an MDI.

TOP TIP!

There are many different types of inhalers available; at the very least you should be familiar with the standard metered dose inhaler for your examinations.

TOP TIP!

It is important to remember that some patients may use a single inhaler that combines both a steroid and bronchodilator in one device.

The standard MDI may also cause problems for young patients who may not be able to operate the device or synchronize their breathing effectively. For this group of patients, the volumatic spacer may be used in conjunction with the inhaler to help the delivery process (see *Chapter 3.15* for more information).

Dry powder inhalers

Dry powder inhalers have no chemical propellant and instead contain the medication in a powdered form. For this reason they are easy to use because the patient only has 'suck in' to receive a dose. There are various different devices available, including the Accuhaler, Turbohaler and Diskhaler. Although they may be useful in patients who are elderly or suffer from arthritis, they may not be suitable for young children who are unable to breathe in with the sufficient degree of force required.

Types of medications

Broadly speaking, inhalers deliver two types of medication; β-agonists, known as relievers, and steroids, known as preventers.

Relievers
Relievers contain bronchodilators such as salbutamol or terbutaline and are taken as required to reduce symptoms of breathlessness and wheeze. They have a rapid onset of action and usually provide relief within 15 minutes of administration. Bronchodilators act by binding to and activating β_2-adrenergic receptors in the airways resulting in relaxation of the bronchial smooth muscle and widening of the airway (bronchodilation). Generally speaking, relievers tend to be put in blue or grey inhalers.

Preventers
Preventers contain a low dose steroid that helps reduce inflammation in the smaller airways. They also reduce the number of bronchial eosinophils that tend to be active in allergic responses. These types of inhalers should be used daily to prevent the development of symptoms – they may take one to two weeks to reach maximal efficacy. Preventer inhalers are usually coloured brown, orange or red to make them easily distinguishable.

3.14.1 **Beginning the procedure**

Start by introducing yourself to the patient, stating your name and job title. Ask the patient their name and age. Check that the patient is well and not in any discomfort before proceeding. It is useful to confirm why the patient needs an inhaler: are they a newly diagnosed asthmatic or has their treatment regime been changed?

Explain the procedure

Most patients who use inhalers suffer from asthma or COPD. Check the patient's understanding of their condition before explaining and demonstrating how to use the inhalers correctly. Since the way in which inhalers work is closely linked with the disease process, eliciting and correcting understanding will work towards improving the patient's compliance with treatment. You may wish to ask the patient: *'I understand that you have been diagnosed with asthma. Could you please tell me what you already know about this condition?'*

Having gained an insight into the patient's level of understanding about their condition, you may wish to correct any inaccuracies they may hold. A useful way of doing this is to explain to the patient what their condition is and how the inhaler works to relieve their symptoms. If the patient suffers from asthma you may wish say: *'Asthma is a condition of the lungs that causes difficulty in breathing. People who suffer with asthma may have sensitive airways that narrow when irritated. Some irritants may include smoke, cold weather, pollen and dust. When the airways narrow, it makes it more difficult for air to move in and out of your lungs and makes you feel short of breath. As the air passes through these narrow tubes, it may make a high-pitched sound known as a wheeze. The blue inhaler contains a drug called salbutamol that works by opening up the airways in the lungs so that air can flow through them more easily.'*

3.14.2 Demonstrating the procedure

Use a new MDI inhaler (standard blue salbutamol) to demonstrate the procedure to the patient. Start by describing the different parts of the device and how they function. Explain the anatomy of the inhaler by pointing out the barrel, mouthpiece and the metal medication canister. Explain to the patient the need to check the expiry date, which is usually located on the container, to ensure that the medication is in-date and usable.

Make sure that the canister is connected securely in the barrel before removing the cap. Now that the inhaler is prepared, shake the device for 5 seconds and hold it upright with your index finger on the top of the container and your thumb supporting the base.

Advise the patient to take a few deep breaths in and out before fully exhaling all the air from their lungs. Make a tight seal around the mouthpiece with your lips ensuring that the inhaler is held correctly such that it is pointing towards the back of the throat. Demonstrate to the patient how to simultaneously press down on the canister to release a dose whilst taking a gradual deep breath in. Warn them that they may experience a cold sensation at the back of the throat which indicates that they have successfully delivered medication.

Ask the patient to hold their breath for 10 seconds before exhaling. This is to allow time for medication to disperse uniformly and act upon the small airways. If the patient requires another puff, advise them to wait 30 seconds before doing so to give time for the medication to reconstitute with the propellant. After finishing using the inhaler, recap the mouthpiece and breathe normally.

Side effects

Patients should be informed about the possible side effects of the medications they have been prescribed. Possible side effects of salbutamol use may include a fast heart rate, shakiness and headaches. Although rare, if the patient notices any of these they should consult their doctor. It may be that the patient is inadvertently overdosing themselves with the medication and may require a preventer.

If the patient was prescribed a steroid inhaler, the most common side effect would be oral mucosal candidiasis. This can easily be prevented by simply rinsing out the mouth after inhaler use or by using a spacer device.

It is important to remember that a course of high dose steroids used over a long period of time can cause stunting of growth in children. Parents should be warned about this and have the child's height regularly checked. All patients on steroids should be offered a steroid card to keep with them at all times, so that they can record the doses, such as 1500 µg daily of beclometasone or 750 µg of fluticasone.

Regularity

Salbutamol inhalers can be taken as two puffs up to four times a day, as and when required. If the patient finds they are using it more than three times a week, then a preventer should be considered. Preventers, on the other hand, should be taken twice a day on a regular basis irrespective of their symptoms.

Seeking help

It is important to tell the patient that if they are not getting relief from their inhalers and that their symptoms are significantly worsening, they may need

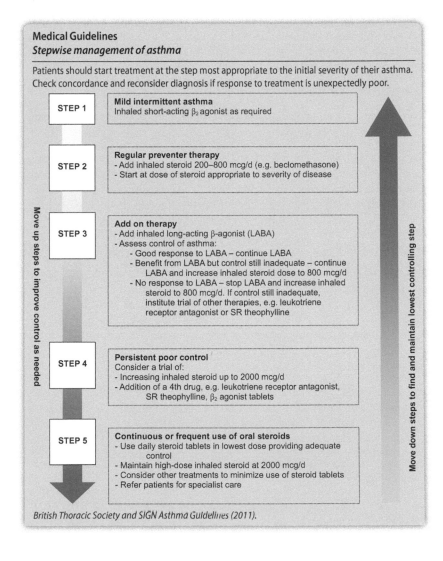

Medical Guidelines
Stepwise management of asthma

Patients should start treatment at the step most appropriate to the initial severity of their asthma. Check concordance and reconsider diagnosis if response to treatment is unexpectedly poor.

STEP 1
Mild intermittent asthma
Inhaled short-acting β₂ agonist as required

STEP 2
Regular preventer therapy
- Add inhaled steroid 200–800 mcg/d (e.g. beclomethasone)
- Start at dose of steroid appropriate to severity of disease

STEP 3
Add on therapy
- Add inhaled long-acting β-agonist (LABA)
- Assess control of asthma:
    - Good response to LABA – continue LABA
    - Benefit from LABA but control still inadequate – continue LABA and increase inhaled steroid dose to 800 mcg/d
    - No response to LABA – stop LABA and increase inhaled steroid to 800 mcg/d. If control still inadequate, institute trial of other therapies, e.g. leukotriene receptor antagonist or SR theophylline

STEP 4
Persistent poor control
Consider a trial of:
- Increasing inhaled steroid up to 2000 mcg/d
- Addition of a 4th drug, e.g. leukotriene receptor antagonist, SR theophylline, β₂ agonist tablets

STEP 5
Continuous or frequent use of oral steroids
- Use daily steroid tablets in lowest dose providing adequate control
- Maintain high-dose inhaled steroid at 2000 mcg/d
- Consider other treatments to minimize use of steroid tablets
- Refer patients for specialist care

Move up steps to improve control as needed

Move down steps to find and maintain lowest controlling step

British Thoracic Society and SIGN Asthma Guidelines (2011).

to go to hospital to receive further treatment in the form of a nebulizer. Most patients with asthma should have an action plan, devised by a physican, which explains what steps to take if their asthma is not being controlled.

3.14.3 **Finishing up**

Once you have explained the technique to the patient, confirm that they understand what you have explained to them and ask that they demonstrate the procedure to you. Compare their technique against your explanation and correct any mistakes they make. Ask if they have any questions or concerns. Every asthmatic patient should have a peak flow meter at home accompanied with a peak flow diary to monitor their condition. Make sure that they measure their peak flow and record it daily so you can assess whether the inhalers are helping settle their symptoms.

You can offer the patient an appropriate follow-up appointment to review their peak flow measurements and their symptoms to make sure that they are on the correct management plan. This will also give you an opportunity to check that they are still using their inhaler correctly.

Advise the patient that if they start to feel worse, they should attend earlier for a review or go to hospital. Thank the patient and confirm again that they have understood what you have told them.

3.14.4 **Common clinical scenarios**

The following are a list of scenarios of patients suffering with asthma. Read the cases carefully and determine the best possible way to treat the patient.

CASE 1

A 37 year old Afro-Caribbean woman has very poorly controlled asthma. She currently uses her short-acting β_2 agonist three times a day, and is using an inhaled steroid inhaler at the maximum dose of 2000 mcg/day. She has tried long-acting β_2-agonists and leukotriene receptor antagonists without success and does not want to consider theophylline tablets.

CASE 2

A 23 year old male student with daily wheeze and nocturnal cough. He currently takes salbutamol three times a day as well as beclometasone 100 mcg two puffs twice a day.

CASE 3

A keen footballer aged 18 using his salbutamol inhaler four times a week. He has been experiencing nocturnal symptoms more than once a week.

CASE 4

A 42 year old woman complains of chest tightness and wheeze. She currently takes her salbutamol inhaler four times a day as well as her beclometasone (200 mcg) inhaler regularly at two puffs twice a day.

CASE 5

A 16 year old boy attends your practice with nocturnal cough and wheeze. His peak flow measurements reveal diurnal variability.

Chapter 3.15
Spacer device explanation

What to do . . .

- Introduce yourself to the patient – establish rapport
- Ask the patient's name and age and confirm the reason why the patient needs a spacer
- Elicit patient's understanding of inhalers and spacer devices
- Explain and demonstrate the procedure to the patient:
    - attach the two ends of the spacer device together correctly
    - remove the cap of the inhaler and shake vigorously; correctly insert into the spacer device
    - take some deep breaths in and out before starting and make a tight seal around the mouthpiece of the spacer
    - press the inhaler canister once to release the medication
    - breathe in deeply and slowly, holding your breath for up to 10 seconds after each breath
    - repeat this for up to 30 seconds; if you require a second puff, wait for a minute and repeat the whole process
- Explain how to clean and store the spacer as well as the need to replace it after 6 months
- Thank the patient and conclude the consultation

Standard inhalers may pose difficulties for particular patient groups such as the young and elderly. They require a degree of hand–breathing co-ordination as well as physical strength to trigger a release of the medication. In such groups, an adjunct device, known as a spacer, can be used to facilitate the process.

A spacer is a cylindrical tube that acts as a holding chamber for the medication once the inhaler has been depressed. It removes the need to synchronize one's breathing with the release of the medication. It provides an environment in which the particles can be evenly spread and inhaled at the patient's leisure. This results in greater deposition of the medication in the peripheral airways and reduces the amount of drug deposited in the oropharynx. In effect, less medication is needed for an effective dose with fewer local and systemic side effects; this property is especially important for inhaled corticosteroids as it will decrease the incidence of adverse effects, such as oral candidiasis.

Spacer devices come in many different shapes and sizes with the most recognizable being the volumatic spacer (*Fig 3.30*), which consists of two plastic cone-shaped ends that click together to form a large chamber. One end consists of a mouthpiece or mask that the patient uses to breathe through, whilst the other end has a slot for the inhaler to be inserted. When the patient presses the inhaler canister a dose of medicine is released into, and contained within, the main chamber by a one-way valve. When the patient breathes in, this triggers the valve to open and allows for the medication to pass into the lungs. Exhalation seals the valve and the contents of the lungs are expired into the surrounding environment.

Other spacer devices, such as the PocketChamber and Aerochamber, use the same principles as described above, but they may require a specific type and shape of inhaler to operate. Try to familiarize yourself with the different spacer models available and their accompanying inhalers.

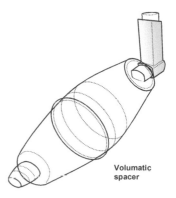

Aerochamber

Volumatic
spacer

Fig 3.30 The two common spacer designs.

> **Medical Guidelines**
> *Use of spacer devices*
>
> There are a few reasons for prescribing a spacer device. NICE recommends that children with chronic asthma and those under the age of 5 should be using spacer devices (with a facemask if necessary). For young children (under 5 years) they should be used for administering both inhaled bronchodilators and corticosteroids, whereas for older children (5–12 years) spacers need only be used with high-dose inhaled corticosteroids (over 800 mcg of beclometasone or equivalent daily).
>
> | Age group | 1st choice device | 2nd choice device | 3rd choice device | Breath-actuated | Dry powder |
> |---|---|---|---|---|---|
> | 0–2 years (inclusive) | MDI + spacer + face mask | MDI + spacer | Nebulizer (rarely needed) | Avoid | Avoid |
> | 3–5 years (inclusive) | MDI + spacer | MDI + spacer + face mask | Nebulizer (rarely needed) | Not proven | Possible use for β_2-agonist but not recommended for corticosteroids |
>
> *NICE Guidelines: Inhaler systems (devices) in children under the age of 5 years with chronic asthma (2000)*

3.15.1 **Beginning the examination**

Start by introducing yourself to the patient, stating your name and job title. Ask the patient, or their responsible adult in the case of a young child, for their name and age. Check if the patient is well and not in any discomfort before proceeding. Confirm the reason why the patient needs a spacer device; the patient may be suffering from arthritis of the hands and has been unable to operate their inhaler correctly, or it may be that a mother is concerned that their child is incapable of co-ordinating their breathing with the inhaler.

Elicit understanding

Once you have established why the patient requires a spacer device, you should go on to explain how it works and how it will be helpful for them. You may wish to say: '*As you suffer from asthma it is important that you use the salbutamol inhaler to relieve your symptoms. However, it seems that you are having some difficulty using the inhaler correctly and therefore I would recommend using a spacer device. This will make it easier to deliver the medicine to your lungs and eliminate the need to co-ordinate use of the inhaler with your breathing. Have you seen or used a spacer before? Do you have any questions about what I have said? I will now show you how to use this device.*'

> **TOP TIP!**
>
> Paediatric spacer devices usually have a small mask that fits onto the mouthpiece of the spacer and which can then be placed over the child's nose and mouth. They are specifically designed for use in babies and toddlers (<3 years of age).

> **TOP TIP!**
>
> If the patient states that they have difficulty using the inhaler, ask them to demonstrate their technique. A simple correction rather than a spacer may be all that is needed.

'A spacer device is a plastic tube that attaches on to your inhaler. It usually comes as two separate pieces that slot together to make a large chamber. At one end you will have a mouthpiece to breathe through, whilst on the other end there is a hole that your inhaler fits into.'

3.15.2 **Demonstrate the procedure**

Tell the patient that you will talk them through the procedure first and that you will ask them to demonstrate it later. Show the patient the different parts of the device so that they can become familiar with them. Bring the two opposing ends of the spacer device together and click them into place. After assembling it, select the appropriate inhaler for the device, checking first that the medication is in date. Shake the inhaler for 5 seconds and remove the cap. Insert the inhaler's mouthpiece into the correct side of the spacer, ensuring a tight fit.

Once you have set up the spacer with the inhaler, advise the patient that they should stand up and take some deep breaths in before beginning. Fully exhale the contents of your lungs before making a tight seal with your lips around the mouthpiece. Make sure that you do not bite the mouthpiece or impede the opening with your teeth. If the patient has been given a spacer device with a face mask, then place the mask over your nose and mouth so that it makes a tight seal. Once you are happy with your positioning of the spacer and/ or mask, press down on the inhaler to release a single puff into the spacer (see *Fig 3.31*).

Breathe in through the mouthpiece deeply and slowly and try to hold your breath for up to 10 seconds or as long as you feel comfortable; if you struggle to do this then breathing normally is acceptable. Then exhale (the one-way value prevents exhaled air entering the spacer chamber) and repeat several times, for up to 30 seconds. If another dose is needed, relax for a minute before administering another dose and repeat the whole process.

It is advisable not to spray more than one puff at a time into the spacer as this may promote the medication to form droplets on the walls of the spacer device, reducing the concentration being inhaled.

Once you have finished demonstrating the procedure, inform the patient that they should dismantle the device and re-cap the inhaler's mouthpiece. Check that they have understood the process and ask them to demonstrate it to you.

Regularity

Explain to the patient that they should continue to use their inhaler as previously prescribed, but with the spacer. Point out that the spacer device should make the medicine delivery more efficient and reduce their symptoms.

Cleaning

It is important to explain to the patient how to clean their spacer correctly. The more the spacer is used, the more medicine residue can build up inside, causing accumulation by attracting further aerosol particles. This reduces the overall effectiveness of the medication.

Advise the patient to clean it once a month in warm water leaving it to 'drip dry'. Avoid using detergents or cloth drying as these can cause static build-up

> **TOP TIP!**
>
> When using the Aerochamber, a whistling sound indicates that you are breathing in too quickly.

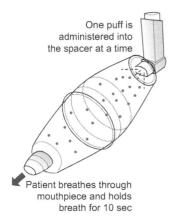

One puff is administered into the spacer at a time

Patient breathes through mouthpiece and holds breath for 10 sec

Fig 3.31 Using the spacer.

inside the spacer and reduce efficacy. The device should be kept in a clean and cool place and great care should be taken to prevent it becoming scratched. Manufacturers recommend that the device should be replaced every 6 months to ensure optimal functionality.

3.15.3 **Finishing up**

Once you have demonstrated the technique to the patient, confirm that they understand what you have explained to them. Ask them if they have any questions or concerns. It may be necessary to reassess the patient's treatment once the spacer has been introduced. In many cases, due to the improved efficiency of delivery, patients experience better symptom control and may need a step down in their asthma treatment.

Chapter 3.16
Setting up a nebulizer

What to do . . .

- Introduce yourself to the patient – establish rapport
- Ask the patient's name and date of birth
- Explain the procedure to the patient:
  - collect all the equipment
  - assemble the nebulizer chamber by screwing the cap to the cup and attaching the tubing to either an oxygen cylinder (for asthma) or air supply (for COPD)
  - attach the face mask or mouthpiece to the nebulizer chamber
  - confirm the correct medication and dose to be given with the drug chart and empty it into the nebulizer chamber; re-attach the cap
  - switch on the compressor or oxygen supply at 5–7 l/min and watch for a mist to indicate that the nebulizer is working
  - place the face mask over the nose and mouth and continue to breathe normally for up to 10 minutes
- Thank the patient and answer any questions they may have; dispose of any waste appropriately

A nebulizer is a machine which administers medication in the form of an aerosol that can be inhaled through a mask or mouthpiece. Compressed air is forced at high velocity through a liquid medium, containing either a β-agonist (salbutamol), anti-cholinergic (ipratropium bromide) or a corticosteroid, to produce a mist. This helps to ensure that a greater proportion of medication is delivered directly into the bronchioles than through a standard inhaler.

Nebulizers are commonly used in the emergency treatment of respiratory conditions such as asthma and COPD. They can be used to provide nebulized antimicrobial drug treatment in cystic fibrosis or bronchiectasis. They also play an important role in the long-term treatment of chronic respiratory conditions and can provide symptomatic relief in the palliative care setting. The British Thoracic Society (1997 Guidelines) also recommends the use of nebulizers when large doses of inhaled drugs are needed, when patients are too ill or otherwise unable to use hand-held inhalers, and when drugs are not available for inhalers.

Nebulizers come in all shapes and sizes, but their mechanisms are all largely based around the same principles. They consist of a basic mechanical compressor that generates high flow air or oxygen (at least 6 l/min), plastic tubing, a medicine reservoir and a facemask. The parts are often found disassembled and must be connected together correctly to make a functioning nebulizer unit. Although in theory a nebulizer should be quite straightforward and simple to set up, in reality they can be quite fiddly to assemble, especially when under pressure.

TOP TIP!

If possible, try to familiarize yourself with the same type of nebulizer used in your medical school to ensure you look confident using it in an exam.

3.16.1 **Beginning the examination**

Start by introducing yourself to the patient, stating your name and job title. Ask the patient for their name and date of birth. Check if the patient is well and not in any discomfort before proceeding. It is useful before you begin to confirm the reason why the patient needs a nebulizer. Try to establish any symptoms they may be having, such as cough, wheeze or shortness of breath. Also look at any observation charts for the respiratory rate, oxygen saturation, temperature and pulse or arterial blood gas results.

Elicit understanding

The most common reason for using nebulizers is for an acute asthma attack and so it may be an idea to clarify with the patient what a nebulizer machine is and when it is indicated. People often feel more at ease when they know what is happening, and this is especially important during an asthma attack when anxiety may exacerbate their symptoms.

3.16.2 **Explain the procedure**

Explain to the patient how a nebulizer machine functions as well as how it may relieve their symptoms. You may wish to say: *'As a result of the wheeze and tightness in your chest you require a short burst of nebulizer therapy. A nebulizer helps deliver medication directly into your lungs where it will relax your airways and help you breathe easier. The nebulizer uses a pump to generate high flow oxygen to do this and as a result may be quite noisy when in use.'*

Preparation

Before you go off to collect the equipment, it is important to check what drug has been prescribed for the patient. Ensure that the drug chart belongs to the patient by cross-referencing their name and date of birth with that on the chart. It is also worth noting whether the patient has been diagnosed with asthma or COPD, particularly in the acute setting. Bear in mind that patients with type 2 respiratory failure may be reliant upon their hypoxic drive to maintain respiration; prolonged exposure to high flow oxygen may inadvertently reduce their respiratory rate, leading to respiratory depression. Consider this fact when deciding to use either air or high flow oxygen for the nebulizer.

Drug chart
Check the prescription chart for the prescribed drug and dosage to be administered. You should be familiar with doses and frequencies for the common nebulized drugs such as salbutamol (2.5 or 5 mg 4–6 hourly) and ipratropium bromide (500 mcg up to qds). Double-check that the patient does not have any allergies before commencing with the medication.

Equipment
Collect the equipment that you will need to set up the nebulizer:
- drug chart
- medication (e.g. salbutamol liquid)
- nebulizer chamber
- plastic tubing
- oxygen (or air) supply
- face mask/mouthpiece (according to patient's preference).

> **TOP TIP!**
>
> Be aware of the common side effects of nebulized medication. Salbutamol can cause fine tremor, headaches, palpitations and tachycardia. Ipratropium bromide can cause dry mouth, sedation, skin flushing and nausea.

> **TOP TIP!**
>
> In the exam you may be offered a range of vials which may include a number of red herrings. Also be aware of the trade and generic names of the common drugs such as Ventolin™ (salbutamol) and Atrovent™ (ipratropium bromide) to avoid confusion when reading the drug chart.

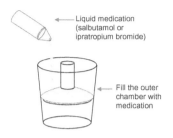

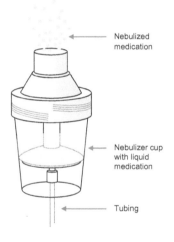

Fig 3.32 Filling the nebulizer cup with medication.

TOP TIP!

Salbutamol nebulizer solution can come in two different strengths: 2.5 mg per 2.5 ml or 5 mg per 2.5 ml; check the vial before diluting.

Fig 3.33 Correctly assembled nebulizer cup connected to compressor.

TOP TIP!

To avoid making patients feel anxious, always inform them when you are about to put the face mask on for them. If the patient feels claustrophobic a mouthpiece may be more suitable.

The procedure

Assembling the nebulizer

Once you have collected the appropriate equipment you should assemble the nebulizer. Start by attaching one end of the plastic tubing onto the nebulizer machine. Unpack the nebulizer cup and attach the lower half (it can be identified as it has a smaller connecting port for the tube at its base as well as a reservoir chamber found on top) to the free end of the plastic tubing.

Identify the correct vial as prescribed on the drug chart. Check its expiry date and confirm these details with a colleague if necessary. Open the vial by twisting the top off and then empty its contents fully into the outer reservoir chamber (*Fig 3.32*). If necessary, dilute the mixture with normal saline solution to make a total volume of 5 ml of solution for optimal delivery.

Once the solution is in place, screw together the two ends of the nebulizer cup. Switch on the compressor to test if it is working by looking for an aerosol mist emerging from the top of the mixing chamber (*Fig 3.33*). If no mist is seen check that the tubing is attached correctly and that the nebulizer cup is appropriately sealed.

Attaching a mask or mouthpiece

The decision to use a mask or mouthpiece largely revolves around the patient's choice or preference. However, it is important to note that if the patient suffers from glaucoma, a mouthpiece should be used when administering ipratropium bromide; this is because there have been reports of acute closed angle glaucoma being triggered by anticholinergics, such as ipratropium, passing on to the eye from the mask. In the emergency situation, face masks are usually preferred because they can be attached quickly and require minimal patient involvement.

Face masks should be tight-fitting to prevent unnecessary wastage of medication. Patients should be advised to breathe steadily and deeply and with an open mouth to ensure optimal delivery. Ask the patient to sit upright when using the nebulizer because this will help increase functional residual capacity. Gently adjust the elastic cord on the mask so that it sits comfortably on the patient. The nebulizer cup should remain in the upright position to allow for optimum treatment.

Flow rate

If you are using an oxygen-driven nebulizer (such as in an acute asthma attack) the flow rate should be set at between 5 and 7 l/min to allow the particles to be dispersed as a mist. If a patient has COPD with type 2 respiratory failure, you should use an air cylinder instead of oxygen but maintain a similar flow rate.

After you have administered the medication, sign the drug chart to document that the nebulizer has been given.

Cleaning advice

Some patients with chronic airway obstruction may require home nebulizer therapy. In such cases it is important to educate the patient about cleaning the device. The face mask and nebulizer chamber must be cleaned regularly to prevent infection. After each usage the nebulizer should be taken apart and all parts (except tubing) should be washed with warm soapy water and rinsed thoroughly. The components should then be dried to prevent build-up of bacteria within a moist environment.

In the hospital setting, the nebulizer's medication cup may be marked as 'single use' or 'single patient use'. Single use means that it should be disposed of after nebulizer treatment has been completed. Single patient use indicates that the chamber can be reused for the same patient at a later date if necessary.

3.16.3 Finishing up

Allow the nebulizer to run for between 5 and 10 minutes. This is to ensure that all the medication is converted into an aerosol and correctly delivered. Using the nebulizer for longer periods without refilling provides no symptomatic benefit for the patient.

Once complete, assess the patient and determine if their symptoms have improved or whether they require further treatment. If they have settled, dismantle the nebulizer and dispose of any waste appropriately. Thank the patient and ask them if they have any questions.

Chapter 3.17
Arterial blood gas sampling and analysis

What to do . . .

- Introduce yourself to the patient – establish rapport
- Ask the patient's name, age and occupation and confirm the reason for the procedure
- Explain the procedure to the patient and position them appropriately
- Gather and prepare equipment; put on gloves
- Palpate for an arterial pulsation – starting with the radial artery in a non-shocked patient
- Feel for the pulsation and insert the needle appropriately
- Allow the syringe to self-fill, collecting an appropriate volume of blood (at least 1 ml)
- Remove the needle and apply pressure to the puncture site with cotton wool or gauze
- Discard the needle in a sharps bin and cover the end of the syringe with a cap
- Put the sample through a blood gas analyser
- Interpret the results in the context of the clinical condition and document them in the patient's notes
- Thank the patient and conclude the consultation

Arterial blood gas (ABG) sampling describes the procedure to take blood from a patient's artery and then analyse the gases contained within the sampled blood. It is often employed in acutely unwell patients, especially those with chronic respiratory conditions, because it provides a rapid and accurate assessment of the oxygenation status that a simple saturation probe cannot achieve. It also provides other information such as the pH status of the blood, partial pressure of oxygen and carbon dioxide as well as bicarbonate and lactate levels; these details can be particularly important in illnesses that may lead to metabolic acidosis, such as liver failure, renal failure, diabetic ketoacidosis and multi-organ failure.

Blood for ABG analysis is usually taken from the radial artery because it is easily accessible and can be compressed to prevent haematoma formation. Occasionally the brachial or femoral artery can be used instead. The blood is extracted using a specially designed heparinized 2 ml syringe that prevents coagulation occurring in the sample. The blood is then transferred as soon as possible to a blood gas analyser where it is immediately processed with a printed result sheet produced for interpretation. Although a single ABG reading may provide information regarding a patient's health, it is more useful to have serial measurements that can reveal improvements or deterioration in their clinical state.

3.17.1 **Beginning the procedure**

Start by introducing yourself to the patient, stating your name and job title. Confirm the patient's name and date of birth as this will ensure that you take blood from the correct patient. This will also help you complete the patient's identifier details when inputting the details into the blood analyser.

Check if the patient is well and not in any discomfort before proceeding with the procedure. In the exam situation, you are more likely to be presented with a simulated manikin arm in lieu of a real patient. In this circumstance, treat the manikin as if it were a patient, maintaining your usual standards of professional courtesy and rapport building.

It may be useful to confirm the reason why the patient is having the ABG so that you can correctly interpret the values in the context of the full clinical picture. The patient may suffer from COPD and run the risk of retaining carbon dioxide if put on high concentration oxygen, or the patient may be a diabetic with diabetic ketoacidosis and in need of an urgent ABG analysis to determine its severity.

Explain the procedure

It is important to explain to the patient the procedure and what it entails. Taking blood from the radial artery can be extremely painful and hence it is of vital importance that you warn them of this in advance. You may wish to say: *'As a result of your difficulty in breathing, we would like to perform a special blood test. This test involves taking a sample of blood from a vessel in your wrist. I must warn you that taking the blood sample can be quite painful.'*

Preparation

Ensure that the patient is seated or lying down comfortably. Roll up any garments so that good access to the wrist area can be achieved. Ensure that any watches or bracelets have been removed so as not to occlude your access. It is usually a good idea to select the non-dominant hand to take blood from because there may be some residual soreness after the procedure.

Rest the hand on a pillow and extend at the wrist joint. If you are having difficulty in palpating a radial pulse, you may wish to consider the brachial or femoral artery for the procedure.

Equipment

Before you start make sure that you have washed your hands and collected all of the equipment that you will require. You will need the following:
- equipment tray/kidney dish
- pair of gloves (non-sterile)
- blood gas syringe with heparin (a 21G or finer needle should be packaged with it)
- sharps box
- cotton wool balls or gauze and alcohol wipes
- tape/plaster

> **TOP TIP!**
>
> If a patient is in shock or cardio-respiratory arrest, go straight for the femoral artery.

Select and prepare the site

If the patient is well enough, begin by assessing the radial artery. Feel for arterial pulsation between the styloid process of the radius and the flexor carpi radialis tendon; this can usually be felt just proximal to the wrist joint. If you are happy with the pulse, you must assess the ulnar collateral supply to the hand using Allen's test. This involves elevating the hand and asking the patient to make a tight fist for 30 seconds. You should then apply pressure over both the radial and ulnar arteries in order to occlude them. Next ask the patient to open their hand and observe for pallor in the fingernails. At this point, release ulnar pressure whilst still occluding the radial artery and observe the fingernails for re-perfusion within 10 seconds. If the hand does not re-perfuse, the ulnar collateral supply to the hand is not adequate and the radial artery should not be punctured.

If you are having difficulty obtaining blood at the radial artery, you should consider moving on to the brachial artery, which is medial to the biceps tendon and best felt under the belly of the biceps muscle. If the patient is well and the brachial pulse is easily palpable, it is preferred to the femoral artery because the groin area can be prone to infection. However, if the brachial artery is unsuitable you will have to consider the femoral artery which is found within the femoral triangle 2 cm below the mid-inguinal point.

Once you have selected the artery, thoroughly disinfect the area by wiping with an alcohol swab. Then put on a pair of non-sterile gloves.

Open the ABG pack and note the presence of the heparinized syringe with needle and cap. In some ABG packs the needle may need to be attached to the syringe and the heparin ejected. When doing so, ensure that you do not aspirate any air back into the syringe. Check whether the syringe contains a vacuum or not – some syringes may need the plunger to be retracted by up to 1 ml to aid filling when inserted.

3.17.2 **The procedure**

Arterial puncture

Use the index and middle finger of your non-dominant hand to locate the patient's radial pulse. Once you have located a good pulse, separate your fingers along the line of the radial artery, ensuring that both pulps can feel the pulsations. Next try to identify where the artery runs between these two points; this should be the spot where you insert the needle.

Take the unsheathed needle and ABG syringe in your dominant hand and hold it as if you were holding a pen. Make sure that the needle is perpendicular to the line of the artery between your two fingers. Warn the patient of a sharp scratch prior to introducing the needle into the skin. Ensure that the bevel of the needle is facing upwards. Push the needle through the skin gently until you see a flash of blood in the hub of the needle. Hold the syringe firm and allow it to fill the chamber under arterial pressure.

Withdrawing the needle

After you have collected up to 2 ml of blood, apply pressure to the artery using a piece of gauze or cotton wool. If provided, stab the end of the needle into a rubber bung to reduce the risk of a needle stick injury. Dispose of the needle in

TOP TIP!

Avoid using your thumb to palpate the radial pulse as you may inadvertently be feeling your own pulse and not the patient's.

TOP TIP!

There are several ways to take blood from an artery: some schools of thought recommend approaching the artery at a 30 degree angle whilst others recommend a 90 degree angle. You should use whichever approach works best for you.

a sharps bin whilst continuing to apply steady pressure. Observe the site for up to 5 minutes for evidence of haematomas or localized swelling.

Expel any air found within the syringe chamber before placing a cap over it. This is an important step to prevent contamination with room air, which would result in abnormally low carbon dioxide levels being found as well as giving falsely reassuring oxygen concentrations. Gently mix the blood with the heparin by turning the syringe upside down a few times; this will help to prevent any clots from appearing. Immediately take the sample to the blood gas analyser for interpretation. If you do not have direct access to such a machine, make sure that the blood sample is kept chilled before being sent to the laboratory for analysis (having been marked with the correct patient's identifier details). Samples that are left at room temperature for long periods of time may give inaccurately low oxygen levels and high carbon dioxide levels.

3.17.3 Finishing up

Print out a copy of the blood gas report for interpretation. Dispose of any gloves and soiled material appropriately. Check for haemostasis over the puncture site and explain the results to the patient in light of the clinical context. Do not forget to wash your hands again at the end of the procedure.

3.17.4 Interpretation

It is important that you adopt a systematic approach when interpreting ABG results so that you do not inadvertently overlook any important information. *Box 3.7* gives the normal ranges for ABG analyses.

Acid–base balance

Start by looking at the pH of the ABG sample. The pH of normal blood ranges from 7.35 to 7.45. A pH of less than 7.35 indicates acidosis, whilst values above 7.45 represent alkalosis. Do not dismiss a normal pH value, particularly in the presence of other abnormal parameters, because this may indicate a 'mixed' picture or a compensatory mechanism at work.

PaO_2 and $PaCO_2$

Next assess the PaO_2 levels on the gas report. This will help determine whether the patient is suffering from hypoxaemia or is in respiratory failure. The normal partial pressure of oxygen in room air is between 11 and 13 kPa. Values between 8 and 10.7 indicate hypoxaemia, while values below 8 are significant and suggest that the patient is in respiratory failure.

Look at the $PaCO_2$ levels to determine whether the patient is in either type 1 or type 2 respiratory failure (see *Table 3.10*). A normal $PaCO_2$ ranges from 4.7 to 6 kPa. If the patient is hypoxic but with a normal or low $PaCO_2$ then they

TOP TIP!

If you find yourself having to draw back on the plunger to fill the syringe with blood it is likely that you are aspirating a venous sample. If the syringe is self-filling in a pulsatile manner you have entered the artery.

TOP TIP!

If you are unsuccessful in obtaining an arterial blood sample, you should slowly withdraw the tip of the needle before reinserting it. You should never probe for the artery with the needle *in situ* as this may cause repeated puncturing and increase the risk of haematomas or damage to the artery.

TOP TIP!

The blood gas analyser will not accept less than 0.3 ml of blood. Make sure that you have collected at least this amount.

TOP TIP!

Most machines require codes before they can be used for analysis of a sample. Find someone who knows the code and can show you how to use the machine. It is not so uncommon for an error to occur during introduction of a sample and you do not want to be in a position where you need to repeat the procedure.

TOP TIP!

If the PaO_2 reading exceeds 14 kPa it is highly likely that the patient is receiving supplementary oxygen.

BOX 3.7 **Normal range values**

pH	7.35–7.45
PaO_2	11–13 kPa
$PaCO_2$	4.7–6.0 kPa
HCO_3^-	22–26 mmol/l

Table 3.10 Causes of type 1 and type 2 respiratory failure	
Type 1	**Type 2**
COPD	COPD
Pulmonary oedema	Severe asthma attack
Asthma	Respiratory centre depression, e.g. drug overdose or head injury
Pneumonia	Respiratory muscle weakness, e.g. myasthenia gravis
Pulmonary embolism	

are in type 1 respiratory failure. However, if they have hypoxaemia with a high $PaCO_2$ (> 6 kPa) then they are considered to be in type 2 respiratory failure. It is important to bear in mind that carbon dioxide is an acidic substance and therefore low $PaCO_2$ levels are associated with alkalosis, whilst high levels result in acidosis.

Bicarbonate levels

The bicarbonate levels help to distinguish between a true respiratory or metabolic cause. Normal bicarbonate values range from 22 to 26 mmol/l. Because bicarbonate is an alkalotic agent, values below 22 will result in acidosis while results above 26 will result in alkalosis.

Assessing the acid–base status

Having looked at all the parameters you should be in a position to determine the cause of the patient's acid–base disturbance (see *Table 3.11*).

Look at the pH and determine if the patient is acidotic or alkalotic. Then look at the $PaCO_2$ and HCO_3^- in conjunction to establish the cause:
- If the pH is acidotic (< 7.35) and the $PaCO_2$ is raised then the patient is considered to have respiratory acidosis
- If the pH is alkalotic (> 7.45) with a low $PaCO_2$ then the patient has a respiratory alkalosis
- If the pH is acidotic with a low HCO_3^- level then the patient is considered to have a metabolic acidosis
- If the pH is alkalotic with a raised HCO_3^- then they are in metabolic alkalosis.

Table 3.11 Interpreting an ABG analysis				
	pH	$PaCO_2$	HCO_3^-	Possible causes
Respiratory acidosis	↓	↑	Normal	Asthma, COPD, central depression (head injury, drug overdose), respiratory muscle weakness (myasthenia gravis), pneumothorax, pulmonary oedema
Respiratory alkalosis	↑	↓	Normal	Asthmatic attack, panic attack, stroke
Metabolic acidosis	↓	Normal	↓	Renal failure, ketoacidosis, lactic acidosis, salicylate intoxication, severe diarrhoea
Metabolic alkalosis	↑	Normal	↑	Persistent vomiting, diuretic therapy

Compensation mechanism

The above explanation describes the acid–base status in the acute setting whereby an insult or illness has just taken place. However, over a prolonged period of time the body will employ compensatory mechanisms to restore the pH back towards normal parameters. The body attempts to reverse any acid–base derangements caused by a particular system, i.e. the respiratory system, by compensating within another system, i.e. the metabolic system. To judge which system is at fault and which system is compensating, the degree of change within each parameter must be considered. For example, in respiratory acidosis with metabolic compensation you would expect to have a very high $PaCO_2$ and a slightly raised HCO_3^-. Likewise, in metabolic acidosis with respiratory compensation you would expect to have a very low bicarbonate level but a slightly reduced $PaCO_2$ concentration.

3.17.5 Common clinical scenarios

Read the clinical scenarios and, in conjunction with the ABG results, describe the acid–base disturbance taking place and its possible cause.

CASE 1

An anxious 29 year old woman complains of palpitations for 1 hour with a respiratory rate of 30 and feelings of impending doom. Her blood gas results reveal:

pH	7.5
PaO_2	13 kPa
$PaCO_2$	3.1 kPa
HCO_3^-	24 mmol/l

CASE 2

A 34 year old man, who is a known asthmatic on home nebulizers, presents with acute onset of shortness of breath. On examination he is fatigued, unable to complete sentences and has a silent chest. He is unable to provide a peak flow reading. His blood gas analysis shows:

pH	7.27
PaO_2	7.9 kPa
$PaCO_2$	6.9 kPa
HCO_3^-	26 mmol/l

CASE 3

A 16 year old boy known to have type 1 diabetes mellitus presents with history of thirst, polyuria, abdominal pain, heavy laboured breathing and reduced consciousness. His urine dipstick shows glucose 3+ and ketones 3+. His blood gas analysis shows:

pH	7.20
PaO_2	12.5 kPa
$PaCO_2$	4.9 kPa
HCO_3^-	15 mmol/l

CASE 4

A 29 year old woman who is 8 weeks pregnant presents with persistent vomiting since the morning. Her urine dipstick shows 2+ ketones and normal BP. Her ABG results were:

pH	7.52
PaO_2	11.2 kPa
$PaCO_2$	5.4 kPa
HCO_3^-	34 mmol/l

CASE 5

A 58 year old woman with chronic kidney disease (stage 5) complains of feeling generally unwell for 5 days. She is due to undergo dialysis later on in the week. Her ABG analysis shows:

pH	7.3
PaO_2	12.7 kPa
$PaCO_2$	4.1 kPa
HCO_3^-	13 mmol/l

CASE 6

A 55 year old man with known COPD complains of a 1 day history of shortness of breath and wheeze. His blood gas analysis shows:

pH	7.3
PaO_2	9 kPa
$PaCO_2$	7.4 kPa
HCO_3^-	30 mmol/l

Chapter 3.18
Nasogastric intubation

What to do . . .

- Introduce yourself to the patient – establish rapport
- Ask the patient's name and date of birth and confirm why they need a nasogastric (NG) tube
- Explain the procedure to the patient and gain consent
- Gather and prepare equipment, put on gloves
- Position the patient sitting upright
- Examine nostrils for deformity to determine best site of insertion
- Measure the tubing from nose to earlobe and then measure to the midpoint between xiphoid process and umbilicus; mark the tube to indicate the approximate length required
- Lubricate the tip of the NG tube and apply anaesthetic spray to pharynx and/or nostril
- Pass the tube parallel to nasal floor, past pharynx and ask the patient to tilt head forward and swallow/sip water; advance the tube with each swallow until the mark is reached
- Withdraw the tube if the patient coughs or is in respiratory distress
- Secure the tube with tape
- Check placement by obtaining aspirate with 50 ml bladder syringe and placing sample onto pH indicator paper: pH should be 5.5 or less before commencing feed
- If unsure about position obtain chest X-ray
- Attach to suction or spigot if clinically indicated
- Dispose of rubbish and document in notes
- Thank the patient and conclude the consultation

A nasogastric (NG) tube is a thin flexible plastic tube that is introduced into the stomach through the nasal passages via the oesophagus. They have a number of clinical indications that broadly fall into two categories: feeding and aspiration.

Perhaps the most commonly known use for NG tubes is for providing enteral feeds or nutritional substances to a patient who may:
- be unconscious – patients who are unconscious for a prolonged period of time require nutrition that can be received via an NG tube
- be unable to swallow – patients who have dysphagia (swallowing disorders), such as in strokes or motor neurone disease, will have poorly co-ordinated swallowing and will be at risk of aspiration pneumonia; in these cases, an NG tube provides a safe means for nutritional support in the short to medium term

- have nutritional needs that are not being met orally – patients who have feeding disorders such as anorexia nervosa, or have difficulty establishing feeds such as neonates, can also benefit from the insertion of an NG tube.

In the surgical or emergency setting, NG tubes provide an essential role in draining the stomach's content in bowel obstruction and other gastric immotility disorders (gastric paresis). They act to release trapped air as well as any excessive gastric secretions that can accumulate in such circumstances. An NG tube can also be used to aspirate ingested toxic substances in the acute setting, such as in an intentional overdose.

Anatomy

A basic understanding of the local structures in the throat as well as the upper thorax will help ensure safe insertion and passage of the NG tube into the stomach.

The oral pharynx is the chamber to which the oesophagus and trachea are connected. If both passages are opened simultaneously then a person may aspirate air into the stomach as well as food into their lungs. To prevent this, whenever a person swallows, the epiglottis and larynx work in conjunction to close off the trachea to prevent food from entering the respiratory tract. This is an important fact to consider when inserting the NG tube. Simply asking the patient to swallow repetitively as you advance the tube should help prevent the NG tube going into the trachea and potentially harming the patient.

Types of tube

NG tubes are manufactured from polyurethane, silicone or PVC, with each type being able to be left *in situ* for different lengths of time. Their sizes are described in French units with 3 Fr units equal to 1 mm; they commonly range from 8 Fr (fine bore) to 18 Fr (wide bore).

NG tubes that are used for feeding are also known as Ryle's tubes. They are usually fine bore tubes (8 Fr) that also allow for the administration of medications. Fine bore tubes are generally more comfortable and because of their size are less likely to cause stricture formation or oesophageal irritation. Large bore tubes are less well tolerated by the patient and should only be considered for the drainage or aspiration of the stomach content, i.e. in bowel obstruction. Large bore tubes tend to be left *in situ* for less than a week whereas fine bore tubes can remain in place for up to 6 weeks.

Risks

Although NG tubes have a number of important roles to play in a patient's care, because of the way they have to be inserted they may not be suitable for everyone. Patients who have suffered trauma to the head, particularly to the maxillofacial areas, or have sustained a basal skull fracture, should not be offered an NG tube. An attempt to insert an NG tube in such patients may inadvertently end up in the intracranial space instead of the oropharynx. Patients with oesophageal disorders such as strictures or varices should also not have an NG tube inserted, to prevent traumatic complications such as bleeding.

As with any procedure, the possibility of post-procedural complications exists. The most serious one to consider is perforation of the oesophagus which may occur secondary to aspiration of the stomach contents or as a result of a traumatic insertion. Another complication may include locating the NG tube in the bronchi, causing respiratory distress through airway obstruction or lung collapse (see *Fig 3.34*). Minor complications include sore throat, epistaxis and oesophagitis. Patients should be informed about the possible complications before commencing the procedure.

3.18.1 Beginning the procedure

Start by introducing yourself to the patient, stating your name and job title. Confirm the patient's name and date of birth. Ensure that the patient is well and not in any discomfort before proceeding. It is useful before you begin to confirm the reason why the patient is having the NG tube inserted and whether they have any contraindications for it. This information may help you decide what size and type of NG tube you should use.

Be aware that in the examination situation you are likely to be faced with a manikin instead of a real patient.

Explain the procedure

It is important to explain to the patient what you intend to do so that informed consent can be obtained. Patients may be hesitant to have an NG tube inserted; however, with good communication skills and a brief explanation as to its purpose, most will be persuaded. You may wish to say: *'Following your stroke, you have had some difficulty in swallowing, and there is a real risk that the food that you eat may accidentally go down into your lungs instead of your stomach. To prevent this from happening I plan to pass a thin, flexible tube down into your stomach through your nose. This tube will allow us to give you the vital nutrients that your body needs, in addition to your prescribed medication. The procedure is quick and simple and should not cause any undue pain.'*

Preparation

Ensure that the patient is sitting upright in a chair or on the bed. This will ensure optimal alignment of the oesophagus with the stomach. This may be a good time to inspect the patient's nostrils for any obstructions such as nasal polyps, or for any deformities such as septal deviation, which may impede the procedure. Note whether the patient has any bleeding disorder or is on any medication, such as warfarin. If so, you may wish to check the patient's INR levels prior to proceeding.

Because you will be passing the NG tube down their throat, it will be extremely difficult for the patient to communicate to you any discomfort or pain that they may be suffering. So, before starting the procedure, agree with the patient a gesture such as a raised hand that they can use to stop the procedure instantly.

Equipment

Before you start make sure that you have washed your hands and collected all of the equipment that you will need. It may be an idea to wear non-sterile gloves, eye protection and an apron if you believe there is a high risk that the patient may vomit during the procedure (e.g. if there is a suspected bowel obstruction). Always prepare the equipment before you start because once you have started inserting the NG tube you will have difficulty leaving the patient's side.

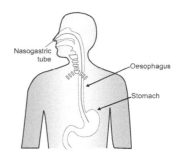

Correctly positioned NG tube

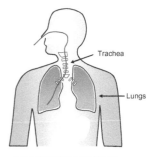

Incorrectly positioned NG tube

Fig 3.34 Correct and incorrect positioning of the NG tube.

Remember the indication for the NG tube insertion because this will determine what size tube you will need.

- gloves (non-sterile)
- NG tube (fine bore for feeding and medication, wide bore for aspiration of stomach contents)
- 50 ml bladder syringe
- 2% xylocaine spray and K-Y jelly
- adhesive tape
- spigot or drainage bag to attach to the tube
- cup of water (unless the patient is dysphagic)
- pH indicator strips
- kidney dish

3.18.2 **The procedure**

Measure

After putting on a pair of gloves, measure the length of the tube required for the patient to ensure that the appropriate length of tube is inserted into the stomach. Hold the tip of the NG tube at the bridge of the nose and align it horizontally across to the earlobe and then down to around halfway between the xiphoid process and the umbilicus. Note down the distance either by marking across the graduations on the tube or by taping around this point.

Prepare the tube

Now that you have measured the length of tube that you will require, you should prepare it for insertion. Place some lubricant jelly on to a piece of gauze and rub it on the distal end of the NG tube. This may help reduce the initial resistance met when introducing it through the nostril. You may also wish to spray some xylocaine at the back of the throat and into the nostril before starting as this will help relieve any initial discomfort.

Prepare the patient

Inform the patient that you are ready to begin. It is important to remind them that the procedure may be uncomfortable and they can gesture to stop at any point if it is intolerable.

Give them clear instructions as to what to do as you pass the NG tube down the back of their throat. You could say: *'I am now going to insert the tube through your nostril and into the back of your throat. As it goes down you may feel the tube at the back of your throat. Once you notice this, tilt your head forward and take small sips of water from this glass and swallow. Doing this will help the tube pass down more quickly. If at any time you are uncomfortable raise your hand to indicate that you wish to stop and, as we agreed, I will stop what I am doing immediately.'*

Insert the NG tube

Pass the tube into the chosen nostril while the patient's head is upright. Continue to gently push the tube along the floor of the nasopharynx. If you encounter any obstruction gently withdraw the tube and reinsert at a slightly different angle to see if you can overcome it. If not, consider removing the tube and introducing it through the other nostril.

TOP TIP!

As a general rule, stiffer tubes are easier to insert and placing them in a cold environment, such as a fridge, may help to achieve this.

TOP TIP!

Remember that if the patient has had a stroke they should not be given water to swallow because they may aspirate it. With such patients you should just tip their head forward and ask them to try to make swallowing movements.

TOP TIP!

When inserting the NG tube never aim upwards through the nostril. Aim to run parallel to the nasal floor, otherwise it can result in intracranial passage!

TOP TIP!

Previously it was advised to confirm the location of the NG tube by injecting air through it and auscultating over the stomach for an increase in gurgling or 'whoosh' sounds. The 'whoosh' test is subjective and not an accurate means of verifying the location of the NG tube and so it is no longer recommended for this purpose.

As the tube approaches the back of the throat, the patient may show signs of discomfort. Tell the patient to tilt their head forward and begin sipping the water. As they swallow, co-ordinate your pushing the tube with each swallow and gently ease the NG tube down the oesophagus; this will ensure that the epiglottis is closed and will prevent the tube from accidentally entering the trachea. If the tube does enter the trachea, the patient may start coughing, gasping for breath or become cyanosed. In such cases, immediately cease your activity and withdraw the tube completely.

Continue advancing the NG tube through the nostril until you reach the end mark that you outlined earlier. After passing the epiglottis you should no longer encounter much resistance. Every so often inspect the patient's mouth to ensure that the tube has not coiled in the oropharynx. If it has, retract it until the NG tube is uncoiled.

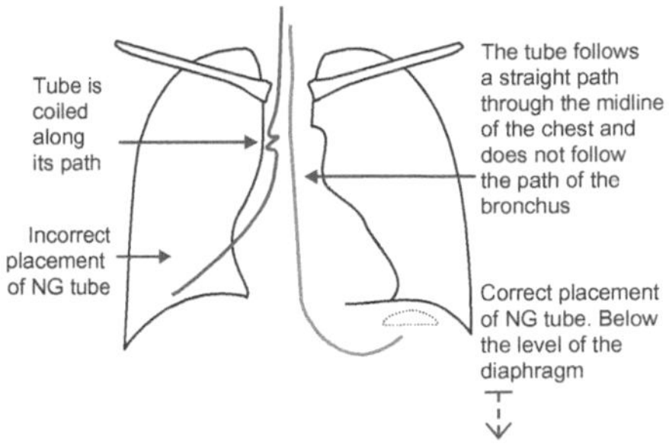

Tube is coiled along its path

Incorrect placement of NG tube

The tube follows a straight path through the midline of the chest and does not follow the path of the bronchus

Correct placement of NG tube. Below the level of the diaphragm

Fig 3.35 X-ray findings of a correctly (green) and incorrectly (red) inserted NG tube.

Check the intra-gastric position

There are two ways of confirming that the tube is in the stomach (particularly important if you are to commence NG feeds, to prevent the risk of aspiration pneumonia): the pH test or by taking an X-ray.

The tube's position must be confirmed not only after the initial insertion, but also before each feed. You should also recheck if the patient starts vomiting or coughing or if the tube is accidentally dislodged.

The pH test
This test utilizes the fact that the stomach contents are highly acidic. Thus, if the NG tube is in the correct location, aspirating fluid and then checking the pH should reveal a low reading. Use a 50 ml bladder syringe to try to aspirate some liquid from the free tip of the NG tube and place it on a pH indicator paper to confirm acidity. It is safe to continue the feed if the pH is 5.5 or below.

Chest X-ray
If you are ever in doubt about the tube's position, it is best practice to request a chest X-ray, and they should always be requested if you obtained an equivocal aspirate test, if the pH is more than 5.5, or if the patient is unconscious. The NG is radio-opaque and should be easy to see on a simple X-ray film (see *Fig 3.35*). Ensure that the tube has passed below the level of the diaphragm and resides comfortably in the stomach. If there is any doubt, replace the NG tube and X-ray again.

3.18.3 Finishing up

Once you have inserted the NG tube and confirmed that it is in the correct position you should attempt to secure it in place to prevent it being accidentally dislodged. Tape the NG tube to the tip of the patient's nose, forehead and side of their face in such a way that is comfortable for the patient.

Dispose of all the rubbish into a clinical waste bin. If you are using an NG tube that has a guide-wire contained within it, remove it once the X-ray has been completed. The guide-wire, if left in, may occlude the foramen of the tube when feeding has been started.

If the NG tube was inserted to aspirate the gastric contents, it should be attached to a suction device. In the emergency setting, such as for a bowel obstruction, up

Medical Guidelines
Checking for misplacement of the NG tube

In 2005 the National Patient Safety Agency published the following guidelines in determining NG tube position:

- Measuring the pH of aspirate using pH indicator strips / paper is recommended
- Radiography is recommended but should not be used 'routinely'
- DO NOT use the 'whoosh' test – this practice must cease immediately
- DO NOT test acidity/alkalinity of aspirate using blue litmus paper
- DO NOT interpret absence of respiratory distress as an indicator of correct positioning

National Patient Safety Agency: Reducing harm caused by the misplacement of nasogastric feeding tubes (2005)

TOP TIP!

Blue litmus paper, which was previously used to test pH, has been shown not to be sensitive enough to differentiate between bronchial and gastric secretions.

TOP TIP!

Some medications such as PPIs and H$_2$ receptor antagonists can alter the pH of the stomach. Milk can also neutralize the stomach's pH. In such cases where you are unsure, it may be wise to check the position of the NG tube by requesting an X-ray.

TOP TIP!

If the NG tube is not attached to a suction device and is not in use then it should remain clamped shut with a spigot.

to one litre of fluid can be aspirated over 4 hours. However, in less severe cases, aspiration rates should usually be one litre over 24 hours.

Document in the notes the reason for the tube insertion, the type and size of tube used, and the nature and amount of any aspirate. You should comment on the colour and pH of the aspirate obtained and state that the insertion was consented and atraumatic. Brown aspirate usually indicates the NG tube is in the bowel and that faecal material is being collected. A yellow aspirate may suggest that the NG tube is located in the small intestine, whilst clear fluid may indicate that the tube is still within the oesophagus.

Make sure you record how you confirmed the position of the NG tube. If the patient was previously nil by mouth and unable to take oral medication, you may wish to consider altering the route of administration from PO to NG on the drug chart if indicated. Consider checking the BNF for more information.

Chapter 3.19
Male catheterization

What to do . . .

- Introduce yourself to the patient – establish rapport
- Ask the patient's name, date of birth and confirm the reason for catheterization
- Explain the procedure to the patient, gain consent and request a chaperone as appropriate
- Gather and prepare equipment on a trolley using aseptic technique
- Position patient appropriately, maintaining privacy and dignity at all times
- Wash hands thoroughly and put on gloves aseptically
- Create sterile field
- Clean penis with 'no touch' technique
- Insert local anaesthetic, allowing 5 minutes to work
- Insert catheter aseptically, with one end in kidney dish; start with penis held vertically then horizontally
- Wait for flow of urine and further advance the catheter before inflating balloon (watch for pain)
- Pull catheter back and tug until balloon reaches bladder neck
- Connect catheter bag and replace foreskin
- Acknowledge patient concerns, replace their clothes and wash hands
- Document procedure in notes and thank the patient

Fig 3.36 Anatomy of the urethra 373

TOP TIP!

It is always important to check that the patient is not allergic to latex prior to catheterizing them. In such cases consider using silicone catheters instead.

Urinary catheterization is the process by which a short plastic tube is inserted under strict aseptic conditions into the patient's bladder via the urethra. In the acute setting it is recommended for the treatment of urinary retention, whereby a patient is unable to pass urine and this is causing them pain and distress. It is also used for treatments such as cytotoxic therapies in bladder cancer or to provide a means for irrigation in gross haematuria. Catheterization is often employed to monitor fluid balance in critically unwell patients, particularly those who are hypovolaemic or in shock. Long-term catheters can be used for the management of severe urinary incontinence or in those with a neuropathic bladder.

Anatomy

The male urethra is approximately 20 cm long, commencing at the neck of the bladder and opening at the end of the penis. The urethra is divided into four parts, each part representing the structure it passes through (*Fig 3.36*).

- The section between the neck of the bladder and the prostate is known as the pre-prostatic urethra.

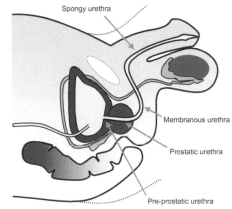

Spongy urethra

Membranous urethra

Prostatic urethra

Pre-prostatic urethra

Fig 3.36 Anatomy of the urethra.

- As the urethra bisects through the prostate it becomes known as the prostatic urethra.
- As the urethra exits the apex of the prostate it passes forwards and goes through the urogenital diaphragm – this is known as the membranous urethra.
- The last part of the urethra is called the spongy (or penile) urethra as it passes through the corpus spongiosum before ending at the external urethral orifice.

Types of catheter

There are several types of catheter available:
- Foley catheters are the most commonly used and consist of a tube with a balloon that can be inflated to secure it within the bladder.
- Nelaton catheters are single-use straight catheters that are used to drain the bladder quickly. They have no balloon because they are not designed to remain *in situ*. They are often used to quickly obtain a urine sample for testing.
- Suprapubic catheters are a special type of Foley catheter that are inserted through the skin into the bladder. They are often used when simple catheterization has failed.
- Three-way haemostatic catheters are thicker than normal catheters and have an extra channel to allow irrigation of the bladder. They are commonly used for bladder washout to prevent blood clots post-operatively.

By accurately assessing the appropriate size, material and balloon capacity required, you can reduce the risk of complications. Short-term catheters should remain *in situ* for less than a month. For this reason they are made from PVC or siliconized latex (a latex catheter with a silicone surface) because latex can irritate the urothelium and cause abrasions. Long-term catheters may stay in place for up to 3 months and are designed to be more resistant to infection. They are usually made from silicone with hydrogel coating to prevent irritation and ulceration.

Catheter diameters are measured in French (Fr); 3 Fr units is equivalent to 1 mm. Choosing the appropriate catheter size depends on a number of different factors including the presence or absence of haematuria or grit, size of blood clots and the turbidity of the urine sample (see *Table 3.12*).

The most commonly used catheter size in adult males is 12 to 14. The reason for this is because these smaller sized catheters allow adequate drainage with minimal irritation to the urothelium.

Table 3.12 Catheter sizes and their indications	
Catheter size (Fr)	**Indications**
12–14	Clear urine, no haematuria, grit or debris
16	Hazy urine with light haematuria (pink tinge), or small amounts of grit
18	Cloudy urine, frank haematuria with moderately sized clots
20	Very cloudy urine with frank haematuria and heavy clots. Large grit and debris particles
22	Severe haematuria and large-sized blood clots

Risks

Despite their benefits, catheters pose an infection risk to the patient. There is a direct relationship between the duration the catheter is left *in situ* and the risk of developing a urinary tract infection. For this reason the continuing need for catheters being left *in situ* should routinely be reviewed. Catheters can also cause other problems such as trauma (bleeding), ulcerations, and urethral stricture formation.

3.19.1 Beginning the procedure

Start by introducing yourself to the patient, stating your name and job title. Confirm the patient's details including their name and date of birth before you begin. It is useful to establish why the patient needs catheterization because this may influence the type of catheter you will use.

In the exams you are likely to be presented with a simulated model in lieu of a patient. You should still act courteously towards it as if you were talking to and treating a real person.

As catheterization involves dealing with intimate parts of the body, it is important to approach this procedure sensitively. You should ensure that you maintain strict privacy and that the patient's dignity is preserved at all times. If you are performing the procedure on the ward you should make sure that you draw across any curtains to prevent any undue embarrassment.

> **TOP TIP!**
>
> It is important to ask the patient if they would prefer the procedure to be performed by a doctor of the same gender – this may make the patient feel less anxious and embarrassed.

Explain the procedure

Explain the procedure to the patient, informing them what you intend to do and the purpose of the procedure. As it is an intimate procedure, the patient may have a number of anxieties. Attempt to elicit these and address them sensitively in your explanation. You may wish to say: *'As a result of your inability to pass urine, I would recommend that we pass a catheter through your penis to relieve the pressure. The catheter is a flexible thin plastic tube that helps drain urine from your bladder. Although it may sound alarming this is a common procedure that we undertake. We always use local anaesthetic gel before we begin in order to reduce any discomfort.'*

After you have explained the procedure to the patient, it is important to check that they have understood what you have said and given you verbal consent to proceed. At this point you should offer them the opportunity to ask any questions.

Chaperone

Once the patient has consented to the procedure, you may wish to offer them a chaperone – this is particularly appropriate if you are a female doctor intending to catheterize a male patient.

Equipment

Before you start make sure that you have washed your hands thoroughly with soap and water and collected all of the equipment which you require. Always prepare the equipment before you expose the patient because it can be embarrassing and undignified to leave them exposed for longer than necessary. You will need the following equipment:

- procedure trolley
- sterile catheterization pack
- pair of sterile gloves
- disposable pad
- catheter bag
- lignocaine gel 2% or Instillagel (this is sometimes included in the catheter pack)
- Foley catheter (12 or 14 Fr)
- antiseptic solution
- 10 ml sterile water in a pre-filled syringe
- adhesive tape
- 10 ml saline solution
- three plastic prongs
- apron

Once you have collected your equipment and washed your hands, clean the procedure trolley with antiseptic solution and put on an apron.

Preparation

Ensure that the patient is lying comfortably. Ask the patient to remove their lower garments and change into a hospital gown. It may be an idea to provide them with a sheet to cover themselves with so that the patient is never exposed unnecessarily. Place a disposable pad on the bed and ask the patient to lie down in a supine position with their legs extended.

Sterile field

You will need to set up a sterile field on the trolley before commencing. This is essential to maintain an aseptic technique to reduce the risk of any contamination.

First peel off the outer plastic covering of the sterile catheter pack and slide it onto the trolley. Grab hold of a corner of the catheter pack and expand the sheet to cover the entire trolley, creating a sterile field. From this point onward be careful what you introduce into this area. Take the yellow waste bag from the catheter pack and attach it to the end of the trolley. This will help you dispose of waste material appropriately.

Open the sterile gloves, plastic prongs, catheter and the Instillagel into the sterile field. Pour the sterile water into the small receptacle found inside the catheter pack which usually contains three swabs within it.

3.19.2 The procedure

You are now ready to begin the procedure. Ask the patient to expose themselves from the umbilicus to their knee. Ask them to retract their own foreskin if present. Put on a pair of sterile gloves. This will now allow you to handle equipment in the sterile field. It may be useful at this point to remove both ends of the plastic cover around the catheter and massage the end of the catheter out of it by a few centimetres. This will prepare it for use later on.

Drape the patient

Locate the drape within the sterile field and tear a hole in the centre. Bring it over to the patient and ensure that the penis passes through the hole so that the surrounding areas are covered. Wrap a gauze (found in the pack) around the shaft of the penis and grasp this with your non-dominant hand. This hand is now considered to be non-sterile and should not be used to touch the equipment in the sterile field.

Cleaning

Using your dominant hand (sterile), pick up a plastic prong with a wet swab from the receptacle and wipe the left side of the glans with a single wipe. Immediately dispose of the swab and prong into the yellow waste bag. Take a new prong and wet swab and wipe the right side of the glans in a similar fashion and dispose. Finally take another wet swab and prong and wipe over the meatus of the penis, disposing as before.

Anaesthetic

Now is the time to anaesthetize the penis. It is important to inform the patient that this part of the procedure may be slightly uncomfortable but that it will help to reduce the pain for the remainder of it. Warn them that they may feel a stinging sensation as the gel is inserted.

Hold the anaesthetic gel with your dominant hand and squirt a small amount into the kidney dish inside your catheter pack. Dip the tip of the catheter into the gel as this will lubricate it upon insertion.

Hold the penis upright with your non sterile hand and insert the anaesthetic gel into the urethral meatus with your dominant hand. Gently squeeze up to 5 ml into the urethra and apply gentle pressure to the shaft of the penis. Hold this position for up to 5 minutes to allow time for the anaesthetic to take effect.

Catheter insertion

Place the catheter in the cardboard kidney dish between the patient's legs. The dish will act as a reservoir to collect the initial urine outflow that will occur when the catheter is inserted.

Having prepared the patient appropriately and given the anaesthetic gel time to take effect, you should now be ready to insert the catheter into the penis. Despite the anaesthetic, this part of the procedure can still be quite uncomfortable for the patient. It is therefore important to remind the patient of this fact and ask them to warn you if the discomfort is unbearable.

It is essential to maintain an aseptic technique throughout the procedure, and particularly so at this point. Remember that the catheter is a conduit between the outside world and the body's inner environment, breaching the body's natural barrier against infection. For this reason a catheter, contaminated due to poor technique, may introduce infection into the urinary tract system.

Inform the patient that you are about to insert the catheter. During insertion, glance back at the patient's face to ensure that they are not grimacing or suffering undue discomfort. Start by holding the penis vertically, with your non-dominant hand, as this will straighten the first curve of the urethra. Insert the catheter through the urethra with your dominant hand by massaging it through the plastic cover, ensuring that you do not touch it directly. Continue pushing the catheter in until you encounter some resistance. This often means that you have reached the second curvature of the urethra. Lower the penis to a horizontal

TOP TIP!

When using the one hand technique remember that you must NOT use the non-sterile hand to touch the equipment in the sterile field. It must remain holding the gauze around the shaft of the penis at all times! If you accidentally touch the equipment you must remove your gloves and put on a new pair.

TOP TIP!

Make sure the foreskin remains retracted throughout the procedure otherwise the meatus will no longer be aseptic.

TOP TIP!

In the examination setting do not forget to tell the examiner that you would normally wait for 5 minutes for the local anaesthetic to work prior to catheter insertion.

TOP TIP!

Always use sterile water to fill the catheter balloon. Saline solution may crystallize over time and make deflation of the balloon problematic. Using air instead of fluid may cause the balloon to act as a 'float' causing urinary by-passing or poor drainage.

TOP TIP!

Different manufacturers have different guidelines as to how much water should be used to inflate the balloon. Always check the guidelines before you do this.

TOP TIP!

NEVER inflate the balloon if you do not see any urine flowing from the catheter as you may not be in the bladder. Seek assistance and advice from a senior doctor.

TOP TIP!

ALWAYS make sure the foreskin is replaced to avoid paraphimosis.

TOP TIP!

You may wish to send off a urine sample to Microbiology for culture and sensitivity analysis.

position to help overcome and negotiate the curvature whilst maintaining gentle pressure. Never force the catheter through any firm resistance as this may cause trauma to the urethra.

As the tip of the catheter enters the bladder you should notice a flashback of urine into the kidney dish. Continue to insert the catheter a further 5 cm to ensure the balloon section inflates safely beyond the neck of the bladder. Now take the prefilled 10 ml syringe and attach it to the injection port of the catheter. Gently introduce 1 ml of sterile water into the balloon and fill it slowly. Check that the patient is not experiencing any pain whilst doing so to make sure that the balloon is not accidentally inflating in the urethra. If there is no pain, continue inflating with the remaining 9 ml of sterile water. It is important to fill the balloon with an adequate volume because under-inflation can cause poor drainage, urinary by-passing and damage to the urethra. Over-filling, on the other hand, can cause bladder spasm through detrusor muscle irritation, erosion and haematuria.

Upon completion, gently pull on the catheter to confirm that the balloon settles over the neck of the bladder and is stabilized.

Catheter bag

Attach the catheter drainage bag to the end of the catheter and secure it comfortably either to the patient's leg (leg bag) or onto a stand. Make sure you replace the foreskin (to avoid paraphimosis) or ask the patient to do so. Once you have finished, dispose of any waste and offer the patient an opportunity to get dressed. Thank them for their co-operation and ask them if they have any questions or concerns. Do not forget to wash your hands.

3.19.3 Finishing up

Once you have inserted the catheter, do not forget to record the procedure in the patient's notes. Document the date and time the catheter was inserted, the clinical indication for its insertion, size of the catheter used, amount of water injected into the balloon, the residual volume of urine collected as well as any abnormalities in colour or smell of the urine. There may be a removable sticker found on the outer packaging of the catheter detailing some of this information. It is also important to note if a chaperone was present, the fact that consent was given and that the procedure was performed aseptically.

Once a catheter has been inserted you should monitor the patient for any complications of infection, such as fever, suprapubic tenderness and discharge from the catheter site. Remember that patients with artificial heart valves or valve abnormalities are at risk of infective endocarditis from such a procedure and may require antibiotic prophylaxis.

If the catheter is for short-term use only, then its clinical indication should be reviewed on a regular basis. There is evidence to show that the longer a catheter remains *in situ*, the greater the risk of developing a urinary infection. Hence, a catheter should be removed as soon as the clinical indication has ceased.

Answers to Common clinical scenarios

Section 1: History taking skills

Chapter 1.1

Case 1: Angina
Case 2: Myocardial infarction
Case 3: Aortic dissection
Case 4: Pulmonary embolism
Case 5: Pericarditis
Case 6: GORD
Case 7: Musculoskeletal pain

Chapter 1.2

Case 1: Heart failure
Case 2: Palpitations due to exertion
Case 3: Anxiety/panic attacks
Case 4: Pregnancy
Case 5: Thyrotoxicosis
Case 6: AF secondary to pneumonia

Chapter 1.3

Case 1: Tuberculosis
Case 2: Lung cancer
Case 3: Heart failure
Case 4: Pulmonary embolism secondary to pregnancy
Case 5: Asthma
Case 6: Legionnaires' disease
Case 7: Coal miner's pneumoconiosis

Chapter 1.4

Case 1: Asthma
Case 2: Pulmonary embolism
Case 3: Carcinoma of the lung
Case 4: Chronic bronchitis
Case 5: Pneumonia

Chapter 1.5

Case 1: Appendicitis
Case 2: Pancreatitis

Case 3: Gastric ulcer
Case 4: Bleeding duodenal ulcer
Case 5: Crohn's disease
Case 6: Viral hepatitis
Case 7: Renal colic
Case 8: Ectopic pregnancy

Chapter 1.6

Case 1: Brain tumour
Case 2: Diabetic ketoacidosis
Case 3: Opioid-related nausea and vomiting
Case 4: Gastroenteritis
Case 5: Pregnancy
Case 6: Vestibular neuritis
Case 7: Migraine

Chapter 1.7

Case 1: Oesophageal (Schatzki's) ring
Case 2: Pharyngeal pouch
Case 3: Oesophageal web (Plummer–Vinson syndrome)
Case 4: Achalasia
Case 5: Scleroderma

Chapter 1.8

Case 1: Viral hepatitis
Case 2: Gilbert's syndrome
Case 3: Alcoholic liver disease
Case 4: Ascending cholangitis
Case 5: Pancreatic cancer

Chapter 1.9

Case 1: Urinary tract infection
Case 2: Polycystic kidney disease
Case 3: Renal colic due to renal stones
Case 4: Renal tumour
Case 5: Benign prostate hypertrophy

Chapter 1.10

Case 1: Sinusitis
Case 2: Tension headache
Case 3: Cluster headaches
Case 4: Migraine
Case 5: Raised intracranial pressure due to pituitary tumour
Case 6: Temporal arteritis
Case 7: Subarachnoid haemorrhage
Case 8: Trigeminal neuralgia
Case 9: Cervical spondylosis

Chapter 1.11

Case 1: Vasovagal syncope
Case 2: Postural hypotension
Case 3: Vertebrobasilar insufficiency
Case 4: Epilepsy
Case 5: Aortic stenosis
Case 6: Hypoglycaemic
Case 7: Carotid sinus hypersensitivity

Chapter 1.12

Case 1: Closed angle acute glaucoma
Case 2: Retinal vein occlusion
Case 3: Optic neuritis
Case 4: AMD
Case 5: Retinal detachment secondary to trauma

Chapter 1.13

Case 1: Acute glaucoma
Case 2: Conjunctivitis
Case 3: Anterior uveitis in Behçet's disease
Case 4: Episcleritis in Crohn's disease
Case 5: Corneal abrasion

Chapter 1.14

Case 1: Otitis media
Case 2: Otosclerosis
Case 3: Acoustic neuroma
Case 4: Ménière's disease
Case 5: Presbycusis
Case 6: Osteogenesis imperfecta

Chapter 1.15

Case 1: Depression
Case 2: Bipolar disorder
Case 3: Bereavement disorder
Case 4: Severe depression with psychosis

Chapter 1.16

Case 1: High risk
Case 2: Low risk

Chapter 1.17

Case 1: 11.5 units of alcohol a week; within government limits
Case 2: 75 units of alcohol a week; CAGE score 4
Case 3: 15 units of alcohol a week; just above the government recommendations but higher risk as a binge drinker

Chapter 1.18

Case 1: Schizophrenia
Case 2: A variant of post-traumatic stress disorder (PTSD) – Gulf War syndrome
Case 3: Bipolar disorder with psychotic symptoms

Section 2: Examinations

Chapter 2.1

Case 1: Mitral stenosis
Case 2: Mitral regurgitation secondary to ruptured papillary muscle resulting in heart failure
Case 3: Aortic stenosis
Case 4: Aortic regurgitation secondary to infective endocarditis
Case 5: Mechanical aortic valve

Chapter 2.2

Case 1: Spontaneous pneumothorax (left sided)
Case 2: Right lobar pneumonia
Case 3: Asthma
Case 4: Right pleural effusion secondary to bronchial carcinoma
Case 5: Right lung collapse secondary to foreign body

Chapter 2.3

Case 1: Chronic liver disease (alcohol)
Case 2: Liver tumour
Case 3: Appendicitis
Case 4: Chronic myeloid leukaemia (splenomegaly)
Case 5: Aortic aneurysm
Case 6: Kidney transplant

Chapter 2.4

Case 1: Strangulated femoral hernia
Case 2: Indirect inguinal hernia
Case 3: Incisional hernia
Case 4: Haematocele
Case 5: Testicular cancer
Case 6: Varicocele

Chapter 2.5

Case 1: BPH
Case 2: Prostate cancer with bone metastasis
Case 3: Haemorrhoids – grade 4 prolapse
Case 4: Anal fissure
Case 5: Inflammatory bowel disease (Crohn's disease)

Chapter 2.6

Case 1: Bell's palsy
Case 2: Horner's syndrome secondary to pancoast tumour
Case 3: Acoustic neuroma affecting the V and VIII nerves
Case 4: Pseudobulbar palsy due to MS
Case 5: Facial nerve palsy – Ramsey Hunt syndrome

Chapter 2.7

Case 1: Right-sided lacunar infarct (pure motor stroke)
Case 2: Left-sided brain tumour
Case 3: Carpal tunnel syndrome
Case 4: Myasthenia gravis
Case 5: Radial neuropathy (Saturday night palsy due to slouching in a chair causing compression to the brachial plexus)

Chapter 2.8

Case 1: Hemiplegia due to right-sided ischaemic stroke
Case 2: Spinal cord compression secondary to cancer
Case 3: Multiple sclerosis
Case 4: Motor neurone disease
Case 5: Proximal myopathy

Chapter 2.9

Case 1: Radial nerve palsy
Case 2: Contralateral hemisensory loss due to right-sided stroke
Case 3: Syringomyelia
Case 4: C7 radiculopathy secondary to osteophytes
Case 5: Peripheral neuropathy (glove and stocking) due to alcohol

Chapter 2.10

Case 1: Diabetic neuropathic arthropathy (Charcot's foot)
Case 2: Spinal cord compression secondary to bony metastasis from prostate cancer

Chapter 2.11

Case 1: Antalgic gait secondary to OA of right hip
Case 2: High stepping gait secondary to common peritoneal nerve palsy
Case 3: Festinating Parkinsonian gait
Case 4: Cerebellar ataxic gait secondary to a cerebellopontine angle tumour
Case 5: Midline vermis lesion

Chapter 2.12

Case 1: Malignant hypertension
Case 2: Mild non-proliferative diabetic retinopathy
Case 3: Closed angle glaucoma
Case 4: Papilloedema secondary to subarachnoid haemorrhage
Case 5: Right eye cataract

Chapter 2.13

Case 1: Presbycusis
Case 2: Otitis media
Case 3: Otitis externa
Case 4: Cholesteatoma
Case 5: Perforation following trauma

Chapter 2.14

Case 1: Intermediate claudication (IIb – Fontaine classification) due to peripheral arterial disease
Case 2: Acute limb ischaemia

Chapter 2.15

Case 1: Varicose vein affecting the short saphenous vein
Case 2: Varicose vein affecting the long saphenous vein with sapheno–femoral junction incompetence

Chapter 2.16

Case 1: Lipoma
Case 2: Sebaceous cyst
Case 3: Ganglion
Case 4: Boil/furuncle
Case 5: Iatrogenic AV fistula

Chapter 2.17

Case 1: Physiological goitre
Case 2: Hypothyroidism and goitre (Hashimoto's thyroiditis)
Case 3: Thyroglossal cyst
Case 4: Thyroid carcinoma
Case 5: Branchial cyst

Chapter 2.18

Case 1: Infectious mononcleosis (rash caused by inappropriate use of amoxicillin in EBV infection)
Case 2: Breast carcinoma
Case 3: Lymphadenopathy secondary to leg ulcer in a newly diagnosed diabetic
Case 4: Hodgkin's lymphoma
Case 5: Tuberculosis

Section 3: Procedures

Chapter 3.1

Case 1: Wash your hands with alcohol gel
Case 2: Liquid soap
Case 3: Disposable paper towel
Case 4: Alcohol gel

Chapter 3.4

Case 1: Treat BP
Case 2: Reassess in 5 years
Case 3: Treat immediately
Case 4: Treat BP (target 130/80)
Case 5: Reassess in 1 year
Case 6: Suspected co-arctation; requires specialist intervention

Chapter 3.5

Case 1: BMI 27 (overweight – preobese)
Case 2: BMI 32.9 (obese – class I)
Case 3: BMI 16.3 (underweight – moderate thinnest)
Case 4: BMI 53 (very obese – class III)

Chapter 3.6

Case 1: Atrial fibrillation
Case 2: Atrial flutter
Case 3: Ventricular tachycardia
Case 4: Ventricular fibrillation
Case 5: Mobitz type 1 (Wenckebach) heart block

Case 6: Complete heart block
Case 7: Sinus bradycardia

Chapter 3.7

Case 1: Hypoglycaemia; give 50 ml 50% dextrose IV stat in a large vein
Case 2: Hypoglycaemia in a conscious patient, oral sugary drink
Case 3: Type 2 insulin-dependent diabetic with infection; increase dose of insulin and regular BM monitoring
Case 4: Suspected newly diagnosed diabetic; patient needs fasting (> 7) or random venous glucose (> 11.1) blood test to confirm diagnosis
Case 5: Suspected diabetic ketoacidosis; patient will need a urine dipstick for ketones and an ABG to check for acidosis

Chapter 3.8

Case 1: Renal stones
Case 2: UTI
Case 3: Pre-eclampsia
Case 4: Newly diagnosed DM with diabetic ketoacidosis
Case 5: Dehydration
Case 6: Patient taking rifampicin for tuberculosis

Chapter 3.9

Case 1: Diabetes mellitus; grey top bottle for glucose
Case 2: Giant cell arteritis/polymyalgia rheumatica; black top bottle for ESR (you may also use purple top bottle)
Case 3: Anaemia; purple top bottle for FBC
Case 4: Liver disease; yellow top bottle for LFTs
Case 5: Warfarin treatment; blue top bottle for INR
Case 6: Hypothyroidism; yellow bottle for TFTs

Chapter 3.12

Case 1: Red blood cells
Case 2: Platelets
Case 3: Fresh frozen plasma (FFP)
Case 4: Albumin
Case 5: Group O RhD -ve blood
Case 6: Group O RhD -ve blood

Chapter 3.13

Case 1: Newly diagnosed asthmatic
Case 2: Acute severe asthma
Case 3: Moderate asthma
Case 4: Life-threatening asthma

Chapter 3.14

Case 1: Steroid tablets in lowest dose providing adequate control

Case 2: Increase inhaled steroids to 800 mcg daily

Case 3: Add an inhaled steroid at a dose of 400 mcg daily

Case 4: Add inhaled long-acting beta2 agonist (LABA)

Case 5: Trial course of short-acting beta2 agonist

Chapter 3.17

Case 1: Respiratory alkalosis (hyperventilation – panic attack)

Case 2: Respiratory acidosis (life-threatening asthma attack)

Case 3: Metabolic acidosis (diabetic ketoacidosis)

Case 4: Metabolic alkalosis (persistent vomiting)

Case 5: Compensated metabolic acidosis (renal failure)

Case 6: Compensated respiratory acidosis (COPD)

Index

Main entries are highlighted in **bold**